LOWER LIMB AMPUTATIONS:
A GUIDE TO REHABILITATION

LOWER LIMB AMPUTATIONS:
A GUIDE TO REHABILITATION

GLORIA T. SANDERS, B.S., M.S., R.P.T.

Major, U.S.A.R.
Private Practitioner
Jacksonville, North Carolina
Formerly, Associate Professor
Department of Physical Therapy
School of Allied Health Professions
East Carolina University
Greenville, North Carolina

WITH CONTRIBUTIONS BY

BELLA J. MAY, Ed.D., R.P.T.

Professor
Department of Physical Therapy
School of Allied Health Sciences
Medical College of Georgia
Augusta, Georgia

CONSULTANTS

RICHARD HURD, JR., M.D.
Orthopedic and Hand Surgery
Atlanta, Georgia

JOHN MILANI, B.S., C.P.O.
Veterans Administration Prosthetic Center
New York, New York

F.A. DAVIS COMPANY 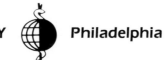 Philadelphia

Library of Congress Cataloging in Publication Data

Sanders, Gloria T.
   Lower limb amputations.

   Bibliography: p.
   Includes Index.
   1. Amputations of foot. 2. Amputations of leg.
3. Hemipelvectomy. 4. Amputees—Rehabilitation.
5. Artificial limbs. I. May, Bella J. II. Title.
RD560.S26 1985   617'.58   85-10439
ISBN 0-8036-7723-5

TO THREE SPECIAL MEMBERS OF MY FAMILY

My grandmother
Pauline Mattocks Sanders
(1890–1982)

My nephew
William Sanders Heller
(b. Feb. 28, 1981)

My niece
Sarah Randal Heller
(b. May 18, 1983)

PREFACE

The primary initial effort in every case of disease or injury should be to save the extremity. Amputation is seldom necessary following bone and joint injuries. More often, it is an admission of defeat in the medical management of the patient with vascular disease. In such cases, it should be performed only as a last resort. The longest possible lever arm, consistent with primary healing, should be maintained for maximum proprioceptive and kinesthetic feedback and thus rehabilitation potential.

If the limb cannot be saved by utilizing the most advanced medical and surgical resources available, then it becomes the obligation of the medical team to ensure that each amputee is afforded a means to regain maximum functional recovery. It is my belief that the likelihood of maximum functional recovery for each amputee is greatly enhanced by a thorough understanding of the entire process by each professional who will interact with the amputee. For example, the surgeon can enhance the functional potential of the amputee by understanding the functional demands of the prosthesis and gait process. Likewise, the therapist can be more effective in developing an exercise program by understanding the surgery that has taken place. Yet, it is not enough just to save a life or provide a prosthesis. We must also afford the amputee a means to a functional reintegration into society.

It is the purpose of this book to provide a guide for these involved, instrumental health care professionals through the complex process of rehabilitation of the amputee.

ACKNOWLEDGMENTS

There have been many talented and knowledgeable people who have been generous with their time and have shared their expertise to help make this book a reality. First and foremost, I would like to thank Richard Hurd, Jr., M.D., orthopedic surgeon, Atlanta; and John Milani, orthotist/prosthetist, VA Prosthetic Center, New York, for editing most of this manuscript; and Joan Edelstein, physical therapist, New York University, for contributing to the editing of this manuscript. I am especially indebted to Bella J. May, Ed.D., R.P.T., for her valuable contributions and assistance in seeing this book to completion.

It is my pleasure and honor to introduce three very talented illustrators who have so ably brought "life" and clarity to this manuscript. They are Angie Britt, Lori Leeds, and Allison Gale. I owe a special thanks to G. vonDrasek Ascher for permission to use her ingenious illustration of Baron von Münchausen in Chapter 4, and Grady Mullis for overlays.

I was very privileged to have received the editorial comments of Thomas Wolff, M.D., Louisville, Kentucky, on Chapter 4, and of Colleen Coulter O'Berry, pediatric physical therapist, on Chapter 23.

Several of my former physical therapy students at East Carolina University have assisted in proofreading and editing this manuscript. Amanda Holliday, Mary Wood Hurdle, and Shawne Soper are due special recognition. Appreciation also to Nancy Urbscheit, Ph.D., for moral support and editorial comments.

This book would have taken many more years to complete if it had not been for the prompt, friendly, and thorough responses of the staff of the Health Sciences Library and the Center for Medical Communication at East Carolina University to my many requests. In particular, I would like to thank Donna Flake, Paul Bredderman, and Mike Dodge of the Health Sciences Library, and John Artois, photographer.

To the wonderful staff at F.A. Davis Company, including Bob Martone, Micaela Palumbo, and especially my copy editor and almost-daily phone correspondent, Zena Sandler Gordon, a special thanks for your support, confidence, ability to keep me on schedule, and most importantly, for your sense of humor, which has made an otherwise laborious process a pleasure.

The task of writing a book of this nature would probably never be undertaken if it were not for the years of inspiration from dedicated, knowledgeable, and talented teachers in our past. I am especially indebted to the teachers at Swansboro Elementary and High School, Swansboro, N.C., who impressed upon me at an early age that education is a privilege and not just a job, and to the faculties at North Carolina Wesleyan College and the Medical College of Virginia, for the high standards and quality they bring to these fine institutions. I am also indebted to Larry Means, Ph.D., my graduate advisor and professor, Department of Psychology, East Carolina University, who by example taught me that friendship and professorship are not mutually exclusive and that education can be a very tough yet pleasurable experience, even at the graduate level. Thanks Larry!

To my former students in the Department of Physical Therapy at East Carolina University, thanks for your friendship and for making my years of teaching such a wonderful experience. To Becky Latham and Barbara James, thanks for the hours of typing.

To my family and friends, thanks for tolerating my semiseclusion for 6 years. To my parents, thanks for providing me with the means to obtain a good education. To my Aunt Helen, thanks for helping with the typing in the early days when the going was rough. To my sister, Sarah Heller, R.P.T., who said "I can't believe you did it." I did it!

Gloria T. Sanders

CONTENTS

UNIT 1
GENERAL CONSIDERATIONS

tomy
Hemi
cor.
por.
ec.
GRITTI-STOKES
KIRK
CALLANDER
(AK)
KNEE
SYME
TERMINAL
HIP DISARTICULATION
ankle
SYME
Mid-thigh
Ph,complete
TOE
Metatarsal Ray
LEG
Resection
(BK)
HEMIPELVECTOMY

CHAPTER 1

NOMENCLATURE

AMPUTATION LEVELS

OPERATIVE PROCEDURES

    GUILLOTINE AMPUTATION

    OPEN AMPUTATION

    CLOSED AMPUTATION

PROSTHESIS

TYPES OF PROSTHESES

PREPARATORY, PROVISIONAL, INTERMEDIATE, OR TEMPORARY

PYLON

PERMANENT OR DEFINITIVE

EXOSKELETAL DESIGN

CRUSTACEAN DESIGN

ENDOSKELETAL DESIGN

MODULAR SYSTEM

AMPUTATION LEVELS

In 1974, the Task Force on Standardization of Prosthetic-Orthotic Terminology of the International Society for Prosthetics and Orthotics met on two occasions to develop a standardized nomenclature for prosthetics. It was hoped that the new terminology would offer more consistency in the use of terms, would lend itself to easier translation, and would enhance processes such as statistical preparation, retrieval, and billing.

The proposed new nomenclature was based on the terminology developed at an international workshop in Dundee, Scotland, in 1973, for congenital limb deficiencies. The two major categories of congenital limb deficiencies identified at Dundee were transverse and longitudinal. Because amputation owing to trauma or disease is, in form and management, essentially the same as transverse congenital deficiencies, the nomenclature for transverse congenital defects was adopted for all acquired amputations (Table 1-1).

TABLE 1-1. LOWER LIMB AMPUTATION LEVELS

Old Terms	Proposed New Terms	Abbreviations
Syme Terminal Toe	Phalangeal, partial	Ph, partial
Toe (digital, disarticulation at metatarsophalangeal joint)	Phalangeal, complete	Ph, complete
Metatarsal Ray Resection Transmetatarsal	Metatarsal, partial	MT, partial
Lisfranc	Metatarsal, complete	MT, complete
Chopart Pirogoff Boyd	Tarsal, partial	Ta, partial
Ankle Disarticulation (through-the-ankle) Syme	Tarsal, complete	Ta, complete
Below Knee (BK) 　Long 　　(lower-third, distal-third) 　Medium 　　(mid-third, standard) 　Short 　　(upper-third, proximal-third)	Leg, partial (Lower $1/3$) (Middle $1/3$) (Upper $1/3$)	Leg, partial (Lower $1/3$) (Middle $1/3$) (Upper $1/3$)
Knee Disarticulation (through-the-knee, thru-knee, at the knee joint, exarticulation, amputation in contiguity) Transcondylar/Supracondylar (at the knee) Gritti-Stokes Kirk Callander	Leg, complete	Leg, complete

TABLE 1-1. *Continued*

Old Terms	Proposed New Terms	Abbreviations
Above Knee (AK)	Thigh, partial	Th, partial
Long	(Lower 1/3)	(Lower 1/3)
(lower-third, distal-third)		
Mid-thigh	(Middle 1/3)	(Middle 1/3)
(middle-third)		
Short	(Upper 1/3)	(Upper 1/3)
(upper-third, proximal-third)		
Hip Disarticulation	Thigh, complete	Th, complete
(femoral exarticulation, through-the-hip)		
Hemipelvectomy	Hip, complete	Hip, complete
(hindquarter, interinnomino-abdominal amputation, interiliosacropubic amputation, sacroiliac disarticulation, exarticulation through the sacroiliac joint, interpelvi-abdominal amputation, transiliac amputation, disarticulation of the innominate bone, interilio-abdominal amputation, lower quarterectomy, transischiosacropubic disarticulation)		
Hemicorporectomy	Pelvic, complete	Pel, complete
(translumbar amputation, paracorporectomy, lumbosacral amputation, transvertebral)		

The new terminology system is structured to designate the most proximal segment that is missing, or the level at which the limb terminates. For example, "thigh, complete" means that the complete thigh is missing, or amputation through the hip joint. "Thigh, partial (upper 1/3)" means that the limb terminates in the proximal, or upper 1/3, of the thigh (Fig. 1-1).

In cases of amputation close to a joint, the epiphyseal growth plate is used as the reference line. For example, if the amputation is just proximal to the distal femoral epiphyseal line, then the amputation would be considered a "thigh, partial (lower 1/3)." If the amputation is at the distal femoral epiphyseal growth plate or between the distal femoral epiphyseal growth plate and the knee joint, it would be a "leg, complete" (Fig. 1-2).

OPERATIVE PROCEDURES

Lower extremity amputations are classified not only according to the level, but also by the type of operative procedure.

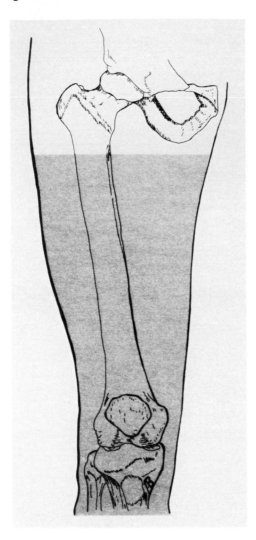

FIGURE 1-1. A thigh (Th), partial (upper ⅓), or short above-knee amputation.

GUILLOTINE AMPUTATION

The name guillotine amputation was given to the technique of Leonard Botalli, surgeon to Charles IX, King of France in the 16th century. In this amputation, all of the tissues were divided at the same level in one stroke of the blade, and the bleeding vessels were immediately sealed with heated irons or oils.

OPEN AMPUTATION

Open amputations are performed in cases of spreading infection or when all devital-ized tissue has not been removed by débridement. The skin is usually incised in a circular fashion around the circumference of the limb. Curved skin flaps, which are used in closed amputations, are usually contraindicated in open amputations because

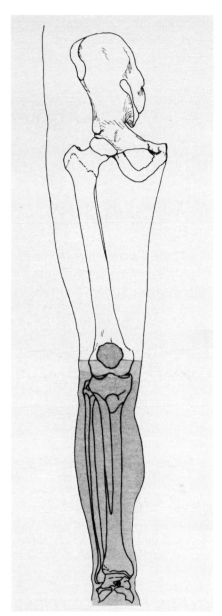

FIGURE 1-2. A leg, complete, or transcondylar amputation.

they often obstruct drainage. Subcutaneous tissue, muscle, and bone are incised at the most distal feasible level. No attempt is made to shape the bone. The periosteum is not stripped from the end of the bone. Loose portions of the periosteum are removed to avoid bone spur formation. A dressing is applied to the open wound. The time required for the primary amputation is less than for a closed amputation.

Skin traction (usually 2.7 to 3.6 kg [6 to 8 lb] for above-knee amputations and 1.8 to 2.7 kg [4 to 6 lb] for below-knee amputations) is applied continuously to bring the skin and muscle down over the end of the bone until the wound heals. If traction is not used, the soft tissue will retract and the bone will protrude, making skin closure difficult and increasing the risk of osteomyelitis.

When the open technique is used, the wound takes longer to heal; asepsis and nitrogen and electrolyte balance are difficult to maintain; and postoperative pain is greater. The limb, if end-bearing, may not be satisfactory because an excessive amount of scar tissue forms on the distal end. Osteomyelitis with sequestration of portions of the bone and adherence of the skin to the bone are also frequent problems. A revision operation, which prolongs hospitalization, is often needed to shape the bone and other tissues before a prosthesis can be fitted.

In the presence of infection, an open amputation reduces the possibility of septicemia, reduces generalized toxicity, and may result in an improvement in overall health. It can be a lifesaving emergency procedure.

CLOSED AMPUTATION

In the closed amputation, skin flaps are shaped for primary closure. Vessels and nerves should be neatly cut, and the muscles and bone should be shaped properly. Myoplasty may be done. Rounded skin flaps cover the residual limb without tension or redundancy. Most amputations are performed using the closed method as the primary operation. This procedure should not be used in cases where infection is inevitable.

PROSTHESIS

In the technical sense, a prosthesis is an artificial replacement, worn in situ, for a lost or absent body part. For example, a wig worn by a person with hair is not considered to be a prosthesis. A wig worn by a bald person is considered to be a prosthesis. Artificial eyes, legs, and dentures are familiar prostheses.

More liberal usage of the word prosthesis has included application to any device that aids or augments performance of a natural function, such as a hearing aid or eyeglasses. Confusion is created by this broad definition, which could include external ambulatory aids (crutches, canes, walkers) and many orthotic devices that also aid or augment performance of a natural function. The term prosthesis is most commonly used in reference to an artificial limb, which will be its subsequent usage in this text.

TYPES OF PROSTHESES

Some of the terms used to designate general types of artificial limbs are defined below.

PREPARATORY, PROVISIONAL, INTERMEDIATE, OR TEMPORARY

This is a cosmetically unfinished prosthesis that has been fitted and aligned to a particular patient using sound biomechanical principles. Because it is less expensive than a permanent prosthesis, it is often prescribed when an amputee's ability to wear a prosthesis is in doubt. With a preparatory prosthesis, the clinic team can determine without question whether a definitive prosthesis is indicated. The residual limb usually decreases in size after ambulation with a prosthesis begins. If a temporary prosthesis is used initially, the residual limb will be less edematous and will have a better contour, thus enabling a longer acceptable fit with the permanent prosthesis. A temporary prosthesis is usually worn only for a limited evaluation period, but it can be used for an indefinite period of time.

PYLON

A pylon is a narrow vertical support. If the amputation is well above the knee, one pylon connects the socket to the knee unit and a second pylon connects the knee unit to the ankle/foot assembly. If the amputation is below the knee, the pylon connects the socket to the ankle/foot assembly. Pylons are usually used for preparatory or temporary prostheses, especially for immediate or early postsurgical fittings. In cases of immediate postoperative fittings, the support can usually be disconnected from the socket when the amputee is in bed, so that the rigid socket remains on the residual limb. Pylons are also used for permanent endoskeletal systems. Early pylons for above-knee amputees did not have a knee joint or an ankle joint. These hingeless supports were called peg legs.

PERMANENT OR DEFINITIVE

A permanent prosthesis is the final prosthesis that has been fitted and aligned for the individual amputee. It should be durable, comfortable, cosmetic in appearance, and should provide adequate function for the missing part. The permanent prosthesis can be either the exoskeletal or endoskeletal type, or it may be partly endoskeletal and partly exoskeletal.

EXOSKELETAL DESIGN

A prosthesis where the outside of the structure provides the required support is an exoskeletal prosthetic design.

CRUSTACEAN DESIGN

This term is often used interchangeably with exoskeletal. Crustacean means outer shell, whereas exoskeletal connotes external support.

ENDOSKELETAL DESIGN

An internal skeleton (pylon) supports the load in an endoskeletal prosthetic design. This is not to be confused with an endoprosthesis, which means a prosthesis lying inside the body.

MODULAR SYSTEM

Interchangeable components that can be assembled easily and quickly into a prosthesis comprise a modular system. It should allow alignment of one module to another, as needed. Most modular systems are of the endoskeletal design.

BIBLIOGRAPHY

CANTY, TJ: *Amputations and recent developments in artificial limbs.* US Armed Forces Med J 3:1147–1152, 1952.

CARNES, EH: *Amputations, stumps and prostheses.* War Med 1:656–663, 1941.

DENNIS, FS: *The general principles involved in amputation, with a consideration of some points in the technique.* JAMA 8:505–509, 1887.

FAXON, HH: *Major amputations for advanced peripheral arterial obliterative disease.* JAMA 113:1199–1204, 1939.

JANES, JM AND JACKSON, AE: *Open-flap amputation.* Surg Clin North Am 29:1049–1064, 1949.

KAY, HW: *A proposed international terminology for the classification of congenital limb deficiencies.* Orth Pros 28:33–48, 1974.

KAY, HW: *A proposed nomenclature for limb prosthetics.* Orth Pros 28:37–47, 1974.

KIRK, NT AND MCKEEVER, FM: *The guillotine amputation.* JAMA 124:1027–1030, 1944.

MEYER, NC: *Guillotine amputation modified to preserve skin flaps.* US Nav M Bull 46:1844–1847, 1946.

MURDOCH, G: *Amputation surgery in the lower extremity.* Prosthet Orthot Int 1:72–83, 1977.

PETERSON, LT: *The Army amputation program.* J Bone Joint Surg 26:635–637, 1944.

SHEA, JD: *Surgical techniques for lower extremity amputation.* Orthop Clin North Am 3:287–301, 1972.

SILBERT, S: *Amputation below the knee for gangrene in the diabetic: Preliminary report.* Am J Dig Dis 11:394–401, 1944.

SILBERT, S AND HAIMOVICI, H: *Results of midleg amputation for gangrene in diabetics.* JAMA 144:454–458, 1980.

SMITH, BC: *Amputation through lower third of leg for diabetic and arteriosclerotic gangrene.* Arch Surg 27:267–295, 1933.

THOMPSON, RG: *Amputation in the lower extremity.* J Bone Joint Surg 45A:1723–1734, 1963.

VANDEN BRINK, KD AND WARING, TL: *A new technique of open amputation: Use of the rolled flap.* Clin Orthop 123:70–72, 1977.

WHITE, WL: *The open amputation stump: Its management, advantages and disadvantages.* US Nav M Bull (Suppl) 46:20–36, 1946.

WILSON, AB, JR: *Recent advances in above-knee prosthetics.* Artificial Limbs 12:1–27, 1968.

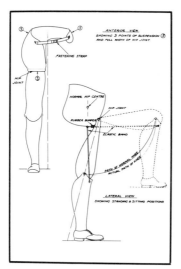

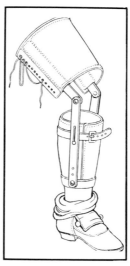

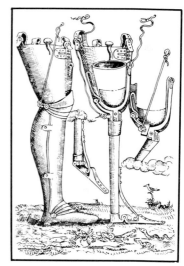

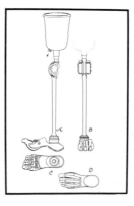

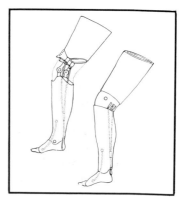

Although undertaken for the purpose of saving lives, the earliest amputations usually resulted in death from shock owing to blood loss or septicemia in those who survived the operation itself. Emphasis was naturally placed on speed in completing the amputation. It was not until the mid-nineteenth century, when antisepsis, asepsis, and anesthesia came into use, that emphasis could be focused on care in the surgical procedure and conservation of tissue. Technical advances in artificial limbs led to consideration of the functional aspects of the residual limb and had an effect on the type and level of amputation performed by the surgeon. Legislation profoundly affected the field of prosthetics by providing prostheses to amputees and financial support for research.

The history of prosthetics has included many notable individual prostheses such as the Verduyn and Anglesey legs. Also of historical interest are anecdotes regarding amputees. One, reported by McCord in an article on the early history of artificial limbs, came from a paragraph originating in *Knickerbocker Birthday: A Sesquicentennial History of The New York Historical Society, 1804–1954,* by R.W.G. Vail, 1954:

> The most curious and one of the most interesting museum pieces to come to us in many a day has just arrived as this is being written. It is none other than the original wooden leg of Honorable Gouverneur Morris (1752–1816), which came as the gift of one of his direct descendants. Morris was one of the two great men of New York to wear a wooden leg, the other, as you very well know, being old Peter Stuyvesant. But Morris appears to have lost his leg in a romantic rather than a military encounter, as did the redoubtable Peter. However, there seem to be two schools of thought as to the manner in which Gouverneur Morris came by his timber toe. One group of historical students maintains he lost his balance and then his leg in falling from a carriage; the other asserts that the accident happened as he was precipitately fleeing from the wrath of a jealous and outraged husband. Be that as it may, the loss of the leg seems to have had no permanent effect on his later diplomatic or undiplomatic career.

Listed below are highlights of recorded history that mark the ongoing international progress in amputation surgery and prosthetics.

3500 to 1800 BC	The Vedas, written in Sanskrit in India, are reported to contain the first recorded instance of amputations and prosthetic replacement. The Rig-Veda, the oldest of the Vedas, is claimed to have been composed between 3500 and 1800 BC. It contains the account of Queen Vishpla, whose leg was amputated in battle. After Queen Vishpla's limb healed, she was fitted with an iron leg to enable her to walk and return to the battlefield.
484 BC	The classic *History,* by the father of history, Herodotus, contains an early record of a prosthesis. A Persian soldier, Hegesistratus, escaped from prison by cutting off part of his foot, which he replaced with a wooden filler in his shoe.
	The author of *On Joints,* who may have been Hippocrates or Herodotus, recommended amputation for gangrene of the joint below the boundaries of blackening as soon as the joint was fairly dead and had lost its sensibility.
300 BC	The oldest prosthesis (an artificial leg constructed of bronze and iron with a wooden core) to be displayed in a museum was unearthed from a tomb in Capua, Italy, in 1858. It was dated about 300 BC and was destroyed when the Museum of the Royal College of Surgeons in London was bombed during World War II.
Birth of Christ	Celsus described amputation through healthy tissue between the sound and diseased parts, as well as ligation of vessels at the time of amputation.
100 AD	Archigenes and Heliodorus began to perform amputations for ulcers, tumors, injuries, and deformities, not just as a last resort for gangrene as had been done previously.
Dark Ages	There was a return to the use of cautery and hot oil to prevent hemorrhage.
1517	Hans von Gersdorff of Strassburg described the use of a tourniquet along with compression or cauterization to control bleeding. He also recommended covering an amputated limb with muscle from a cow or pig bladder, and dressing the wound with warm—not boiling—oil. Gersdorff's *Field-Book of Wound Surgery* contains the first known illustration of an amputation.
1529	Ambroise Paré (1510–1590), a French Army surgeon, reintroduced the use of ligatures, originally set forth by Hippocrates. This technique was more successful than crushing the amputation limb, dipping it in boiling oil, or any other means of cautery that had been used during the Dark Ages to stop bleeding. An artificial leg, invented by Paré in 1561 for above-knee amputees, was constructed of heavy metals and was the first artificial leg known to employ articulated joints (Fig. 2-1). Paré was the first to describe phantom sensation.

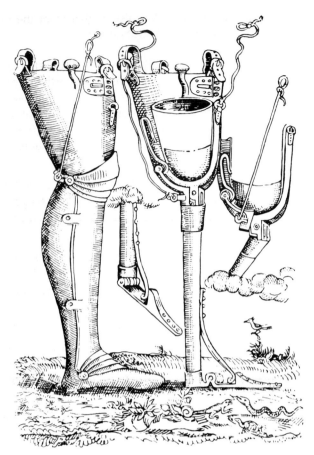

FIGURE 2-1. An above-knee artificial leg invented by Ambroise Paré (middle sixteenth century). (From Pare, A: *Oeuvres Completes,* Paris, 1840. From the copy in the National Library of Medicine. From Wilson, AB, Jr: *Limb prosthetics: 1970.* Artificial Limbs 14:2, 1970, with permission.)

1593	Wilhelm Fabry (Fig. 2-2), in a monograph on gangrene, also recommended amputation above the diseased part. He devised a tourniquet—a ligature tightened by a stick of wood—to stop circulation before surgery. Fabry has been recognized as the first educated and scientific German surgeon.
1596	The first English reference to ligation of arteries in amputations appeared in the *Discourse of the Whole Art of Chyrurgerie* by Peter Lowe, a Scottish army surgeon.
1674	Etienne J. Morel, a French army surgeon, reintroduced the use of the tourniquet, which led to an increase in limb amputations as a surgical procedure.
1679	Yonge was the first to describe an amputation that included a flap to facilitate closure.

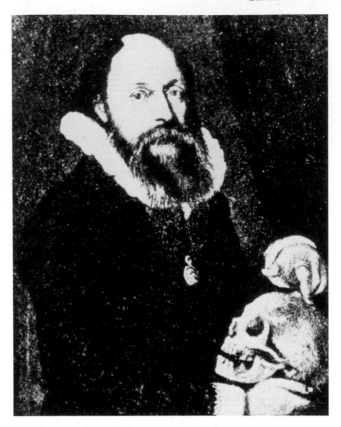

FIGURE 2-2. Wilhelm Fabry of Hilden (1560–1642), a leading German surgeon. (From Garrison, FH: *An Introduction to the History of Medicine.* **WB Saunders, Philadelphia, 1929, p 275, with permission.)**

1696	Pieter Andriannszoon Verduyn (Verduin), a Dutch surgeon, introduced the first known below-knee prosthesis with an unlocked knee joint. In concept, it resembled the thigh-corset below-knee prosthesis used today (Fig. 2-3). A thigh cuff bore part of the weight. It was connected by external hinges to a leg piece whose socket was made of copper and lined with leather. The leg piece terminated in a wooden foot.
1782	Edward Alanson, an English surgeon, described a surgical amputation method in which the skin and muscles were cut in a circular manner so that the amputation limb was shaped like a hollow cone, utilizing flaps.
1803	Dominique-Jean Larrey (Fig. 2-4), Napoleon's personal surgeon, tried refrigeration to dull the pain of amputation surgery. He was one of the first to amputate at the hip joint. He was said to have performed as many as 200 amputations in 24 hours and is recognized as the inventor of the "flying ambulances" with which he gathered the wounded during battle rather than compelling them to wait until the end of the conflict.

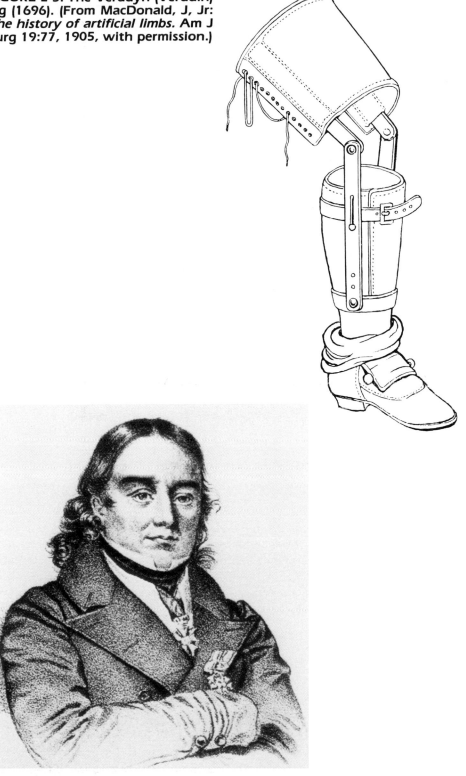

FIGURE 2-3. The Verduyn (Verduin) leg (1696). (From MacDonald, J, Jr: *The history of artificial limbs.* Am J Surg 19:77, 1905, with permission.)

FIGURE 2-4. Dominique-Jean Larrey (1766–1842). (From Garrison, FH: *An Introduction to the History of Medicine.* WB Saunders, Philadelphia, 1929, p 488, with permission.)

1810   Johann Georg Von Heine of Würzburg, the founder of German ortho-
        pedics, introduced an artificial leg that utilized a ball joint at the ankle
        and was suspended by a corset about the trunk.

1815   Jacques Lisfranc of France devised a disarticulation amputation of the
        foot at the tarsometatarsal articulation: Lisfranc's amputation.

        George Guthrie, an English military surgeon, performed a successful
        amputation at the hip joint while at Waterloo. His most important
        book was *Treatise on Gunshot Wounds of the Extremities Requiring
        Amputation*. He, as well as Larrey, advocated primary amputation as
        soon after injury as possible. This produced a lower operative mortal-
        ity, a lower incidence of wound infection, and fewer cases of recur-
        rent hemorrhage than waiting the prescribed 3 weeks after injury for
        secondary amputation.

1816   James Potts of London introduced an above-knee prosthesis with a
        wooden shank and socket, a steel knee joint, and an articulated foot
        with artificial tendons connecting the knee to the ankle. This enabled
        dorsiflexion (toe lift) whenever the wearer flexed the knee. The device
        was known as the "Anglesey (Anglesea) leg" because it was used by
        the Marquis of Anglesey following the loss of his leg in the Battle of
        Waterloo (Fig. 2-5).

1818   Professor Antenrieth suspended wooden legs by a waist belt and a
        strap over the opposite shoulder.

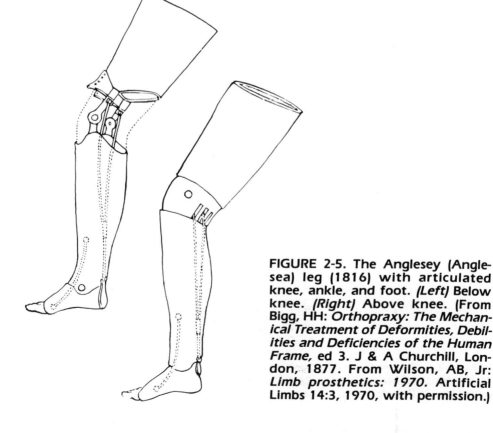

FIGURE 2-5. The Anglesey (Angle-
sea) leg (1816) with articulated
knee, ankle, and foot. *(Left)* Below
knee. *(Right)* Above knee. (From
Bigg, HH: *Orthopraxy: The Mechanical Treatment of Deformities, Debil-
ities and Deficiencies of the Human
Frame*, ed 3. J & A Churchill, London, 1877. From Wilson, AB, Jr:
Limb prosthetics: 1970. Artificial
Limbs 14:3, 1970, with permission.)

1824   Nathan Smith, who in 1797 became the first professor of his own medical school at Dartmouth and in 1813 moved to Yale Medical Institute, performed the first knee disarticulation in America.

1826   The Verduyn prosthesis, designed to maximize support at the thigh rather than at the knee, was reintroduced by Serre.

        Albert Ludwig Dornblüth constructed a prosthesis with a right-angled knee position for below-knee amputees. The artificial knee joint was located below the anatomic knee joint.

1831   Jean-Gaspard-Blaise Goyrand was the first to report the use of the ischial tuberosities for weight-bearing.

1839   The Anglesey leg (see Fig. 2-5) was introduced in the United States by the Englishman William Selpho, a protégé of Potts. Selpho modified the leg by inserting a rubber plate at the ankle to reduce jarring and adding a rubber sole to provide elasticity and reduce slippage. With alterations by American prosthetists, it became known as the "American leg."

1842   James Syme (Fig. 2-6) of Edinburgh performed the first successful Syme amputation at the ankle joint. He also advocated thigh amputation through the cancellous bone of the condyles or the trochanters.

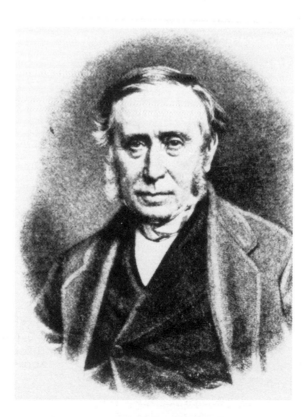

FIGURE 2-6. James Syme (1799–1870), author of *Excision of Diseased Joints* (1831). (From Garrison, FH: *An Introduction to the History of Medicine.* WB Saunders, Philadelphia, 1929, p 483, with permission.)

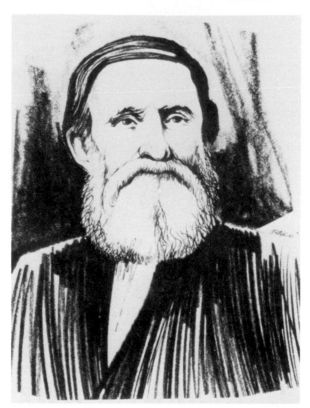

FIGURE 2-7. Crawford Williamson Long (1815–1878) of Georgia, who graduated from the University of Pennsylvania School of Medicine. (From Talbott, JH: *A Biographical History of Medicine: Excerpts and Essays on the Men and Their Work.* Grune & Stratton, New York, 1970, p 1000, with permission.)

Crawford Long (Fig. 2-7), who practiced in Athens, Georgia, was the first physician to use sulfuric ether for surgical anesthesia.

Ferdinand Martin and Joseph François Benoit Charrière of France displaced the artificial knee joint behind the limb axis for alignment stability.

1846   William Morton (Fig. 2-8), a dentist, was the first to proclaim the use of ether for general anesthesia.

Dr. Benjamin F. Palmer of Philadelphia, who himself wore an artificial limb made by William Selpho, obtained the first patent for an artificial leg from the United States government after seeking to improve the Selpho leg. He received an honorable citation for the artificial limb at the World's Fair in London in 1851. The Palmer leg was made of wood and had movable knee and ankle joints that were controlled by artificial tendons.

1847   Pierre Jean Marie Flourens, a French physiologist, discovered the anesthetic properties of chloroform. The increasing availability of ether and chloroform led to improved surgical procedures and more functional amputation limbs.

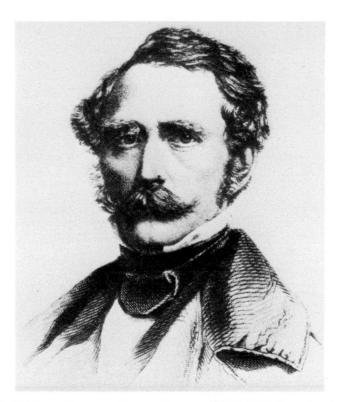

FIGURE 2-8. William Thomas Green Morton (1819–1868), a dentist from Massachusetts. (From Talbott, JH: *A Biographical History of Medicine: Excerpts and Essays on the Men and Their Work.* Grune & Stratton, New York, 1970, p 1002, with permission.)

1850	Unna's paste, a compound of zinc oxide, gelatin, glycerin, and calamine, was invented by P.G. Unna, a German dermatologist.
1852	Plaster of Paris bandages were introduced by Anthony Mathijsen of Holland. This material was used in the construction of peg legs.
1853	The Marks Artificial Limb Company was founded in New York City.
1854	Nikolai Ivanovitch Pirogoff, a Russian, described an amputation at the foot in the Russian *Journal of Military Medicine.*
	D.B. Marks obtained a patent on an artificial limb. He also introduced the use of rawhide to cover the surface of the wooden parts, which improved their durability.
1857	Rocco Gritti of Milan described an amputation through the knee using the patella in an osteoplastic flap.
1858	Ball-and-socket ankle joints were devised by Dr. Douglas Bly of New York. Leather straps limited motion, and soft rubber in the joints prevented jarring.
1859	A leg manufactured by Amasa A. Marks in 1856, which had knee, ankle, and toe movements with adjustable articulations, received the Highest Award at the American Institute Exhibition.

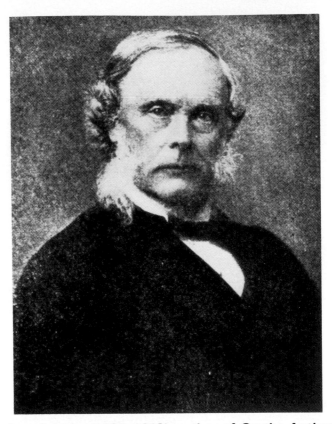

FIGURE 2-9. Joseph Lister (1827–1912), author of *On the Antiseptic Principle in the Practice of Surgery*. (From Garrison, FH: *An Introduction to the History of Medicine*. WB Saunders, Philadelphia, 1929, p 589, with permission.)

1860	Joseph Lister (Fig. 2-9) became Regius Professor of Surgery at the University of Glasgow. His principles of antiseptic surgery were soon discovered (1865) and published (1867). These principles made amputation a less fatal operation. Lister married the daughter of his chief, James Syme. Lister also experimented with using catgut as a ligature (1880) rather than silk or hemp, which were not absorbed by body tissues and often caused inflammations and severe hemorrhage.
American Civil War 1861–1865	Interest in artificial limbs and amputation surgery increased because of the increased number of amputees (30,000 in the Union army alone) and the commitment of the federal and state governments to pay for artificial limbs for veterans. J.E. Hanger, a Southerner who lost a leg during the Civil War, replaced cords of the American leg with rubber bumpers at the ankle to control plantarflexion and dorsiflexion.
1861	The J.E. Hanger Company opened in Richmond, Virginia.
1862	The first law providing free prostheses to people who lost limbs in warfare was enacted by the United States Congress.
1863	The suction socket (Fig. 2-10), which employed the concept of using pressure to suspend an artificial limb, was patented by an American,

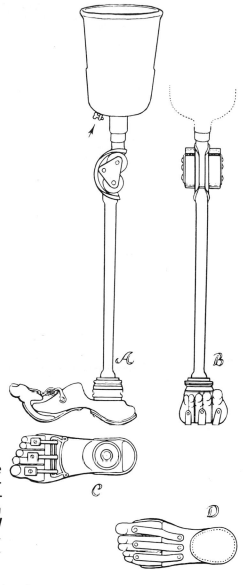

FIGURE 2-10. The D.D. Parmelee prosthesis with suction socket, patented in 1863. (From *Historical development of artificial limbs*. In *Orthopaedic Appliances Atlas, Vol 2, Artificial Limbs*. JW Edwards, Ann Arbor, Michigan, 1960, p 11, with permission.)

Dubois D. Parmelee, who also invented a polycentric knee unit and a multiarticulated foot.

The first rubber foot, invented in 1861, was patented by Amasa A. Marks.

1867   The Beaufort limb, which had an automatic knee lock, was described in Paris.

1868   Dr. August Gustav Hermann of Prague wrote the treatise, *Mechanism of Gait With an Artificial Leg and a New Construction of an AK and BK Prosthesis*. He also introduced the use of aluminum to replace the steel in a prosthesis.

1870   Congress passed a law that not only supplied artificial limbs to all honorably discharged persons from the military or naval service who had lost a limb while in the United States service, but also entitled them to receive one every 5 years.

William Stokes published a modification of Gritti's amputation at the knee.

1871	Silas Weir Mitchell, an American neurologist, described phantom limbs.
1877	Captain Gerard of the United States returned from England and reported Lister's antiseptic method to the Surgeon General. Listerian principles were adopted by the American military surgeons.
1880	A new foot that reinforced the rubber foot with layers of canvas at the toes to prevent them from turning upward was patented and called the "laminated foot."
1885	Heather Bigg of London published a book, *Amputations and Artificial Limbs,* which included anatomic studies on the alignment of prosthetic parts.
1891	Additional pension laws enacted by the United States Congress enabled receipt of a new prosthesis every 3 years, as well as transportation to and from the manufacturer to have a limb fitted.
1893	August Bier introduced an osteoplastic procedure in which a flap of cortical bone and attached periosteum is used to cover the cut end of the bone to reduce distal limb sensitivity. This is the same principle as Gritti's amputation at the knee and Pirogoff's at the ankle.
1895	Charles Girard of Berne, Switzerland, performed the first successful hemipelvectomy.
1909	Joseph Ransohoff in Cincinnati, Ohio, performed the first successful complete hemipelvectomy in the United States.
1912	Marcel Desoutter, an Englishman, introduced the first all-aluminum lightweight prosthesis. He also introduced the concept of pelvic suspension.
World War I 1914–1918	The number of American amputees was relatively small (4,403) when compared to the British (42,000) or to total amputations (approximately 100,000) in all of the armies of Europe. Consulting relationships developed between prosthetists and surgeons. During this time (1917), the Artificial Limb Manufacturers Association was formed.
1918	Dr. Martin of Paris described the Belgian artificial limb, which was founded on scientific principles derived from intensive studies of the anatomy and physiology of the leg. Dr. Martin sought to improve on the American leg by attempting to reproduce the natural static and aesthetic qualities of the lower limb. The Belgian limb could be made from proper measurements and projections along with a cast of the sound limb and residual limb.
1928	Sir Alexander Fleming, of St. Mary's Hospital in London, discovered penicillin.

1930s	Because of the economic depression, progress in prosthetics in the United States was minimal.
1935	C. Latimer Callander described an amputation in the distal thigh.
1940	Sir Howard Walter Florey, Ernst Boris Chain, and associates at Oxford concentrated penicillin to a solid product suitable for therapeutic use. The results of animal studies (1940) and trials on humans (1941) were published showing penicillin to be the most effective chemotherapeutic agent for controlling infection. Fleming, Florey, and Chain were jointly awarded a Nobel Prize in 1945 for the discovery and therapeutic development of penicillin.
	Selman Abraham Waksman, who was a Russian immigrant to the United States, and H.B. Woodruff isolated the active antibiotic actinomycin. In 1944, Waksman isolated streptomycin, for which he received a Nobel Prize in 1952.
1945	Norman Kirk, Surgeon General of the Army, requested that the National Academy of Sciences investigate the provision of artificial limbs to war veterans.
	Dr. Philip D. Wilson, Chairman of the Panel on Amputations of the Committee on Surgery, Division of Medical Sciences, National Research Council, recommended the initiation of a research program. Contracting with universities and industrial laboratories began.
	The Army established a research laboratory at Walter Reed Army Medical Center; the Navy established one at Mare Island, California (later at Oakland Naval Hospital).
1946	A commission of engineers and surgeons was sent to Europe by the Surgeon General of the United States Army to study the state of the art. They recommended a re-evaluation of the suction socket.
	The leaders of the Artificial Limb Manufacturers Association invited the orthopedic brace fabricators to join them, which they did. The name was changed to Orthopedic Appliance and Limb Manufacturers Association, and a full-time executive director was appointed.
1947	The Veterans Administration (VA) established a prosthetics research laboratory in New York.
	It soon became apparent that the design and engineering of components (the mechanical aspect) needed to be paralleled by fundamental research in limb function (biomechanics). Laboratories were established at the University of California at Berkeley for lower limb study and the University of California at Los Angeles for upper limb study.
	Harold Boyd at the Campbell Clinic, Memphis, described a method of anatomic disarticulation at the hip.
	Research involving the suction socket by the National Academy of Sciences was transferred to the University of California at Berkeley and San Francisco.

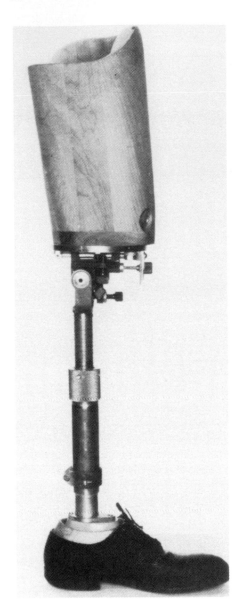

FIGURE 2-11. An early version of the above-knee suction socket and the University of California adjustable leg. (From Wilson, AB, Jr: *The modern history of amputation surgery and artificial limbs.* Orthop Clin North Am 3:271, 1972, with permission.)

From 1947 to 1953, educational workshops were held for suction socket prescription and construction (Fig. 2-11).

1948   Public Law 729, which supported the VA as the sole sponsor of governmental contractual research in limb prosthetics, was passed.

1949   The American Board for Certification of the Prosthetic and Orthopedic Appliance Industry, Inc., was formed to certify those who met its standards and to approve facilities for serving the amputee.

H.J. Seddon and J.T. Scales described an above-knee amputation with enucleation of the remaining femur and replacement with an internal femoral prosthesis.

1951	The International Society for Rehabilitation of the Disabled (from 1939 to 1960 called The International Society for the Welfare of Cripples, since 1972 known as Rehabilitation International) created the Committee on Prostheses, Braces and Technical Aids, which has sponsored international courses and symposia to encourage world-wide cooperation.
1952	Dr. Felix Mondry reported a myoplastic technique for below-knee amputations in which the flexors and extensors are sutured together creating a stronger limb with better circulation.
1954	The Vocational Rehabilitation Act provided authority to the Office of Vocational Rehabilitation of the Department of Health, Education, and Welfare to support research seeking improved management procedures and devices for the physically handicapped.
	The Children's Bureau began research support for the physically handicapped child.
	The Canadian hip-disarticulation prosthesis, designed at Sunnybrook Hospital, Toronto, was introduced by Colin McLaurin. This prosthesis allows standing and walking without a locked hip joint (Fig. 2-12).
1955	The Canadian Syme prosthesis, also designed at Sunnybrook Hospital, was introduced. It combined the use of plastic laminates and the solid rubber foot. This prosthesis revived the Syme procedure.
1956	The solid-ankle–cushion-heel (SACH) foot was introduced by the Biomechanics Laboratory at the University of California.
	The National Academy of Sciences organized the Committee on Prosthetics Education and Information to encourage the inclusion of prosthetics in the curricula for physicians and therapists.
	The University of California at Los Angeles and New York University initiated postgraduate courses in above-knee prosthetics for physicians, prosthetists, and therapists.
	The Committee on Prosthetics Research and Development established a standing Subcommittee on Child Prosthetics Problems (SCPP). Charles H. Frantz, M.D., served as the first chairman until 1965, when he was succeeded by George T. Aitken, M.D.
	The Child Prosthetics Studies program was created at New York University under the direction of Sidney Fishman.
1957	The Lower-Extremity Amputee Research Project (later, Biomechanics Laboratory) at the University of California was requested to study the problems of the below-knee amputee.
1958	Michel Berlemont, in France, demonstrated immediate postsurgical fitting of prostheses.
1959	The patellar-tendon-bearing (PTB) prosthesis was first introduced at the University of California at Berkeley.
	The name of the Orthopedic Appliance and Limb Manufacturers Association was changed to the American Orthotics and Prosthetics As-

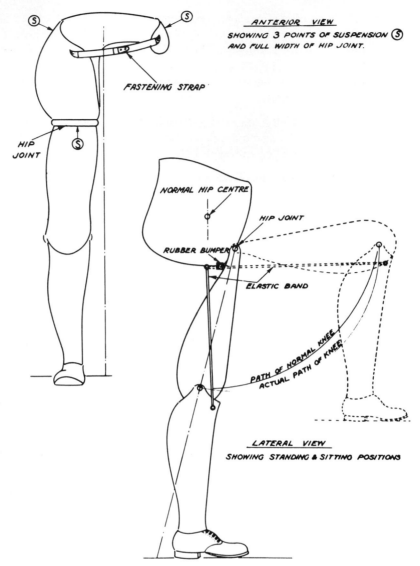

ANTERIOR VIEW
SHOWING 3 POINTS OF SUSPENSION Ⓢ
AND FULL WIDTH OF HIP JOINT.

FASTENING STRAP

HIP
JOINT

NORMAL HIP CENTRE

HIP JOINT

RUBBER BUMPER

ELASTIC BAND

PATH OF NORMAL KNEE
ACTUAL PATH OF KNEE

LATERAL VIEW
SHOWING STANDING & SITTING POSITIONS

FIGURE 2-12. A schematic drawing of the Canadian hip-disarticulation prosthesis. (From Wilson, AB, Jr: *The modern history of amputation surgery and artificial limbs.* **Orthop Clin North Am 3:275, 1972, with permission.)**

sociation (AOPA). The name of the American Board for Certification of the Prosthetic and Orthopedic Appliance Industry, Inc., was changed to the American Board for Certification in Orthotics and Prosthetics, Inc.

1959–1960   The "thalidomide tragedy" led to government-supported research, particularly in Germany, Canada, and the United States.

1960   The Stewart-Vickers unit became commercially available as the Hydra-Cadence leg (Fig. 2-13). This unit, which was developed by Jack Stewart of the Vickers Corporation, was a complete leg prosthesis that achieved knee stability by weight-bearing through the ball of the

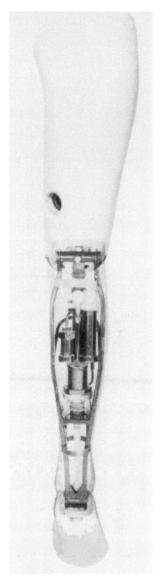

FIGURE 2-13. A cutaway view of an early model of the Stewart-Vickers hydraulic leg. With modifications, it became the Hydra-Cadence leg. (From Wilson, AB, Jr: *The modern history of amputation surgery and artificial limbs.* Orthop Clin North Am 3:278, 1972, with permission.)

foot; plantarflexion control by a hydraulic cylinder; and coordinated knee and ankle motion during swing phase for a greater vertical clearance.

1961   The chairman of the SCPP proposed the creation of a bulletin to exchange information among child amputee clinics. To this end, the first issue of the Inter-Clinic Information Bulletin was published.

1962   At Duke University, investigators began a study on early fitting of all levels of lower limb amputees. They found that early fitting of a temporary, well-fitted and well-aligned prosthesis reduced rehabilitation time and postsurgical problems and enabled the amputee to return to work earlier, which offset the extra cost.

The first successful complete human limb (an arm) replantation was reported by Ronald Malt and Charles McKhann in Boston.

The first successful hemicorporectomy amputation was reported by Bradley Aust and Karel Absolon at the University of Minnesota.

1963   Marian Weiss of Poland reported his experience with immediate post-surgical fittings of lower limb prostheses.

The first undergraduate curriculum leading to a Bachelor of Science degree in Prosthetics and Orthotics was inaugurated at New York University.

Guy Fajal of France developed the prosthèse-tibiale-supracondylienne (PTS), the PTB prosthesis with suprapatellar/supracondylar suspension.

1964   Two below-knee amputees were fitted with temporary prostheses immediately postsurgically at the University of California. This prompted investigators at the Navy Prosthetics Research Laboratory to begin a study of the technique; Ernest Burgess in Seattle, Washington, to evaluate the procedure in a VA-initiated program; and Augusto Sarmiento in Miami, Florida, to begin independent investigation.

1965   Congress passed Public Law 89-97, the Medicare Bill, which provided artificial limbs at a minimal cost to people 65 or older or those who are medically indigent at any age.

The "Hermes" hydraulic knee unit was made available.

The elastic-liner Syme prosthesis was developed at the University of Miami Prosthetic-Orthotic Laboratory.

1966   Dr. Götz-Gerd Kuhn of Münster, West Germany, introduced the Kondylenbettung Münster below-knee prosthesis. This was brought to the United States (1967) and refined by Carlton Fillauer of Chattanooga, Tennessee, as the wedge suspension socket.

Kurt Marschall and Robert Nitschke introduced the PTS prosthesis in the United States.

1968   The Henschke-Mauch "Hydraulic" Swing-N-Stance (S-N-S) system was commercially introduced. This unit, designed by Dr. Ulrich Henschke and Hans Mauch, offers both hydraulic swing and stance control.

Leigh A. Wilson, Eric Lyquist, and Charles W. Radcliffe designed and developed the air-cushion socket for the PTB prosthesis at the Biomechanics Laboratory, University of California at San Francisco.

1969   Clinical trials began on the PTB suction prosthesis, which was developed in Sweden.

1970   The International Society for Prosthetics and Orthotics was founded to improve communication between researchers and clinicians throughout the world.

A pneumatic piston cylinder unit was developed at the University of California.

1971   Endoskeletal prostheses with an adjustable tubular structure encased by a foam-plastic material and covered by an elastic hose were introduced by the Otto Bock Orthopaedic Industry (Fig. 2-14).

         The first commercially available axial rotator unit, the Weber-Watkins design, was introduced.

1974   An axial rotator unit, the Shank Torque Ankle Rotator (STAR), developed at Rancho Los Amigos Hospital in conjunction with United States Manufacturing Company, was introduced.

         The Hosmer modulorotator, the lightest of the available rotator units at that time (weighing approximately 300 g), was introduced.

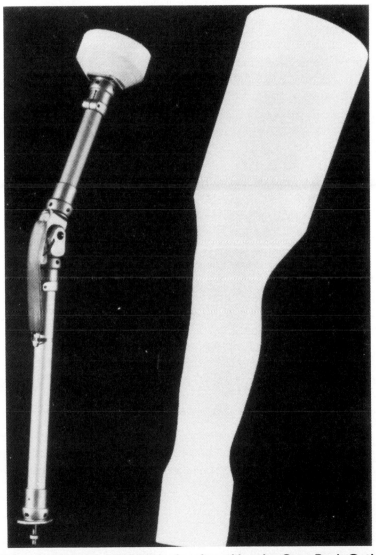

FIGURE 2-14. A modular prosthesis developed by the Otto Bock Orthopaedic Industry for above-knee amputees. The soft cosmetic cover is shaped by the prosthetist and covered by a cosmetic stocking. (From Wilson, AB, Jr: *The modern history of amputation surgery and artificial limbs.* Orthop Clin North Am 3:283, 1972, with permission.)

| 1976 | Another rotator, the Rochester Orthopedic Laboratories (ROL) unit, was introduced. It offered quick, easy replacement of components, rather than total unit replacement as with former designs, as well as adjustment of torque. |
| 1980 | The Stationary Attachment Flexible Endoskeletal (SAFE) prosthetic foot was introduced by John Campbell and Charles Childs of California. |

BIBLIOGRAPHY

ALLEN, RW AND VERHOFF, JR: *Supracondylar suspension patellar tendon bearing prosthesis: Its evaluation in unselected cases.* South Med J 63:59–61, 1970.

CARNES, EH: *Amputations, stumps and prostheses.* War Med 1:656–663, 1941.

DALE, WA AND JACOBS, JK: *Lower extremity amputation: Results in Nashville, 1956–1960.* Ann Surg 155:1011–1021, 1962.

DEDERICK, R: *Stump correction by muscle-plastic procedure.* In *Prosthetics International, Proceedings of the Second International Prosthetics Course, Committee on Prostheses, Braces and Technical Aids, International Society for the Welfare of Cripples.* Copenhagen, 1960, pp 59–61.

DEDERICK, R: *Technique of myoplastic amputations.* Ann R Coll Surg Engl 40:222–227, 1967.

DURAISWAMI, PK, ORTH, MS, AND TULI, SM: *5000 years of orthopaedics in India.* Clin Orthop 75:269–280, 1971.

FICARRA, BJ: *Amputations and prostheses through the centuries.* Med Rec 156:94–97, 154–156, 239–240, 1943.

FLIEGEL, O AND FEUER, SG: *Historical development of lower-extremity prostheses.* Arch Phys Med Rehabil 47:275–285, 1966.

FRANTZ, CH: *An evolution in the care of the child amputee.* Artificial Limbs 10:1–4, 1966.

FRIEDMANN, IW: *Amputations and prostheses in primitive cultures.* Bull Prosthet Res (17):105–138, 1972.

FRIEDMANN, LW: *Amputation in pre-Columbian America.* Arch Phys Med Rehabil 54:323–325, 1973.

GARRISON, FH: *Prosthetic appliances in war-time (historical resumé).* Mil Surgeon 39:507–509, 1916.

GARRISON, FH: *An Introduction to the History of Medicine.* WB Saunders, Philadelphia, 1929.

JANES, JM AND JACKSON, AE: *Open-flap amputation.* Surg Clin North Am 29:1049–1064, 1949.

KAY, HW: *The children's prosthetics and orthotics program.* Artificial Limbs 15:6–10, 1971.

LECONTE, RG: *New war methods in amputations, stumps, and prosthesis of the lower limbs.* US Nav M Bull 13:244–254, 1919.

LITTLE, EM: *Notes on artificial limbs for sailors and soldiers.* Amer J Orthop Surg 15:596–602, 1917.

LOON, HE: *Below-knee amputation surgery.* Artificial Limbs 6:86–99, 1962.

MACDONALD, J, JR: *The history of artificial limbs.* Am J Surg 19:76–80, 1905.

MAJOR, RH: *A History of Medicine, Vol I & II.* Charles C Thomas, Springfield, Illinois, 1954.

MCCORD, CP: *Cork legs and iron hands: The early history of artificial limbs.* Indust Med Surg 32:102–112, 1963.

McLAURIN, CA: *The evolution of the Canadian-type hip disarticulation prosthesis.* Artificial Limbs 4:22–28, 1957.

MURPHY, EF: *Projects, programs, and perspectives.* Artificial Limbs 14:I–IV, 1970.

Orthopaedic Appliances Atlas, Vol 2, Artif Limbs. JW Edwards, Ann Arbor, Michigan, 1960.

PETERSON, LT: *The army amputation program.* J Bone Joint Surg 26:635–637, 1944.

PUTTI, V: *Historic Artificial Limbs.* Paul B Hoeber, New York, 1930.

RACETTE, W AND BREAKEY, JW: *Clinical experience and functional considerations of axial rotators for the amputee.* Orth Pros 31:29–33, 1977.

RANG, M: *Anthology of Orthopaedics.* Churchill Livingstone, Edinburgh, 1966.

SCHMIDT, JE: *Medical Discoveries: Who and When.* Charles C Thomas, Springfield, Illinois, 1959.

SHUFELDT, RW: *Improvements in artificial limbs since the Civil War: As seen in examples in the Army Medical Museum.* Med Rev 24:643–649, 1918.

SINGER, C AND UNDERWOOD, EA: *A Short History of Medicine.* Oxford University Press, New York, 1962.

SMITH, BC: *Amputation through lower third of leg for diabetic and arteriosclerotic gangrene.* Arch Surg 27:267–295, 1933.

STEINDLER, A: *Artificial limbs.* Mil Surgeon 86:560–564, 1940.

TALBOTT, JH: *A Biographical History of Medicine: Excerpts and Essays on the Men and Their Work.* Grune & Stratton, New York, 1970.

THOMPSON, RG: *Amputation in the lower extremity.* J Bone Joint Surg 45A:1723–1734, 1963.

VAN DERWERKER, EE, JR: *A brief review of the history of amputations and prostheses.* Inter-Clinic Info Bull 15:15–16, 25, 1976.

VITALI, M, ET AL: *Amputations and Prostheses.* Baillière Tindall, London, 1978.

WAGENSTEEN, OH, SMITH, J, AND WANGENSTEEN, SD: *Some highlights in the history of amputation reflecting lessons in wound healing.* Bull Hist Med 41:97–131, 1967.

WAGENSTEEN, OH AND WAGENSTEEN, SD: *Military surgeons and surgery, old and new: An instructive chapter in management of contaminated wounds.* Surgery 62:1102–1124, 1967.

WEISS, AA: *The phantom limb.* Ann Intern Med 44:668–677, 1956.

WHITTAKER, AH: *Inter-innomino-abdominal amputation.* Indus Med 2:1–3, 1942.

WILSON, ABK: *Hand and foot prostheses.* Practitioner 201:759–766, 1968.

WILSON, AB, JR: *Limb prosthetics: 1970.* Artificial Limbs 14:1–52, 1970.

WILSON, AB, JR: *The modern history of amputation surgery and artificial limbs.* Orthop Clin North Am 3:267–285, 1972.

77% to 23%

RATIO

9.2 to 1

GLATTLY Study

CPOE Study

CPRD–CPOE Study

72% to 28%

9.2 to 1

percent-age %

CHAPTER **3**
STATISTICS

In 1964, Dr. Harold W. Glattly published the results of a survey of new amputees conducted from October 1, 1961 to January 31, 1963. With the assistance of the American Orthotic and Prosthetic Association (AOPA), data were obtained from more than 12,000 amputees. In 1975, Hector W. Kay and Jane D. Newman published the results of a study conducted from 1973 to 1974 by the Committee on Prosthetics Research and Development and the Committee on Prosthetic-Orthotic Education (CPRD-CPOE) based on 5830 cases. The CPRD-CPOE study was conducted identically to the Glattly study so that characteristics of the two amputee populations could be compared. Many of the data presented here were gathered in these surveys.

INCIDENCE OF AMPUTATION SURGERY

In 1964, amputations of the lower extremity (3962) comprised 1.9 percent of all the operations (210,444) performed in the Veterans Administration Hospitals. During this same year, the rate in the United States (US) was estimated to be 1.7 amputees per 1000 people, or 300,000 individuals who were missing part or all of one or more of their extremities. Public Health Service statistics revealed that about 33,000 lower extremity amputees were discharged from short-stay hospitals in 1965 in the US. The number of noninstitutionalized civilian amputees was estimated to be 274,000 in 1971 and 358,000 in 1977. In 1979, estimates from the National Health Interview Survey based on household interviews of the civilian noninstitutionalized population indicated the number of individuals with absence of extremities or parts of extremities (excluding tips of fingers or toes only) to be 1,849,000 at a rate of 8.6 per 1000 persons in the US.

After World War I, there were 26,262 British service casualties with resulting amputations who were treated at Roehampton. The total number of amputees in England and Wales was approximately 70,000 in 1963 and 80,000 in 1964. The Department of Health statistics for 1970 indicated that 4559 new patients attended limb-fitting centers in England. By 1978, there were about 5000 new patients each year. In 1973, there were more than 70,000 amputees in England and Wales, with 15,485 war pensioners, 5,074 of whom were from World War I.

CAUSES OF AMPUTATION

In the Glattly and CPRD-CPOE reports, the causes of amputation were categorized into four groups: (1) congenital, (2) tumor, (3) trauma, and (4) disease. The data indicate that in both studies the majority of amputations were due to disease, with trauma being the second most frequent cause (Table 3-1). It is interesting to note that the percentage of amputation due to trauma has decreased. One could hypothesize that this is due to improved medical care of traumatized limbs and improved work safety conditions.

Other authors have reported even higher percentages of amputation for disease. Hansson (1964) reported 85 percent lower extremity amputation for peripheral vascular disease in 586 amputees in Sweden from 1947 to 1963. Warren and Kihn (1968), in a 1964 study of Veterans Administration Hospitals, reported that 76 percent of the amputations were for vascular insufficiency. Vascular disease and infection were the reasons for amputation in 98 percent of 172 cases between 1964 and 1968 reported by Burgess (1969). Of 165 cases, 71 percent were found to be due to vascular disease in a study by Weiss and Janeczek (1973), 85 percent in a study of 194 amputees by Kerstein

TABLE 3-1. PERCENTAGE DISTRIBUTION OF AMPUTATIONS BY CAUSE

Cause of Amputation	Glattly Study (1961–1963)	CPRD-CPOE Study (1973–1974)
Congenital	4.3	2.8
Tumor	4.5	4.5
Trauma	33.2	22.4
Disease	58.0	70.3

and associates (1974), and 95 percent of 292 below-knee amputations reported by Murray (1965).

The data reported by Rosenberg and associates (1970) on 176 cases of lower extremity amputations for vascular insufficiency between 1948 and 1969 revealed gangrene to be the predominant indication for amputation (159 limbs). The increased frequency of amputation for peripheral vascular disease probably reflects the increasing geriatric population.

BY AGE

- Tumor. The percentage of amputation owing to tumor was largest in the 11 to 20 age group (Table 3-2) in both the Glattly and CPRD-CPOE studies.
- Trauma. In the Glattly study, the largest percentage of amputation owing to trauma was in the 41 to 50 age group; while in the later study, it was in the 21 to 30 age group (see Table 3-2).
- Disease. Amputation resulting from disease was greatest in the 61 to 70 age group in both studies (see Table 3-2), with over half being found in the combined 61 to 80 age groups (Glattly, 56.2 percent; CPRD-CPOE, 60.7 percent).

TABLE 3-2. PERCENTAGE OF AMPUTATIONS DUE TO TUMOR, TRAUMA, AND DISEASE, BY AGE

Age Group	TUMOR		TRAUMA		DISEASE	
	Glattly Study (1961–1963)	CPRD-CPOE Study (1973–1974)	Glattly Study (1961–1963)	CPRD-CPOE Study (1973–1974)	Glattly Study (1961–1963)	CPRD-CPOE Study (1973–1974)
0–10	4.9	2.7	3.6	4.2	1.1	0.1
11–20	28.3	33.5	11.0	19.7	1.3	0.9
21–30	12.1	13.8	17.4	25.7	1.3	0.8
31–40	14.0	10.0	18.8	16.9	3.7	2.1
41–50	13.4	11.5	20.7	14.2	10.0	7.7
51–60	13.6	12.7	15.7	10.4	22.6	21.7
61–70	9.1	10.0	9.2	6.8	35.9	36.8
71–80	3.8	5.4	3.0	1.8	20.3	23.9
81–90	0.8	0.4	0.6	0.3	3.7	5.7
91 +	0	0	0	0	0.1	0.3

SITE OF AMPUTATION

A comparison of the results of the Glattly and CPRD-CPOE studies shows that there is a trend toward an increase in below-knee and Syme amputations, with a proportionate decrease in above-knee amputations (Table 3-3). Above-knee and below-knee amputations continue to constitute the overwhelming majority of all amputations (Glattly, 80.9 percent; CPRD-CPOE, 86.4 percent). The remaining 14.5 percent (Glattly study) and 8.3 percent (CPRD-CPOE study) are upper extremity amputations.

A study by Sarmiento and Warren in 1969 of above-knee and below-knee amputations performed in the years 1960 to 1963 (297 amputations) and 1964 to 1968 (328 amputations) also shows a trend toward an increase in below-knee amputations.

	Above-knee	Below-knee	Reamputation from below-knee to above-knee
1960-1963	69.3%	30.7%	50.0%
1964-1968	17.0%	83.0%	7.5%

The ratio of lower limb amputations to upper limb amputations shows a greater preponderance of lower limb amputees in both studies (Table 3-4). The increase in this ratio in the CPRD-CPOE study could be due to an increase in the number of elderly lower extremity amputees rather than an actual decrease in the number of upper extremity amputees.

SIDE OF AMPUTATION

The Glattly and CPRD-CPOE studies revealed no significant difference in right- or left-sided amputations in either the upper or lower extremities. This might be expected in the congenital, tumor, and disease groups, in which one would not expect to find laterality preference. Amputations resulting from trauma, however, might be expected to occur more frequently in the dominant extremity, especially upper extremity amputations. The percentages of amputation by side were not grouped according to cause or hand dominance; therefore, this information was not available.

SEX RATIO

The proportion of males undergoing amputation is demonstrably greater than females (Tables 3-5, 3-6).

BILATERAL AMPUTATIONS

About 25 percent to 45 percent of the amputee population has had amputation of both lower extremities (Table 3-7). Most bilateral amputees have either below-knee amputations bilaterally or an above-knee amputation on one side and a below-knee amputation on the other side. Of those amputees who survive, about 10 percent lose the other leg within 1 year, 20 percent within 2 years, and one third within 5 years.

TABLE 3-3. PERCENTAGE OF ALL AMPUTATIONS BY SITE IN THE LOWER EXTREMITY

Lower Extremity Level	Glattly Study (1961–1963)	CPRD-CPOE Study (1973–1974)
Hip disarticulation	1.8	2.0
Above-knee	44.1	32.6
Knee disarticulation	1.1	0.7
Below-knee	36.8	53.8
Syme	1.7	2.6

TABLE 3-4. RATIO OF LOWER LIMB TO UPPER LIMB AMPUTATIONS

	Glattly Study (1961–1963)	CPRD-CPOE Study (1973–1974)
Lower limb	6	11
Upper limb	1	1

TABLE 3-5. RATIO OF MALES TO FEMALES BY STUDY

Study	Ratio of Males to Females
Glattly study (1964) (USA)	77% to 23%
CPRD-CPOE study (1975) (USA)	72% to 28%
Barnett, et al, study (1976) (Australia)	59.5% to 40.5%

TABLE 3-6. RATIO OF MALES TO FEMALES BY CAUSE OF AMPUTATION

Cause	Ratio of Males to Females (Glattly Study, 1964)
Trauma	9.2 to 1
Disease	2.6 to 1
Tumor	1.2 to 1
Congenital	1.2 to 1

TABLE 3-7. PERCENTAGES OF BILATERAL AMPUTEES

Study Author	Year	Total Amputees	Bilateral Amputees AK/AK	BK/BK	AK/BK
McKittrick & Pratt	1934	20%			
Faxon	1939	22%			
Edwards, et al	1953	23%			
Claugus, et al	1958	22%	50%	40%	10%
Goldner	1960	45%			
Bugel & Carlson	1961	21%	66%	4%	30%
Cameron, et al	1964	28%			
Murray	1965	25%			
Baddeley & Fulford	1965	26.5%			
Ecker & Jacobs	1970	42%	21%	30%	32.6%
Kihn, et al	1972	23%			
Najenson & Levy	1972	22%			
Kerstein, et al	1974	23%	25%	50%	25%
Sakuma, et al	1974		49%	21%	28%
Kerstein, et al	1975		19%	60%	17%
Kerstein, et al	1975		20%	60%	20%

AK = above knee, BK = below knee

MORTALITY FROM AMPUTATION SURGERY

Mortality from amputation surgery has shown a marked decline in the antibiotic era (Table 3-8). Although below-knee amputations have been reported to have a lower primary healing rate than above-knee amputations (Table 3-9), the mortality rate after below-knee amputations is lower (see Table 3-8).

The more frequent causes of death following an amputation are myocardial infarction, cerebrovascular accident, kidney disease (uremia), pneumonia, sepsis, pulmonary embolism, gas gangrene, and diabetic acidosis. Factors that contribute to mortality include diabetes mellitus (Table 3-10), obesity, underlying heart disease, advanced age, gangrene with sepsis, and chronic pulmonary disease. When advanced gangrene and toxemia are present, the chance for survival is better if an open amputation is done.

Weiss found that osteosarcoma occurs more frequently in males than in females. The primary tumor is most often located in the distal femur (50 percent), with 72 percent being located in the long bones of the lower extremities. Most patients exhibit the disease during the second decade of life. Pain is the most common symptom. The median time from diagnosis until death for Weiss's group was 10.8 months. The initial metastatic site is usually (52 percent) pulmonary. Recurrence or metastasis was present in 93 percent. The 5-year survival rate following amputation for recurrent melanoma (Table 3-11) is as low as for osteosarcoma (Table 3-12).

POSTOPERATIVE COMPLICATIONS

The most frequent complications after amputations are infection, hematoma or skin necrosis of the residual limb, urinary tract sepsis, pneumonia, myocardial infarction, pulmonary embolism, upper gastrointestinal bleeding, depression or psychosis, decubitus ulcer, and cerebrovascular accident.

DURATION OF HOSPITALIZATION

The average hospitalization for the below-knee amputee is longer than for the above-knee amputee (Table 3-13). This probably reflects the fact that the below-knee amputee is more likely to have postoperative wound complications (less likelihood of primary healing) and is more likely to undergo prosthetic rehabilitation.

AGE AT FITTING WITH A PROSTHESIS

In both the Glattly and CPRD-CPOE studies, most amputees who were fitted with prostheses were in the 61 to 70 age group (Table 3-14). It is interesting to note that the percentage of amputees being fitted with a prosthesis who fall in the 61+ age group increased from 39.7 (Glattly study) to 49.6 (CPRD-CPOE study).

TABLE 3-8. MORTALITY FOR AMPUTATION SURGERY OF THE LOWER LIMB

| Study | | | | | % MORTALITY | | | | |
Author(s)	Year Published	Years Data Collected	Amputations	Cases	AK	BK	Combined	Diabetic	Nondiabetic
Buel	1848	1839–1848	91		26.5%	29.2%	31.66%		
Hayward	1850	to 1840	60	57	26%	22%			
		1840–1850	63		29%	18%	24%		
McKittrick & Pratt	1934	1923–1933	467	396			11.4%		
Levin & Dealy	1935	1930–1935	24		50%			50%	
Taylor	1939	1930–1938	137	117			32%	34.4%	27.7%
Faxon	1939	1929–1939		262			13.1%		
Pearse & Ziegler	1940							32%	
Bickel	1943	1930–1942	110	103		3%			
Mandelberg & Sheinfeld	1946	1934–1943	128		32.2%	34.5%		32.8%	
Silbert	1948	1916–1942		1242	44%			44%	
		1940–1946	151				9.3%	9.4%	8.7%
Perlow & Roth	1949	1936–1938	165				25%	13.3%	
		1939–1944					15.5% } 17.5%		
		1945–1947					11.7%		
Regan, et al	1949	1933–1939		140			35%		
		1940–1944		136			8.8%		
		1945–1948		122			4.1%		
Silbert & Haimovici	1950	1940–1949	213 BK	196			9.4%	9.3%	9.7%

TABLE 3-8. *Continued*

Author(s)	Year Published	Years Data Collected	Amputations	Cases	AK	BK	Combined	Diabetic	Nondiabetic
Kern	1951	1938–1948	74	72			12%	7.5%	
Shumacker & Moore	1951	1946–1951	128 61 BK	113	6%	6.6%	6.25%	2.7%	
Mooney, et al	1951			85		6.5%		6.5%	
Silbert & Haimovici	1954	1939–1954	455 Total 331 BK		12.1%	7%		6.7% (all BK)	7.8% (all BK)
Smith	1956		50	50		12%		12% (all BK)	
Claugus, et al	1958	1946–1956	155	89	7%	0%	6%		
Dale & Capps	1959	1948–1958	284	237			20%	12%	
Schlitt & Serlin	1960	1953–1958	129	96	13%	7%	10.1%		
Harris, et al	1961	1948–1958	52	47		6%			
Perlow	1962	1936–1958	269		21%	3%			
Dale & Jacobs	1962	1956–1960	479	385	14%	1%	8%		
Hoar & Torres	1962	1954–1960		100		7%		7%	
Block & Whitehouse	1963		43	40		0%			
Eraklis & Wheeler	1963		16	15		0%			
Pedersen, et al	1964		60 BK	55		0%			
Otteman & Stahlgren	1965	1955–1960	413	323	42%	30%	29.7%		
Murray	1965		292			6%			

Author	Year	Period	No.	No.	%	%	%	%	%
Tracy	1966		82	77		11.7%			
Lim, et al	1967	1960–1965	103		35%	16%			
Eidemiller, et al	1968	1938–1945			46.8%				
		1946–1950	57		22.8%				
		1952–1967	436		19.7%				
Warren & Kihn	1968	1964	453 240 AK 121 BK	91	28.1%	10.3%	21.8%		
Cranley, et al	1969		101					7% early 56% late	8% early 58% late
Rosenberg, et al	1970	1948–1967	176		21.9%	9.9%	17%	23.6%	10.3%
Ecker & Jacobs	1970	1952–1965	178	103	12.4%	8.7%	23%	23%	
Burgess, et al	1971		193			7%	8%		
Silverstein & Kadish	1973	1967–1972	515	320	35%	35%	34%	45%	
Barnett, et al	1976	1970–1972	119	111			18%		
Berardi & Keonin	1978	1971–1976	163	100	18%	10%	16%		
Malone, et al	1979	1966–1978	142	133		0%			
Fleurant & Alexander	1980	1970–1978	373	353		5%			

AK = above knee, BK = below knee

TABLE 3-9. Successful Healing

Study		AK			BK			TM
Author	Year	Total	Primary	Secondary	Total	Primary	Secondary	
McKittrick	1946							85%
McKittrick, et al	1949							72%
Silbert & Haimovici	1950				97%	70%	27%	63%
Warren, et al	1952							63%
Edwards & Linton	1953				81%			
Silbert & Haimovici	1954				93%	73%	20%	
Haimovici	1955							91%
Pedersen & Day	1956							76%
Kendrick	1956				84%	63%	21%	
Carney & Goldowsky	1957				71%			20%
Kelly & Janes	1957				93%	76%	17%	
Wheelock, et al	1957							83%
Claugus, et al	1958	92%	79%	13%	87%	74%	13%	29%
Schlitt & Serlin	1960	85%			68%			33%
Wheelock	1961							63%
Harris, et al	1961				75%	54%	21%	
Hoar & Torres	1962				90%	82%	8%	
Dale & Jacobs	1962	87%	72%	15%	76%	62%	14%	
Block & Whitehouse	1963				93%			

Study	Year					
Eraklis & Wheeler	1963		82%	63%	19%	
Perry	1963		93%	40%		
Pedersen, et al	1964		84%	47%	37%	
Murray	1965		85%			
Bradham & Smoak	1965	96%	86%			33%
Burgess	1965		82%			
Tracy	1966		90%			
Lim, et al	1967		85%			
Eidemiller, et al	1968	65% (1946–1950) 68% (1952–1967)				
Warren & Kihn	1968	82%	68%			50%
Cranley, et al	1969		83% nondiabetic 98% diabetic			
Ecker & Jacobs	1970	95%	85%			
Schwindt, et al	1973					63%
King, et al	1975		89%	68%	21%	
Effeney, et al	1977					52%
Malone, et al	1979		89%			
Fleurant & Alexander	1980		82.8%	73.3%	9.5%	

AK = above knee, BK = below knee, TM = transmetatarsal

TABLE 3-10. INCIDENCE OF DIABETES IN AMPUTEES

Author(s)	Year	% of Amputees with Diabetes
Holden	1947	69%
Carney & Goldowsky	1957	54%
Dale & Capps	1959	32%
Rosenthal	1961	47%
Harris, et al	1961	60%
Otteman & Stahlgren	1965	33%
Murray	1965	67%
Thompson, et al	1965	44%
Warren & Kihn	1968	39%
Sarmiento & Warren	1969	
	1960–1963	49%
	1964–1968	69%
Najenson & Levy	1972	67%
Wray, et al	1972	36%
Silverstein & Kadish	1973	65%
Malone, et al	1979	66%

TABLE 3-11. SURVIVAL FOLLOWING AMPUTATION FOR RECURRENT MELANOMA

Study	5 years
McPeak, et al (1963) (46 cases)	35%
Pack, et al (1952) (1190 cases—1917–1950)	27% for females 16% for males
Turnbull (1973) (43 pts—1950–1964)	40% after hip disarticulation (20 pts) 9% after hemipelvectomy (23 pts)
Cox (1974) (13 pts—1946–1966)	29% for females 0% for males

TABLE 3-12. SURVIVAL IN CASES OF OSTEOSARCOMA

Author	Year	5 Years	10 Years
Coventry & Dahlin	1957	19.3% (353 cases)	15.3% (294 cases)
Taft	1966	16% (163 children)	
Johnson, et al	1971	10% (50 cases)	
Sutow, et al	1976	56% (12–61 months, 43 cases) 67% (12–26 months, 30 cases)	
Weiss, et al	1978	12% (50 cases)	

TABLE 3-13. AVERAGE HOSPITALIZATION FOR AMPUTATION

STUDY		AMPUTATION LEVEL			
Author	Year	AK	BK	TM or Ray	All
McKittrick, et al	1949			30 days postop	
Carney & Goldowsky	1957	43 days			
Chapman, et al	1959				147 days* 90 days from amputation to discharge
Ecker & Jacobs	1970	177 days	201 days	69 days	
Schwindt, et al	1973			Postoperative days for those who healed 50 days diabetics 65 days nondiabetics	
Weaver & Marshall	1973	56 days	83 days		
Kerstein, et al	1974				189 days

*43 more days from amputation to discharge for those who received a prosthesis
AK = above knee, BK = below knee, TM = transmetatarsal

TABLE 3-14. PERCENTAGE OF AMPUTEES FITTED WITH A PROSTHESIS, BY AGE

Age	Glattly Study	CPRD-CPOE Study
1–10	5.1	3.4
11–20	6.6	6.9
21–30	7.2	7.1
31–40	9.1	5.7
41–50	13.3	9.1
51–60	19.0	18.2
61–70	24.3	27.8
71–80	13.0	17.5
81–90	2.4	4.1
91 +		0.2

PROSTHETIC USAGE

There is a greater potential for functional prosthetic usage by a below-knee amputee than by an above-knee amputee (Table 3-15). Because the below-knee amputee is a better rehabilitation candidate, it is important for the knee to be saved, if possible.

TABLE 3-15. PROSTHETIC USERS

STUDY		AK		BK		AK/BK
Author	Year	Unilateral	Bilateral	Unilateral	Bilateral	
Bickel	1943			80% of those fitted		
Edwards & Linton	1953			92% of those who healed		
McKenzie	1953	49% of those amputated	37%	58% of those amputated	100%	33%
Smith	1956			72% of those surviving	48%	
Watkins & Liao	1958		71%		87%	54%
Erlacher	1958		0%			
Bertelsen & Rønn	1960	60% (elderly)		80% (elderly)		
Russek	1960		12%		61%	38%
Hoar & Torres	1962			63%		
Hansson	1964				27%	25%
Cameron, et al	1964	80% of those fitted 36% of those amputated		78% of those fitted 30% of those amputated		
Baddeley & Fulford	1965	60% of those fitted 32% of those amputated		58% of those fitted 38% of those amputated		

Author	Year					
Smith	1965			72% of those surviving	48%	
Murray	1965			60% of those fitted 25% of those amputated		
Warren & Kihn	1968		19% of those amputated	40% of those amputated		
Cranley, et al	1969			87% of nondiabetics 77% of diabetics		
Ecker & Jacobs	1970	55%	0%	96%	100%	83%
McCollough	1972		0%			
Sakuma, et al	1974		15%	66%		29%
Malone, et al	1979			100%	93%	
Jensen, et al	1983	47% of those surviving		69% of those surviving		
Volpicelli, et al	1983		6% (only traumatic amputees)	67%		22%

AK = above knee, BK = below knee

TABLE 3-16. REHABILITATION OF LEFT VERSUS RIGHT LOWER LIMB AMPUTEES

Rehabilitation Status	Prosthesis Worn on	
	Left	Right
Full restoration	41%	34%
Partial restoration (required cane for ambulation)	36.3%	45.6%

Bilateral amputees are less likely to be prosthetic users than unilateral amputees of the same level. The bilateral below-knee amputee, however, is more likely to be a functional prosthetic user than a unilateral above-knee amputee.

Left lower extremity amputees are more likely to be independently ambulatory without an external ambulatory aid than their counterpart right lower extremity amputees (Table 3-16). Left lower extremity amputees not only make better progress in rehabilitation, but they do so in less time than the right lower extremity amputee. This suggests that maximum potential is generally better if the nondominant lower extremity is amputated. It has been estimated that half of the geriatric lower extremity amputees who receive an artificial limb discard it within 6 months.

BIBLIOGRAPHY

ANDERSON, AD, ET AL: *The use of lower extremity prosthetic limbs by elderly patients.* Arch Phys Med Rehabil 48:533–538, 1967.

BADDELEY, RM AND FULFORD, JC: *A trial of conservative amputations for lesions of the feet in diabetes mellitus.* Br J Surg 52:38–43, 1965.

BARNETT, AJ, TWIST, E, AND BALFE, A: *Lower limb amputation in a general hospital: A comparative review.* Med J Aust 2:14–18, 1976.

BERARDI, RS AND KEONIN, Y: *Amputations in peripheral vascular occlusive disease.* Am J Surg 135:231–235, 1978.

BICKEL, WH: *Amputations below the knee in occlusive arterial disease.* Surg Clin North Am 23:982–994, 1943.

BICKEL, WH AND GHORMLEY, RK: *Amputations below the knee in occlusive arterial disease.* Proc Mayo Clinic 18:361–367, 1943.

BLOCK, MA AND WHITEHOUSE, FW: *Below-knee amputation in patients with diabetes mellitus.* Arch Surg 87:682–689, 1963.

BRADHAM, RR AND SMOAK, RD: *Amputations of the lower extremity: Used for arteriosclerosis obliterans.* Arch Surg 90:60–64, 1965.

BRICE, GB: *Rehabilitation of the elderly vascular amputee: A ten year survey.* J Assoc Phys Ment Rehab 18:138–140, 1964.

BUEL, HW: *Statistics of amputations in the New York Hospital: From January 1, 1839 to January 1, 1848.* Am J Med Sci 16:33–43, 1848.

BUGEL, HJ AND CARLSON, RI: *A study of lower extremity amputees.* Am J Phys Med 40:93–95, 1961.

BURGESS, EM: *The below-knee amputation.* Inter-Clinic Info Bull 8:1–22, 1969.

BURGESS, EM AND MARSDEN, FW: *Major lower extremity amputations following arterial reconstruction.* Arch Surg 108:655–660, 1974.

BURGESS, EM, ET AL: *Amputations of the leg for peripheral vascular insufficiency.* J Bone Joint Surg 53A:874–890, 1971.

CAMERON, HC, LENNARD-JONES, JE, AND ROBINSON, MP: *Amputation in the diabetic: Outcome and survival.* Lancet 2:605–607, 1964.

CARNES, EH: *Amputations, stumps and prostheses.* War Med 1:656–663, 1941.

CARNEY, WI AND GOLDOWSKY, SJ: *Amputations in peripheral vascular disease.* Am J Surg 93:795–797, 1957.

CHAPMAN, CE, ET AL: *Follow-up study on a group of older amputee patients.* JAMA 170:1396–1402, 1959.

CLAUGUS, CE, ET AL: *Amputations of the lower extremity for arteriosclerosis.* Arch Surg 76:992–996, 1958.

COVENTRY, MB AND DAHLIN, DC: *Osteogenic sarcoma: A critical analysis of 430 cases.* J Bone Joint Surg 39A:741–758, 1957.

COX, KR: *Survival after amputation for recurrent melanoma.* Surg Gynecol Obstet 139:720–722, 1974.

CRANLEY, JJ, ET AL: *Below-the-knee amputation for arteriosclerosis obliterans: With and without diabetes.* Arch Surg 98:77–80, 1969.

CUMMINGS, V, ET AL: *The elderly medically ill amputee.* Arch Phys Med Rehabil 44:549–554, 1963.

DALE, WA AND CAPPS, W, JR: *Major leg and thigh amputations: Ten-year survey of results.* Surgery 46:333–342, 1959.

DALE, WA AND JACOBS, JK: *Lower extremity amputation: Results in Nashville, 1959–1960.* Ann Surg 155:1011–1022, 1962.

DAVIES, EJ, FRIZ, BR, AND CLIPPINGER, FW: *Amputees and their prostheses.* Artificial Limbs 14:19–48, 1970.

DEDERICH, R: *Stump correction by muscle-plastic procedure.* In *Prosthetics International, Proceedings of the Second International Prosthetics Course, Committee on Prostheses, Braces and Technical Aids, International Society for the Welfare of Cripples.* Copenhagen, 1960, pp 59–61.

ECKER, ML AND JACOBS, BS: *Lower extremity amputation in diabetic patients.* Diabetes 19:189–195, 1970.

EDWARDS, EA, McADAMS, AJ, AND CRANE, C: *Events leading to major amputation in patients with arteriosclerosis.* N Engl J Med 249:514–519, 1953.

EDWARDS, WS AND LINTON, RR: *Closed lower leg amputations in arterial insufficiency.* Surgery 34:688–692, 1953.

EFFENEY, DJ, LIM, RC, AND SCHECTER, WP: *Transmetatarsal amputation.* Arch Surg 112:1366-1370, 1977.

EIDEMILLER, LR, AWE, WC, AND PETERSON, CG: *Amputation of the ischemic extremity.* Am J Surg 34:491–493, 1968.

ELIASON, EL AND WRIGHT, VWM: *Diabetic and arteriosclerotic gangrene of the lower extremities: Analysis of one hundred cases of amputation.* Surg Gynecol Obstet 42:753–768, 1926.

ERAKLIS, A AND WHEELER, HB: *Below-knee amputations in patients with severe arterial insufficiency.* N Engl J Med 269:938–943, 1963.

ERDMAN, WJ, II AND MAXWELL, EL: *Analysis of results of training 400 A/K amputees.* Arch Phys Med 36:209–211, 1955.

FALKEL, JE: *Amputation as a consequence of diabetes mellitus.* Phys Ther 63:960–964, 1983.

FAXON, HH: *Major amputations for advanced peripheral arterial obliterative disease.* JAMA 113:1199–1204, 1939.

FLEURANT, FW AND ALEXANDER, J: *Below knee amputation and rehabilitation of amputees.* Surg Gynecol Obstet 151:41–44, 1980.

FREED, MM AND CHARETTE, EE: *Rehabilitation after amputation of the lower extremity for malignancy.* Arch Phys Med Rehabil 45:564–570, 1964.

FURSTÉ, W AND HERRMANN, LG: *Value of transmetatarsal amputations in the management of gangrene of toes.* Arch Surg 57:497–512, 1948.

GILLIS, L: *Amputations including congenital abnormalities.* Practitioner 193:626–633, 1964.

GLATTLY, HW: *A preliminary report on the amputee census.* Artificial Limbs 7:5–10, 1963.

GLATTLY, HW: *A statistical study of 12,000 new amputees.* South Med J 57:1373–1378, 1964.

GOLDNER, MG: *The fate of the second leg in the diabetic amputee.* Diabetes 9:100–103, 1960.

HAIMOVICI, H: *Criteria for and results of transmetatarsal amputation for ischemic gangrene.* Arch Surg 70:45–51, 1955.

HARRIS, PD, SCHWARTZ, SI, AND DEWEESE, JA: *Midcalf amputation for peripheral vascular disease.* Arch Surg 82:381–383, 1961.

HAYWARD, G: *Statistics of the amputations of large limbs that have been performed at the Massachusetts General Hospital: From its establishment to Jan 1, 1850.* Boston Med Surg J 43:169–181, 1850.

HICKEY, WF, JR AND ROSSE, AA: *Providing prostheses after amputation for malignancy.* J Rehabil 21:9–10, 1955.

HOAR, CS AND TORRES, J: *Evaluation of below-the-knee amputation in the treatment of diabetic gangrene.* N Engl J Med 266:440–443, 1962.

HOLDEN, WD: *Arteriosclerotic ischemic necrosis of the lower extremities.* Surgery 22:125–128, 1947.

JAMIESON, CW AND HILL, D: *Amputation for vascular disease.* Br J Surg 63:683–690, 1976.

JANSEN, K: *Amputation: Frequency and cause.* In Prosthetics International, Proceedings of the Second International Prosthetics Course, Committee on Prostheses, Braces and Technical Aids, International Society for the Welfare of Cripples. Copenhagen, 1960, pp 105–107.

JENSEN, JS, MANDRUP-POULSEN, T, AND KRASNIK, M: *Prosthetic fitting in lower limb amputees.* Acta Orthop Scand 54:101–103, 1983.

JOHNSON, RJ, BONFIGLIO, M, AND COOPER, RR: *Osteosarcoma.* Clin Orthop 78:314–322, 1971.

KAY, HW AND NEWMAN, JD: *Amputee survey, 1973–74: Preliminary findings and comparisons.* Orth Pros 28:27–32, 1974.

KAY, HW AND NEWMAN, JD: *Relative incidences of new amputations: Statistical comparisons of 6,000 new amputees.* Orth Pros 29:3–16, 1975.

KELLY, PJ AND JANES, JM: *Criteria for determining the proper level of amputation in occlusive vascular disease: A review of 323 amputations.* J Bone Joint Surg 39A:883–891, 1957.

KENDRICK, RR: *Below-knee amputation in arteriosclerotic gangrene.* Br J Surg 44:13–17, 1956.

KERN, HM: *Amputation of lower extremities in the aged.* Amer J Surg 82:479–484, 1951.

KERSTEIN, MD, ET AL: *Amputations of the lower extremity: A study of 194 cases.* Arch Phys Med Rehabil 55:454–459, 1974.

KERSTEIN, MD, ET AL: *Associated diagnoses complicating rehabilitation after major lower extremity amputation.* Angiology 25:536–547, 1974.

KERSTEIN, MD, ET AL: *Associated diagnoses which complicate rehabilitation of the patient with bilateral lower extremity amputations.* Surg Gynecol Obstet 140:875–876, 1975.

KERSTEIN, MD, ET AL: *Rehabilitation after bilateral lower extremity amputation.* Arch Phys Med Rehabil 56:309–311, 1975.

KERSTEIN, MD, ET AL: *What influence does age have on rehabilitation of amputees?* Geriatrics 30:67–71, 1975.

KERSTEIN, MD, ET AL: *Successful rehabilitation following amputation of dominant versus nondominant extremities.* Am J Occup Ther 31:313–315, 1977.

KEY, JA: *Amputation for chronic osteomyelitis.* J Bone Joint Surg 26:350–355, 1944.

KIHN, RB, WARREN, R, AND BEEBE, GW: *The geriatric amputee.* Ann Surg 176:305–314, 1972.

KING, B, MCINTYRE, R, AND MYERS, K: *Below-knee amputation in peripheral arterial disease.* Aust NZ J Surg 45:301–304, 1975.

KOHN, KH: *Use of lower-extremity prostheses in geriatric amputees.* Arch Phys Med Rehabil 51:99–104, 1970.

LEMPKE, RE, ET AL: *Amputation for arteriosclerosis obliterans.* Arch Surg 86:406–413, 1963.

LEVIN, CM AND DEALY, FN: *The surgical diabetic: A five year survey.* Ann Surg 102:1029–1039, 1935.

LIM, RC, JR, ET AL: *Below-knee amputation for ischemic gangrene.* Surg Gynecol Obstet 125:493–501, 1967.

LITTLE, JM: *Amputation of the leg: A dull topic revisited.* Med J Aust 2:442–445, 1973.

LOWENTHAL, M, POSNIAK, AO, AND TOBIS, JS: *Rehabilitation of the elderly double above-knee amputee.* Arch Phys Med 39:290–295, 1958.

MALONE, JM, ET AL: *Therapeutic and economic impact of a modern amputation program.* Bull Prosthet Res 10–32:7–17, 1979.

MANDELBERG, A AND SHEINFELD, W: *Diabetic amputations: Amputation of lower extremity in diabetics—analysis of 128 cases.* Am J Surg 71:70–76, 1946.

MAZET, R, JR: *The geriatric amputee.* Artificial Limbs 11:33–41, 1967.

MCCOLLOUGH, NC, III: *The dysvascular amputee.* Orthop Clin North Am 3:303–321, 1972.

MCKENZIE, DS: *The elderly amputee.* Br Med J 1:153–156, 1953.

MCKITTRICK, LS: *Recent advances in the care of the surgical complications of diabetes mellitus.* N Engl J Med 235:929–932, 1946.

MCKITTRICK, LS, MCKITTRICK, JB, AND RISLEY, TS: *Transmetatarsal amputation for infection or gangrene in patients with diabetes mellitus.* Ann Surg 130:826–842, 1949.

MCKITTRICK, LS AND PRATT, TC: *The principles of and results after amputation for diabetic gangrene.* Ann Surg 100:638–653, 1934.

MCPEAK, CJ, ET AL: *Amputation for melanoma of the extremity.* Surgery 54:426–431, 1963.

MOONEY, V, ET AL: *Comparison of postoperative stump management.* J Bone Joint Surg 53A:241, 1951.

MURDOCH, G: *Levels of amputation and limiting factors.* Ann R Coll Surg Engl 40:204–216, 1967.

MURRAY, DG: *Below-knee amputations in the aged: Evaluation and prognosis.* Geriatrics 20:1033–1038, 1965.

NAJENSON, T AND LEVY, M: *Rehabilitation of amputees with progressive vascular disease.* Rheumatology and Physical Medicine 11:250–259, 1972.

OTTEMAN, MG AND STAHLGREN, LH: *Evaluation of factors which influence mortality and morbidity following major lower extremity amputations for arteriosclerosis.* Surg Gynecol Obstet 120:1217–1220, 1965.

PACK, GT, GERBER, DM, AND SCHARNAGEL, IM: *End results in the treatment of malignant melanoma: A report of 1190 cases.* Ann Surg 136:905–911, 1952.

PEARSE, HE AND ZIEGLER, HR: *Is the conservative treatment of infection or gangrene in diabetic patients worthwhile?* Surgery 8:72–78, 1940.

PEDERSEN, HE, LAMONT, RL, AND RAMSEY, RH: *Below-knee amputation for gangrene.* South Med J 57:820–825, 1964.

PERLOW, S: *Amputation for gangrene because of occlusive arterial disease: Results in 312 amputations.* Am J Surg 103:569–574, 1962.

PERLOW, S AND ROTH, HA: *Amputations for gangrene due to occlusive arterial disease.* Surgery 25:547–555, 1949.

PERRY, T, JR: *Below-knee amputations.* Arch Surg 86:199–202, 1963.

PRATT, GH: *Amputation after surgical sympathectomy for obliterative vascular disease: Incidence after 309 sympathectomies.* Surg Gynecol Obstet 100:43–50, 1955.

RECORD, EE: *Surgical amputation in the geriatric patient.* J Bone Joint Surg 45A:1742–1749, 1963.

REEVES, MM AND QUATTLEBAUM, FW: *The lateral flap technique in supracondylar amputations.* Surg Gynecol Obstet 102:751–756, 1956.

REGAN, JS, BOWEN, BD, AND FERNBACH, PA: *Reduction in mortality and loss of limbs in diabetic gangrene and infection.* Arch Surg 59:594–600, 1949.

ROSENBERG, N, ET AL: *Mortality factors in major limb amputations for vascular disease: A study of 176 procedures.* Surgery 67:437–441, 1970.

ROSENTHAL, AM: *The case for below-knee amputation.* J Einstein Med Cent 9:233–234, 1961.

SAKUMA, J, ET AL: *Rehabilitation of geriatric patients having bilateral lower extremity amputations.* Arch Phys Med Rehabil 55:101–111, 1974.

SARMIENTO, A AND WARREN, WD: *A re-evaluation of lower extremity amputations.* Surg Gynecol Obstet 129:799–802, 1969.

SCHLITT, RJ AND SERLIN, O: *Lower extremity amputations in peripheral vascular disease.* Am J Surg 100:682–689, 1960.

SCHMITT, HJ, JR AND ARMSTRONG, RG: *Wounds causing loss of limb.* Surg Gynecol Obstet 130:682–684, 1970.

SCHWINDT, CD, LULLOF, RS, AND ROGERS, SC: *Transmetatarsal amputations.* Orthop Clin North Am 4:31–42, 1973.

SHUMACKER, HB, JR AND MOORE, TC: *Leg and thigh amputations in obliterative arterial disease.* Arch Surg 63:458–465, 1951.

SILBERT, S: *Amputation below the knee for gangrene in the diabetic: Preliminary report.* Am J Dig Dis 11:394–401, 1944.

SILBERT, S: *Mid-leg amputations for gangrene in the diabetic.* Ann Surg 127:503–512, 1948.

SILBERT, S AND HAIMOVICI, H: *Results of midleg amputations for gangrene in diabetics.* JAMA 144:454–458, 1950.

SILBERT, S AND HAIMOVICI, H: *Criteria for the selection of the level of amputation for ischemic gangrene.* JAMA 155:1554–1558, 1954.

SILVERSTEIN, MJ AND KADISH, L: *A study of amputation of the lower extremity.* Surg Gynecol Obstet 137:579–580, 1973.

SMITH, BC: *A twenty-year follow-up in fifty below-knee amputations for gangrene in diabetics.* Surg Gynecol Obstet 103:625–630, 1956.

SMITH, HG: *Amputation above or below knee for primary peripheral vascular disease.* J Bone Joint Surg 32B:392–395, 1950.

STERN, PH AND SKUDDER, PA: *Amputee rehabilitation. I. Lower-limb amputations.* NY State J Med 77:1436–1440, 1977.

SUTOW, WW, ET AL: *Multidrug chemotherapy in primary treatment of osteosarcoma.* J Bone Joint Surg 58A:629–633, 1976.

TAFT, CB: *Survival and prosthetic fitting of children amputated for malignancy.* Inter-Clinic Info Bull 5:9–28, 1966.

TAYLOR, FW: *Arteriosclerotic gangrene: Relation of the amputation stump to morbidity and mortality.* JAMA 113:1196–1198, 1939.

THOMPSON, RC, JR, DELBLANCO, TL, AND MCALLISTER, FF: *Complications following lower extremity amputation.* Surg Gynecol Obstet 120:301–304, 1965.

THURSBY, PF AND DUNN, RM: *Amputations of the lower limb in a repatriation hospital.* Med J Aust 1:161, 1970.

TOLSTEDT, GE AND BELL, JW: *Failure of below-knee amputation in peripheral arterial disease: Use of arteriography in determining site of election.* Arch Surg 83:934–936, 1961.

TRACY, GD: *Below-knee amputation for ischemic gangrene.* Pacif Med Surg 74:251–253, 1966.

TURNBULL, A, SHAH, J, AND FORTNER, J: *Recurrent melanoma of an extremity treated by major amputation.* Arch Surg 106:496–498, 1973.

VANKKA, E: *Study on arteriosclerotics undergoing amputations.* Acta Orthop Scand 104:1–98, 1967.

VEAL, JR: *The prevention of pulmonary complications following thigh amputations by high ligation of the femoral vein.* JAMA 121:240–244, 1943.

VITALI, M: *Rehabilitation of the amputee.* In *Recent Trends in Limb Fitting.* Proc R Soc Med 59:1–3, 1966.

VOLPICELLI, LJ, CHAMBERS, RB, AND WAGNER, FW: *Ambulation levels of bilateral lower-extremity amputees: Analysis of one hundred and three cases.* J Bone Joint Surg 65A:599–605, 1983.

WARREN, R, ET AL: *The transmetatarsal amputation in arterial deficiency of the lower extremity.* Surgery 31:132–140, 1952.

WARREN, R AND KIHN, RB: *A survey of lower extremity amputations for ischemia.* Surgery 63:107–120, 1968.

WATKINS, AL AND LIAO, SJ: *Rehabilitation of persons with bilateral amputation of lower extremities.* JAMA 166:1584–1586, 1958.

WEAVER, PC AND MARSHALL, SA: *A functional and social review of lower-limb amputees.* Br J Surg 60:732–737, 1973.

WEISS, AB: *Cooperative study on osteogenic sarcoma.* J Med Assoc State Ala 44:179–186, 1974.

WEISS, AB, ET AL: *Osteosarcoma: A review of 50 patients treated at the University of Alabama in Birmingham Medical Center between 1944 and 1975.* Clin Orthop 135:137–147, 1978.

WHEELOCK, FC: *Transmetatarsal amputation and arterial surgery in diabetic patients.* N Engl J Med 264:316–320, 1961.

WHEELOCK, FC, JR, MCKITTRICK, JB, AND ROOT, HF: *Evaluation of transmetatarsal amputation in patients with diabetes mellitus.* Surgery 41:184–189, 1957.

WHITEHOUSE, FW, JURGENSEN, C, AND BLOCK, MA: *The later life of the diabetic amputee: Another look at the fate of the second leg.* Diabetes 17:520–521, 1968.

WILSON, AB, JR: *Limb prosthetics: 1970.* Artificial Limbs 14:1–52, 1970.

WOLTERS, BJ: *Follow-up survey study of a group of elderly above-knee amputees.* Arch Phys Med Rehabil 42:68–74, 1961.

WRAY, CH, STILL, JM, JR, AND MORETZ, WH: *Present management of amputations for peripheral vascular disease.* Am Surg 38:87–92, 1972.

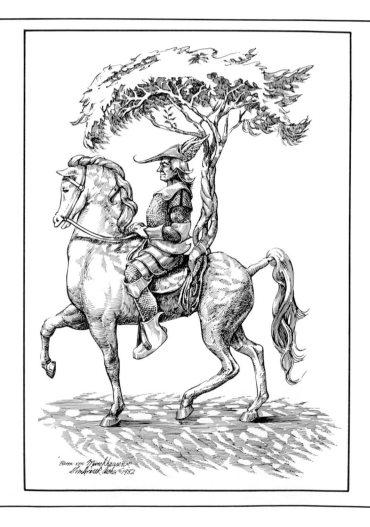

"Baron von Münchhausen"
Ambrose Asher ©1982

REPLANTATION*

*This chapter was written in collaboration with Thomas W. Wolff, M.D., Louisville, Kentucky.

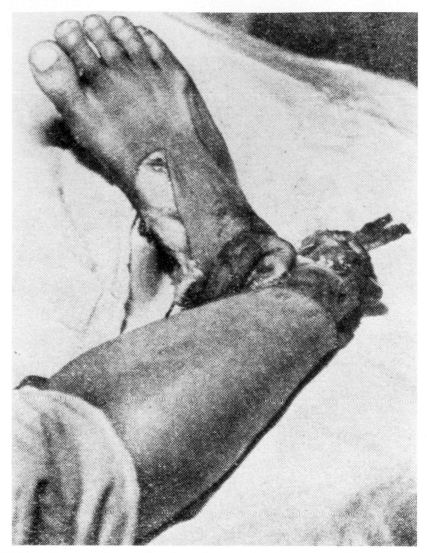

FIGURE 4-1. Traumatic amputation of the right foot at the ankle by a cable. (From Huang, CT, Li, PH, and Kong, GT: *Successful restoration of a traumatic amputated leg.* Chin Med J 84:641, 1965, with permission.)

The frequency of complete traumatic amputation (Fig. 4-1) in highly industrial societies has led to increased interest in replantation of the completely severed limb. Increasing success has been achieved because of microsurgery in vascular anastomoses. Better emergency care of both the patient and the amputated limb, along with modern high-speed transfer, also makes the conditions for replantation more favorable. Skillful repair of injured osseous, nervous, and soft tissues, as well as vascular tissue, is essential (Fig. 4-2). Factors that enhance recovery include the prevention of (1) ischemic necrosis of the devascularized tissue, (2) thrombus formation, (3) postoperative swelling, (4) infection, and (5) shock or acidosis following replantation. Although viability of the replanted extremity may be achieved, functional return is of paramount importance and is the true measure of success (Fig. 4-3). An essential to remember is that function in the

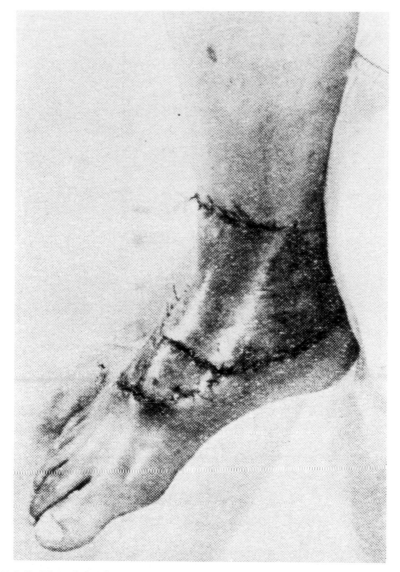

FIGURE 4-2. The right foot on the eighth postoperative day. Skin graft is in place. Edema is evident. (From Huang, CT, Li, PH, and Kong, GT: *Successful restoration of a traumatic amputated leg.* **Chin Med J 84:642, 1965, with permission.)**

replanted limb should be compared with the alternative—prosthetic function—not with normal limb function.

HISTORY

During the Middle Ages and Renaissance, tales were told of successful replantations of noses, ears, fingers, and other bodily parts that had been severed. In 1731, R.J.C. de Garengeot's case of the replantation of the bitten-off nose was published in Paris. He was ridiculed by his contemporaries for his claim.

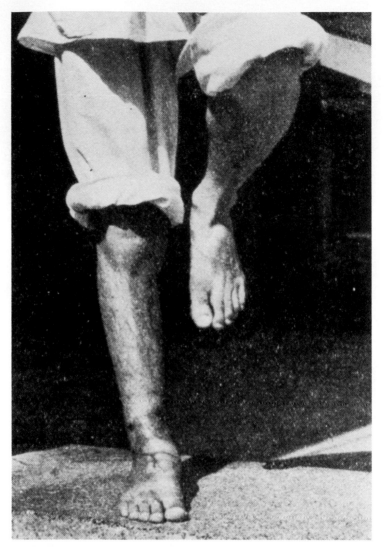

FIGURE 4-3. Seven months after replantation. The patient is able to stand on the replanted foot. (From Huang, CT, Li, PH, and Kong, GT: *Successful restoration of a traumatic amputated leg.* Chin Med J 84:643, 1965, with permission.)

In 1785, *Travels and Campaigns in Russia* by Baron Karl Frederick von Münchausen of Hanover was published. In this work, Baron Münchausen, known for his boastful, ridiculous tales, relates the following delightful story: Following a bloody skirmish, Münchausen discovered that the rear of his battle steed was missing. He rapidly rode the horse to the scene of the accident and retrieved its back portion. His veterinarian, using laurel sprigs, replanted the horse's posterior section, which was still warm, to its anterior section. Soon the two sections of the horse grew together into a happy, synergistic augmentation, as did the laurel sprigs. Later, the Baron was provided with a shaded arbor whenever he mounted his beloved steed (Fig. 4-4).

In 1841, Dr. Balfour successfully reattached the left index finger of an Edinburgh carpenter. Several similar cases were soon reported in the *Edinburgh Medical and Surgical Journal.*

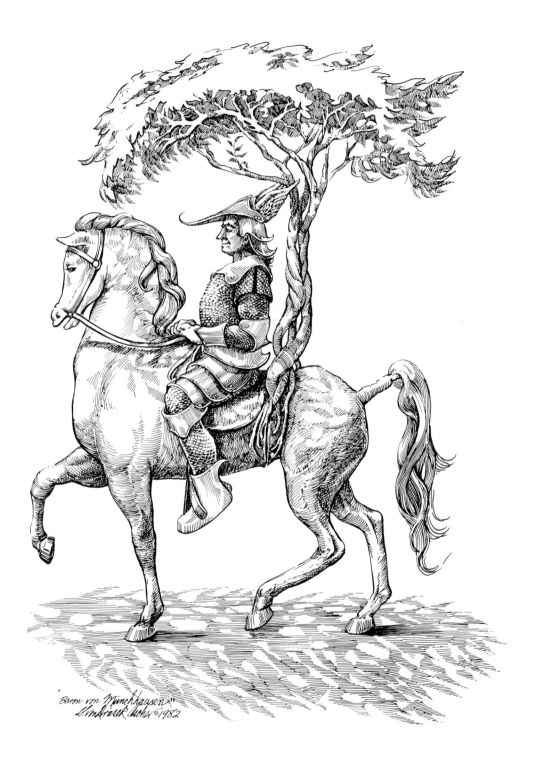

FIGURE 4-4. Baron von Münchausen mounted on his beloved steed. (By permission of the artist, G. vonDrasek Ascher.)

Gottlied Wilhelm Hoffacker, a medical attendant to the student duelists at Heidelberg University, in 1828 published a series of 16 case histories from 1822 to 1827 entitled *Observations on the healing of cut-off portions of the nose and lips*. Hoffacker reported his partial successes and failures, as well as his complete successes.

In 1887, William Halsted of Johns Hopkins University successfully translocated the hind leg of a dog from one side to the other, leaving the femoral artery intact until the tissue had healed in the new position. E. Höpfner, in 1903, reported three attempts at complete transplantation. Alexis Carrel and C.C. Guthrie, in 1906, reported replantation failure owing to venous congestion from constriction by a circular dressing. In 1908, Carrel reported the successful results of limb transplantation from one dog to another. The duration of viability was not mentioned, however. In 1944, Richard Hall of Denver described an operative protocol for the transplantation of the human arm transected in mid-humerus.

The most successful long-term results were reported in 1960 by Anastasy Lapchinsky of Moscow, who described the successful replantation of a dog limb that had been traumatically amputated at the mid-thigh 6 years prior. The dog was still able to stand on its replanted hind leg 6 years after the operation. Of 67 limbs preserved at 2°C and 4°C for up to 28 hours, Lapchinsky reported permanent survival in 16 dogs for 6 years or longer. He also added that following replantation of extremities preserved by cooling alone for 24 hours or more, the dogs usually died. They would first become excited, with an increase in respiratory rate, pulse rate, and intestinal peristalsis. Next, their blood pressure would gradually fall; and 5 to 12 hours postoperatively, respiratory arrest would occur. Post-mortem examination revealed evidence of toxicosis.

Clifford Snyder and associates of Miami reported the successful replantation, in 1960, of a canine limb that had been perfused, via a pump oxygenator, with heparinized autogenous or homologous blood prior to replantation. They noted that with long periods of separation from the host, the pH of the blood being perfused decreased, becoming acidotic.

Although limb replantation requires no novel surgical principles, but rather a synthesis of many well-publicized procedures, it was not until 1964 that Ronald Malt and Charles MaKhann reported the first successful complete human replantation, an arm, done in 1962 in Boston. C.W. Ch'en of Shanghi reported the second successful replacement of an arm in 1963.

THE CHOICE

ANIMAL EXPERIMENTS

Animal experiments indicate that ischemia of a muscle for 4 to 6 hours at normal temperatures results in permanent inability of muscle proteins to produce a contraction; however, nerve tissue, connective tissue, and skin will recover function almost completely even after 12 or more hours of ischemia. The difference is that muscle tissue has a higher metabolic rate and thus is the most vulnerable to ischemia. If an amputated extremity has been without blood flow for 5 to 6 hours, replantation should not be done unless the extremity has been cooled. Hypothermia retards the rate of cell necrosis and thus offers an extension of the critical time for as long as 28 hours. Perfusing the limb with oxygenated blood via a pump oxygenator or storing it in a hyperbaric oxygen chamber may also extend the critical time factor.

SELECTION OF PATIENTS

If surgical replantation is not considered, obviously it will not be performed; however, not all amputated limbs are candidates for replantation. If the patient's general health is good and the amputated part is not too seriously damaged, then the procedure should be considered, assuming that qualified staff and adequate facilities are available.

Before the decision can be made, homeostasis should be restored. There is a morbid curiosity about replantation that may interfere with looking at the whole patient. Internal injuries, other fractures, and other nervous system damage take priority.

If possible, the patient should participate in the decision. Psychological, emotional, economic, and social factors need to be considered.

INDICATIONS

1. No life-threatening injury is present during the critical time for performing the replantation.
2. The amputated limb is intact and adequately preserved.
3. The wound is sharp and clean rather than crushed, dirty, or thermally injured.
4. Nerves are capable of regeneration.
5. Muscles and tendons are capable of functioning.
6. The patient's condition will permit a lengthy operation.
7. The patient is not senile and has no history of vascular disease or diabetes.
8. The patient is young. Those who are less than 30 years old have the best chance for nerve regeneration.
9. Upper limb amputations are given higher consideration than lower limb amputations because shortening of the extremity has a less adverse effect, the chances for nerve regeneration are better, and the prosthetic alternative is much less adequate.
10. The staff and patient recognize the unpredictable course and are willing to commit themselves to a long-term rehabilitation program that may take years and may include subsequent operations and complications.

CONTRAINDICATIONS

1. Poor general health of the patient where surgery would be a significant risk to the patient's life.
2. The presence of multiple major injuries that demand immediate attention.
3. Tissue injury at the amputation site that is too extensive for technical success. If the limb has been severely crushed or burned, or has sustained an explosive type of injury, success is unlikely.
4. If the time since injury has exceeded approximately 6 hours without either hypothermia or perfusion of the limb with oxygenated blood or solution. This critical period varies, being shorter if the amputation is proximal through muscle masses and longer if it is distal through tendons. Muscle masses undergo

irreversible changes sooner than tendons, which are less sensitive to anoxia.

5. If the spinal roots of the limb have been avulsed, or if long segments of peripheral nerve have been stretched.

6. In the lower limb, if there is extensive bone loss.

REPLANTATION OF THE UPPER VERSUS THE LOWER LIMB

Reasons for doing replantation favor the upper limb. Some primary points to consider are listed below:

	Arm	*Leg*
1.	The hand is mechanically irreplaceable, with very poor mechanical substitutes that do not have tactile sensation.	Mechanical substitutes are reasonably satisfactory. Absence of tactile sensation is functionally less critical.
2.	If replanted, the patient could be mobile in a short period of time.	If replanted, the patient would be immobile for an extended period of time.
3.	Moderate shortening is functionally acceptable.	Minimal shortening creates postural and gait problems.
4.	The potential for the return of protective sensory and motor function following proximal lesions is good.	The potential for the return of protective sensory and motor function following proximal lesions is poor.

IMMEDIATE MANAGEMENT

PATIENT

The patient's life is the first concern. Massive hemorrhage should be controlled first by pressure and then by ligation as close to the severed end as possible. Next, the patient should be treated for shock, if present. The patient needs to be transported as soon as possible to a center where evaluation and treatment by specialists, especially in vascular and orthopedic surgery, are available. A sterile dressing should cover the wound. Immediate care should include a blood transfusion, antibiotics, and roentgenograms of the wound and the severed extremity to aid in determining the level and extent of injury. Wound irrigation and débridement should begin at once following transport.

LIMB

The amputated part should be kept moist and cool (Table 4-1). Sterile saline, if available, may be used to cover the open wound. The limb should be wrapped dry in plastic bags to prevent direct contact with the ice. Hypothermia retards autolysis, reduces bacterial growth, and minimizes plasma loss with consequent edema and metabolic acidosis. Arteriovenous flushing precedes replantation. If a major vessel is apparent, a

TABLE 4-1. PROCEDURE TO PRESERVE THE AMPUTATED EXTREMITY

1. Cleanse gross contamination with normal saline.
2. Wrap with moist sterile dressings and place in a plastic bag.
3. Pack in ice (the extremity or digit should be dry to prevent maceration).
4. Get to a medical facility as soon as possible.

cold, sterile, isotonic intravenous solution (e.g., Ringer's lactate) that contains an anticoagulant (heparin) may be instilled by gravity flow perfusion to flush out thrombi within the vessel. Perfusion using a syringe may cause damaging pressures. Dextran (10 percent low molecular weight) is sometimes also used in small amounts to prevent further microthrombi. If the intra-arterial perfusion is precooled (4°C), rapid cooling of the limb can be achieved. Large doses of nonirritating antibiotic may be contained in the perfusate. A manual milking maneuver enhances the return of the perfusate through the veins.

TECHNIQUE

ANIMAL EXPERIMENTS

In animal studies, low-viscosity dextran has been administered to maintain good perfusion by preventing clot formation. Heparin has also been used, but it often resulted in local wound bleeding and hematoma formation. For this reason, and because heparin does not prevent platelet thrombosis, many surgeons do not use it or other anticoagulants systemically following replantation.

SURGICAL REPLANTATION

Massive irrigation and thorough, meticulous débridement, under magnification, of all devitalized tissues of both the amputation stump and the amputated part must be performed (Table 4-2). Bone fixation usually precedes vascular anastomosis to avoid undue bending and twisting of the vessels. The bone is shortened so that there will be less tension on the vessels and nerves. The bone is stabilized using internal fixation, such as intramedullary nails, Kirschner wires, Steinmann's pins, Rush pins, plates, or screws. External fixation with a plaster cast is contraindicated because the limb is anesthetic, but an external fixator might be adequate.

The arteries and veins are sutured after bone fixation, unless the time interval since amputation has been long, in which case restoration of circulation must take priority. In major limb replantations, performing arterial repair first without venous repair will prevent microthrombi from entering the general circulation and will minimize "seeding" the lungs. In digit replantation, performing arterial repair first aids in identifying the very small veins for anastomosis by observing for "bleeding points." Venous continuity is critical for successful replantation; therefore, as many large veins as possible should be repaired. To avoid imbalance, it may be necessary to anastomose

TABLE 4-2. OPERATIVE TECHNIQUE

1. Débridement
2. Bone shortening
3. Fixation of bone
4. Vascular anastomosis
   (a) Mechanical distention (relieve vascular spasm)
   (b) Arterial
   (c) Venous
   (d) Autogenous vein graft, if needed
5. Tendon suture
6. Nerve repair
   (a) Primary
   (b) Secondary
7. Grafts, if necessary, for skin coverage
   (a) Split-thickness
   (b) Pedicle flap
8. Decompression incision
9. Splint for support

two or three veins for every artery, so that venous outflow is ensured in the event of partial venous thrombosis.

Priority is given to arterial anastomosis if there has been a long delay, if the vascular bed has not been washed thoroughly, or if the venous plexus has been extensively damaged. In arterial repair, care is taken to completely excise all of the damaged portion of the vessel because it is a potential cause of postoperative thrombosis. If the bone has not been shortened to reduce tension on the vessels at the site of the anastomosis, then an autogenous saphenous vein graft may be needed to bridge the gap. If the graft is too long the vessel may kink, which would result in thrombosis. Veins go into spasm when removed. The vein may be distended with heparin or normal saline solution to relieve the spasm before suturing. Vascular (arterial or venous) spasm can reduce the lumen to half of the original size in vessels of both the proximal and distal segments of the wound, as well as in grafts. Warming or a sympathetic procaine nerve block may be necessary to relieve the spasm. Mechanical distention may also overcome the spasm. If veins are used for arterial grafts, then they are reversed so the venous valve will not impair blood flow.

Circulation to the muscle is checked following arterial anastomoses. If muscle revascularization has not been achieved, then further débridement may be necessary to remove crushed, devitalized muscle.

Tenorrhaphy of muscles that are innervated above the level of amputation allows for early return of function. Early movement of the muscles about the amputation site reduces the chance of adhesions and may also promote healing of the fracture. Tendons are repaired at the primary operation if possible.

If the amputation is guillotine-like with a clean laceration, then primary repair of the nerve is indicated unless prolongation of the operative time would threaten the patient's life. Return of sensation and movement is usually quicker following primary repair. Delayed nerve repairs (within 3 weeks or as soon thereafter as possible) are performed if there is considerable damage to the nerve or if the extent of the nerve injury is poorly defined. In such cases, the nerve endings are marked for later procedures. The likelihood of developing causalgia may be greater when the repair is delayed.

All devitalized soft tissue must be débrided to avoid sepsis. Late transplant failure is usually due to necrosis and sepsis near the injury site. Dead space should be obliterated by the accurate approximation of soft tissue. If the bone is shortened, there is usually enough soft tissue to cover the anastomoses and to provide a broad surface for capillary and lymphatic regeneration. Split-thickness skin grafts can provide the final epidermal coverage. If soft tissue is lacking, then pedicle flaps that contain a thick layer of subcutaneous tissue may be necessary for essential coverage of the vessel and nerve anastomoses.

If the amputation is at a level that involves muscle, then hemorrhage will be impressive and a transfusion will usually be necessary. A fasciotomy of the anterior and posterior muscle compartments from the knee to the ankle is recommended in cases of replanted thigh amputations. In replantations of the upper extremity, a longitudinal section of the flexor retinaculum overlying the median nerve at the wrist, or a fasciotomy over the dorsum of the hand and/or volar forearm, will usually be necessary. Excessive swelling in the closed fascial compartments will result in muscle necrosis because the tension within the muscle will prevent blood from entering the muscle. Adequate venous return is paramount for preventing edema. The limb is immobilized in a splint.

IMMEDIATE RESULTS

ANIMAL EXPERIMENTS

In animal experimentation, serious complications appeared soon after replantation, including severe local wound infection with abscess formation and dehiscence of the suture line, vascular occlusion, shock, local hematoma formation, and edema of the replanted limb. Later complications included bone infection, pseudarthrosis, kidney infarcts, and severe contracture and atrophy of the muscles. Excessive limb edema may prevent adequate capillary perfusion of the limb and may compress the large vessels, which can result in gangrene. Swelling also puts tension on the suture lines, which, if unable to heal adequately, will be a likely site for infection. In the experimentally replanted limbs, fluid accumulation was 30 percent to 70 percent of the original weight of the limb 6 hours after recirculation and was as high as 95 percent by the sixth postoperative day. The amount of edema was greater with longer durations of ischemia before re-establishment of circulation and was less with hypothermia of the amputated extremity to 4°C during the period of ischemia.

The exact cause of shock following replantation is still unproven. Suggested causes include marked extravasation of fluid into the replanted limb, myoglobin liberated from the damaged muscle, and systemic metabolic acidosis produced by an accumulation of anaerobic metabolites in the anoxic and unperfused tissue. The systemic effect of depression of the cardiovascular system—progressive hypotension—precedes death. Tourniquet shock and crush syndrome—traumatic toxicosis—are similar.

HUMANS

Any postoperative impairment of blood circulation requires immediate treatment. Therefore, the skin temperature, color, and degree of swelling must be observed frequently (Table 4-3).

TABLE 4-3. SIGNS OF CIRCULATORY CONDITION

Good Circulation	Arterial Obstruction	Venous Obstruction
1. Skin temperature slightly higher or the same as the normal side	1. Skin temperature falls rapidly	1. Skin temperature falls slowly
2. Pink color	2. Pale color (pallor) and mottling on elevation	2. Cyanotic (flushed, purple) color with the limb at heart level
3. Fresh red blood emerges when the skin is punctured	3. A prick causes no blood or a small amount of blood of normal color	3. Copious bleeding (thick, cyanosed blood that clots rapidly) if skin is incised
4. No swelling	4. No swelling	4. Swelling and throbbing
5. Normal capillary filling time	5. Capillary reflex is sluggish	5. Capillary reflex is exaggerated and brisk

If circulatory embarrassment occurs, the cause should be determined and treatment begun.

1. *Venous thrombosis:* Venous flow impairment is usually prevented and initially treated by elevation. If circulation does not improve after a short period, then surgical exploration is indicated. Any clots should be removed and damaged vein resected. A vein graft is used if direct reanastomosis is not possible.
2. *Arterial thrombosis:* If color or capillary return does not improve on changing to the dependent position, then the artery should be surgically explored. The thrombus is removed, and the traumatized section of the artery is adequately excised and replaced with a vein graft.
3. *Arterial spasm:* Arterial spasm can be treated with local heat, antispasmodic drugs, or sympathetic procaine nerve blocks. If conservative measures fail, then a thrombus is probably present, requiring immediate surgical exploration.
4. *Excessive pressure proximal to the reattachment:* This may be externally caused by splints or bandages that are improperly applied. Such devices can be removed or properly reapplied. Internal causes include tissue swelling and hematoma formation requiring fasciotomy or evacuation of the hematoma.

Hyperbaric oxygen may be valuable in some cases of marginal circulation in difficult replantations. If circulation has ceased, the employment of hyperbaric oxygen is futile and will only delay exploration.

Cardiac arrest may follow the release of vascular clamps during surgery for major limb replantation as blood suddenly fills the limb's vascular system. Shock had also been reported in the immediate postoperative period. If interstitial plasma loss is not severe enough to cause shock, it may cause hypotension and hypoproteinemia, especially if the replantation is at the thigh. Renal shutdown caused by myoglobinemia and hemoglobinemia is another risk. Metabolic acidosis can be treated with bicarbonates. Systemic measures include restoration of blood volume, maintenance of plasma protein level, and prevention of infection and acute renal failure. For the first few days after surgery, limb movement is kept to a minimum and the dressing is not changed (Table 4-4).

TABLE 4-4. POSTOPERATIVE COMPLICATIONS OF MAJOR REPLANTATIONS

1. Cardiac arrest immediately following restoration of circulation
2. Shock (metabolic acidosis)
3. Hemorrhage causing hematoma formation
4. Infection (septicemia, osteomyelitis)
5. Vascular occlusion (thrombosis, vascular spasm, external pressure)
6. Pseudarthrosis
7. Edema of the replanted limb
8. Contractures
9. Muscle atrophy and weakness
10. Anesthesia or paresthesia

REASONS FOR FAILURE

1. Infection is the greatest single cause of failure. Factors that favor the development of clinical infection in a contaminated wound created by traumatic amputation are a prolonged length of time between amputation and replantation, inadequate débridement of devitalized tissue, edema, and an increase in blood viscosity.
2. The limb is not perfused for an adequate amount of time to flush out existing thrombi.
3. The tissue is not cooled to prolong muscle viability.
4. Bony fixation is not accomplished before vascular anastomosis.
5. Venous circulation is not restored.
6. Débridement of the vascular wall is insufficient, leaving damaged intima that results in thrombus formation and ischemia of the limb.
7. Blood vessels and nerves are inadequately covered with healthy soft tissue.
8. Vascular spasm is not relieved, resulting in thrombus formation.
9. The amputation is so far proximal that there is irrecoverable degeneration of the nerves and the muscles they innervate. If limb viability is achieved, the extent of return of function depends largely upon the extent of nerve injury and the success of its repair.
10. The amputation is through large muscle masses, with resulting metabolic acidosis.
11. The patient is not motivated or guided by an informed, enthusiastic staff to participate in the extensive rehabilitation program.

IMMEDIATE POSTOPERATIVE THERAPY

A program should be conducted to protect and maintain the denervated structures from the time of injury until reinnervation, as well as to create optimum conditions for nerve regeneration (Table 4-5).

EDEMA CONTROL

Elevation of the extremity slightly above heart level is usually necessary if there is swelling. Dressings that are constricting will cause catastrophic results; therefore, cir-

TABLE 4-5. POSTOPERATIVE GOALS

1. Prevent infection
2. Minimize edema
3. Prevent shock
4. Maintain joint mobility
5. Maintain muscle contractility
6. Enhance wound and bone healing

cumferential dressings are contraindicated. If arterial supply is precarious, the limb may need to be lowered. If severe edema with a decrease in local skin temperature develops, then venous outflow is seriously compromised; decompression incisions through the skin and underlying fascia (i.e., fasciotomies) may be necessary to save the extremity. Prevention of infection after decompression is very important.

PASSIVE MOVEMENT

Gentle passive movements of the joints are begun on about the fourth postoperative day, when possible, and are performed daily thereafter. Care should be taken in the first month not to disrupt the anastomoses.

ELECTRICAL STIMULATION

Direct-current stimulation of the denervated muscles on a regular basis will maintain the contractility of the muscles.

NEUROLOGIC TESTING

Electromyography and strength duration curves are valuable for determining the progress of nerve regeneration. Less specific signs such as Tinel's sign, chronaxies, and return of muscle function may also be used to monitor progress. Although sometimes painful, paresthesias and dyesthesias during the recovery period may be indicative of nerve regeneration.

SPLINTS

Static splints are used initially to maintain the limb in a posture that is least conducive to the development of deformities. Later, as peripheral nerve regeneration occurs, dynamic splinting will be necessary to allow functional use of the imbalanced extremity. Special attention must be given to frequent observation of the skin at points of pressure since the extremity is initially completely anesthetic.

TEMPERATURE

The environment should be kept at approximately 25°C. Higher temperatures will lead to further swelling. Although cooling at temperatures appreciably below 25°C decreases local metabolic demands, it does not enhance limb survival.

LONG-TERM RESULTS

ANIMAL EXPERIMENTS

NEUROMUSCULAR SYSTEM

All animals with replanted extremities exhibited some evidence of neurologic deficits, including footdrop, where the animal hops on the sound leg, plantarflexion contractures, and absent ankle reflexes. Pain sensation usually returned by the fourth month, and light-touch sensation by the sixth month. Complete function did not return even 29 months after replantation. Afferent conduction velocity increased from the third to the ninth month after replantation and then showed no further significant increase. The reduction of motor conduction velocity through the area of transection ranged from 40 percent to 80 percent of normal. Histologic examination revealed neuroma formation at the site of replantation in all animals. Some normal nerve fibers were present in all distal nerves. The majority of muscle fibers appeared normal, although degenerating fibers were seen. Although normal fibers were present after reinnervation, normal muscle mass and strength never returned completely. The rate and degree of nerve regeneration were usually better when a microscope was used to repair the nerve.

Factors that may interfere with normal nerve regeneration other than neuroma formation are ischemia, inflammation, and edema. All animals showed a greater defect in the function of the peroneal nerve than the tibial nerve. The peroneal nerve has less blood supply and, thus, is more sensitive to ischemia than the tibial nerve.

CIRCULATORY SYSTEM

Although the anastomosed vessels may be patent, collateral vessels usually do not cross the amputation line. Changes in nails and trophic ulcers on the foot indicate inadequate vascularization.

OSSEOUS SYSTEM

Pseudarthrosis was frequent, although bone healing occurred in some animals. Chronic osteomyelitis at the site of bone division may exist.

HUMANS

NEUROVASCULAR SYSTEM

In the lower limb, nerve damage presents the major obstacle to complete rehabilitation. Natural sensory stimuli often produce pain. Satisfactory motor recovery is unlikely, especially following sciatic nerve section. The foot may be insensitive and painful, with no recovery of the small muscles of the foot.

PSYCHOLOGICAL

Replantation surgery necessitates a prolonged hospitalization, a lengthy rehabilitation program, and often subsequent corrective surgery. Patients who are young and highly motivated tolerate the long and painstaking rehabilitation period better than elderly or unmotivated patients.

PHYSICAL THERAPY

The physical therapy program will likely continue for 2 or more years following replantation surgery.

FURTHER SURGERY

Further corrective surgical procedures that may be performed are tendon transfers and grafts, arthrodesis, release of contractures, and repair of ununited or malunited bone. These procedures are usually performed only if improvement is not obtained by more conservative means.

   Although considerable functional return has been reported following replantation of an extremity, these results are obtained infrequently. Inadequate peripheral nerve regeneration presents the major functional problem.

OSSEOUS SYSTEM

Late-appearing osteomyelitis may be treated by drainage and irrigation with bactericidal antibiotics if there is hope of saving the limb. If the infection is life-threatening, then a proximal open amputation will be required.

BIBLIOGRAPHY

Arms and the man. Br Med J 2:1024–1025, 1966.

BALAS, P: *Replantation of amputated extremities: The necessity for re-evaluation.* Angiology 24:1–2, 1973.

BALAS, P, ET AL:*The present status of replantation of amputated extremities: Indications and technical considerations.* Vasc Surg 4:190–209, 1970.

BOYES, JG, JR: *Reimplantation of extremities by microvascular suture.* NC Med J 35:479–481, 1974.

CARREL, A: *Results of the transplantation of blood vessels, organs, and limbs.* JAMA 51:1662–1667, 1908.

CARREL, A AND GUTHRIE, CC: *Complete amputation of the thigh with replantation.* Am J Med Sci 131:297–301, 1906.

CARREL, A AND GUTHRIE, CC: *Results of replantation of thigh.* Science 23:393–394, 1906.

CH'EN, CW, CH'IEN, YC, AND PAO, YS: *Salvage of the forearm following complete traumatic amputation.* Chin Med J 82:632–638, 1963.

CH'EN, CW, ET AL: *Further experiences in the restoration of amputated limbs: Report of two cases.* Chin Med J 84:225–231, 1965.

CH'IEN, YC, ET AL: *Some problems concerning small vessel anatomosis in the reattachment of complete traumatic amputations.* Chin Med J 85:79–86, 1966.

CHIRSTEAS, N, BALAS, P, AND GIANNIKAS, A: *Replantation of amputated extremities: Report of two successful cases.* Am J Surg 118:68–74, 1969.

CLOSE, MB AND GILBERT, RS: *Replantation of almost completely amputated thigh with recovery.* Am J Surg 118:623–626, 1969.

Editorial. *Replacing limbs.* Br Med J 5413:832–833, 1964.

EIKEN, O, ET AL: *Limb replantation. III. Long-term evaluation.* Arch Surg 88:66–77, 1964.

EIKEN, O, ET AL: *Limb replantation. I. The technique and immediate results.* Arch Surg 88:48–53, 1964.

EIKEN, O, ET AL: *Limb replantation. II. The pathophysiological effects.* Arch Surg 88:54–65, 1964.

EIKEN, O, ET AL: *Fate of limbs following severance and reimplantation.* Surg Forum 14:204–206, 1963.

ENGBER, WD AND HARDIN, CA: *Replantation of extremities: Collective review.* Surg Gynecol Obstet 132:901–916, 1971.

FRANK, GR AND PEDERSEN, T: *A three-year follow-up on a limb reimplantation performed under virtually ideal conditions.* Inter-Clinic Info Bull 7:8–14, 1968.

GIBSON, T: *Early free grafting: The restitution of parts completely separated from the body.* Br J Plast Surg 18:1–11, 1965.

HALL, RH: *Whole upper extremity transplant for human beings: General plans of procedure and operative technic.* Ann Surg 120:12–23, 1944.

HALSTED, WS: *Replantation of entire limbs without suture of vessels.* Proc Nat Acad Sci 8:181–186, 1922.

HALSTED, WS, REICHERT, FL, AND REID, MR: *Replantation of entire limbs without suture of vessels.* Trans Amer Surg Assoc 40:160–167, 1922.

HORN, JS: *Successful reattachment of a completely severed forearm.* Lancet 1:1152–1154, 1964.

HORN, JS: *Some advances in surgery in China with special reference to the reattachment of severed limbs.* Proc Roy Soc Med 59:587–590, 1966.

HORN, JS: *The reattachment of severed extremities.* In APLEY, AG (ED): *Recent Advances in Orthopedics.* J & A Churchill, London, 1969, pp 49–78.

HUANG, CT, LI, PH, AND KONG, GT: *Successful restoration of a traumatic amputated leg.* Chin Med J 84:641–645, 1965.

INOUE, T, ET AL: *Factors necessary for successful replantation of upper extremities.* Ann Surg 165:225–238, 1967.

INOUE, T, ET AL: *Replantation of severed limbs.* J Cardiovasc Surg 8:31–39, 1967.

JAFFE, S, ET AL: *Replantation of amputated extremities: Report of five cases.* Ohio State Med J 71:381–386, 1975.

LAPCHINSKY, AG: *Recent results of experimental transplantation of preserved limbs and kidneys and possible use of this technique in clinical practice.* Ann NY Acad Sci 87:539–569, 1960.

LENDRUM, J: *Alternatives to amputation.* Ann R Coll Surg Engl 62:95–99, 1980.

MACDONALD, GL, JR, TOSE, L, AND DETERLING, RA: *A technique for reimplantation of the dog limb involving the use of a mechanical stapling device and a rapidly polymerizing adhesive.* Surg Forum 13:88–90, 1962.

MAGEE, HR AND PARKER, WR: *Replantation of the foot: Results after two years.* Med J Aust 1:751–755, 1972.

MALT, RA: *Clinical aspects of restoring limbs.* In WELCH, CE (ED): *Advances in Surgery.* Year Book Medical Publishers, Chicago, 1966, pp 19–33.

MALT, RA AND MCKHANN, CF: *Replantation of severed arms.* JAMA 189:716–722, 1964.

MAMAKOS, MS: *Lower extremity replant: A preliminary report.* Ann Plast Surg 4:48–52, 1980.

NCNEILL, IF AND WILSON, JSP: *The problem of limb replacement.* Br J Surg 57:365–377, 1970.

MEHL, RL, PAUL, HA, AND BEATTIE, EJ, JR: *Successful treatment of "shock" after experimental replantation of extremities severed for long periods.* Lancet 1:1419–1420, 1964.

MEHL, RL, ET AL: *Treatment of "toxemia" after extremity replantation.* Arch Surg 89:871–878, 1964.

MORRISON, WA, O'BRIEN, BM, AND MACLEOD, AM: *Major limb replantation.* Orthop Clin North Am 8:343–348, 1977.

MUSTARD, WT: *The technic of immediate restoration of vascular continuity after arterial wounds.* Ann Surg 124:46–59, 1946.

NABSETH, DC, MAYER, RF, AND DETERLING, RA, JR: *Experimental basis of limb replantation.* In WELCH, CE (ED). *Advances in Surgery.* Chicago, Year Book Medical Publishers, 1966, pp 35–57.

O'BRIEN, BM: *Replantation surgery.* In *Clinics in Plastic Surgery.* WB Saunders, Philadelphia, 1974, pp 405–426.

O'DONOGHUE, DH, ET AL: *The management of traumatic amputations.* J Okla Med Assoc 55:419–420, 1962.

ONJI, Y, ET AL: *Experimental surgery on resuscitation and reunion of amputated or nearly amputated leg.* Plast Reconstr Surg 31:151–165, 1963.

ONJI, Y, ET AL: *The possibility of salvaging an amputated extremity.* Clin Orthop 32:87–92, 1964.

ORTNER, AB, BERG, HF, AND LEBENDIGER, A: *Limb salvage through small-vessel surgery.* Arch Surg 83:414–419, 1961.

OTTER, G, DEN: *The clinical problems encountered in replantation of limbs.* Arch Chir Neerl 20:127–139, 1968.

PALETTA, FX: *Replantation of the amputated extremity.* Ann Surg 168:720–726, 1968.

PAUL, HA, ET AL: *Shock in replantation and crush syndrome.* J Trauma 5:349–356, 1965.

POLACEK, MA, PAGEDAS, T, AND WELSH, E: *Emergency room principles in limb amputation and replantation.* Wis Med J 67:147–153, 1968.

RAMIREZ, MA, ET AL: *Reimplantation of limbs.* Plast Reconstr Surg 40:315–324, 1967.

Reattachment of traumatic amputations: A summing-up of experience. China Med 5:392–402, 1967.

REICHERT, FL: *The importance of circulatory balance in the survival of replanted limbs.* Bull Johns Hopkins Hosp 49:86–93, 1931.

Replaced leg or prosthesis? Br Med J 5493:935, 1966.

ROTH, RB: Letter: *Replantation in China.* JAMA 230:1127–1128, 1974.

SHAFTAN, GW, HERBSMAN, H, AND MALT, RA: *Fracture Trauma Conference: Replantation of limbs.* Minn Med 48:1645–1650, 1965.

SHAW, RS: *Treatment of the extremity suffering near or total severance with special consideration of the vascular problem.* Clin Orthop 29:56–71, 1963.

SNYDER, CC AND KNOWLES, RP: *Autoplantation of extremities.* Clin Orthop 29:113–122, 1963.

SNYDER, CC, ET AL: *Extremity replantation.* Plast Reconstr Surg 26:251–263, 1960.

TS'UI, CY, ET AL: *Microvascular anastomosis and transplantation: Experimental studies and clinical application.* Chin Med J 85:610–617, 1966.

WILLIAMS, GR: *Replantation of amputated extremities.* Monogr Surg Sci 3:53–83, 1966.

WILLIAMS, GR: *Replantation of amputated extremities: Present status.* Md State Med J 20:64–68, 1971.

WILLIAMS, GR, ET AL: *Replantation of amputated extremities.* Ann Surg 163:788–794, 1966.

WORMAN, LW, DARIN, JC, AND KRITTER, AE: *The anatomy of a limb replantation failure.* Arch Surg 91:211–215, 1965.

SURGICAL AMPUTATION LEVELS AND ASSOCIATED PROSTHESES

HEALING

LIMB

VIABILITY

ASSESSMENT

Gangrene

Peripheral Circulation

AMBULATION

OPERATIVE

RISK

Operative Technique

AMPUTATION FOR PERIPHERAL VASCULAR DISEASE

SKIN TEMPERATURE AND TISSUE APPEARANCE

CONDITION OF ADJACENT AREA

EXTENT OF GANGRENE

DIABETES

REST PAIN OR CLAUDICATION

PREOPERATIVE SYMPATHECTOMY

ARTERIAL RECONSTRUCTION

MEASUREMENT OF PERIPHERAL CIRCULATION

PERIPHERAL PULSES
ARTERIOGRAPHY
CAPILLARY SKIN BLOOD FLOW AS MEASURED BY RADIOACTIVE XENON 133 (^{133}Xe) CLEARANCE
DIRECTIONAL DOPPLER FLOW DETECTION
PLETHYSMOGRAPHY
OSCILLOMETRY
INTRA-ARTERIAL INJECTION OF RADIOACTIVE (^{99m}Tc) MICROSPHERES
SKIN BLOOD PRESSURE
TRANSCUTANEOUS P_{O_2}
MUSCLE PERFUSION

ONSET OF ARTERIAL OCCLUSION

OPERATIVE RISK

WOUND BLEEDING

PRESENCE OF ISCHEMIC MUSCLE AT THE TIME OF SURGERY

AMPUTATION TECHNIQUE

POSTOPERATIVE FACTORS

INFECTION
EDEMA
TYPE OF POSTOPERATIVE DRESSING

SUMMARY

AMPUTATION FOR TRAUMA

AMPUTATION FOR TUMOR

AMPUTATION FOR DEFORMITY

CONGENITAL LIMB DEFICIENCY REVISION

SURGICAL EXPERTISE

The four major indications for performing a lower extremity amputation are ischemia, trauma, revision of a congenital deformity, and resection of a tumor. The vast majority of lower extremity amputations are performed on dysvascular limbs. The selection of the amputation level has less well-defined criteria for dysvascular cases than for amputations for congenital deformity, trauma, or tumor. The purposes of amputation are to remove dead or diseased tissue, to relieve pain, to obtain healing, and to rehabilitate the amputee. In cases of vascular disease, skin healing is generally more readily obtained with proximal amputations, but ambulation is easier with distal amputations.

Nathan Smith, a professor at Yale Medical Institute, in his lecture notes of 1825 to 1826 said that "as a general rule, you should save all the stump you can." To this end, there is a need for a means of circulatory evaluation at the arteriolar, capillary, and cellular levels to aid in the decision of the lowest amputation that will allow the patient to return to satisfactory health. The emphasis has broadened over the years to include not only survival but also function. Not so many years ago, amputations were performed at several specific sites that were determined largely by the prosthetic considerations of the day. Knee disarticulation and Syme amputations were seldom seen. With the prosthetic capabilities of today, it is possible to fit any level of amputation with a satisfactory prosthesis. Advanced technology makes the words of Nathan Smith even truer today than when spoken in the early 1800s.

Concern has been expressed for the low rate of primary healing of distal amputations (below-knee or lower), resulting in prolonged hospitalization, as compared with proximal amputations (above-knee or higher). There are many criteria used for the prediction of wound healing (Table 5-1). Many surgeons feel that clinical judgment continues to provide the most accurate and reliable information in the level selection process, and they view the various techniques of assessing limb viability as only complimentary to a well-taken history and physical examination.

The philosophy that "the first amputation should be the last" has been interpreted by some to mean "amputate high to be safe." A more precise interpretation would be to amputate at the lowest possible level to obtain satisfactory wound healing.

All health professionals who treat patients with peripheral vascular disease should make every effort to salvage the entire limb. Amputation is performed only when such measures have failed or when the duration of treatment would adversely affect the patient's psyche and socialization.

> He is a good surgeon who can amputate a limb, but he is a better surgeon who can save a limb.
>
> Sir Astley Cooper

AMPUTATION FOR PERIPHERAL VASCULAR DISEASE

Regarding subjective measures:

> When you can measure what you are speaking about and express it in numbers, you know something about it; but when you cannot measure it, when you cannot express it in numbers, your knowledge is a meagre kind.
>
> Lord Kelvin
> (On the Royal College of Surgeon's building in London)

TABLE 5-1. LIMB VIABILITY ASSESSMENT*

I. Extremity blood flow
  A. Venous filling time
  B. Plethysmography, wave form analysis, and pulse volume recording
    1. Volume plethysmography
    2. Circumference plethysmography
    3. Photoplethysmography
  C. Noninvasive electromagnetic flowmetry
  D. Isotope scans
II. Arterial blood flow
  A. Pulses by palpation
  B. Arteriography
  C. Doppler effect
  D. Invasive electromagnetic flowmetry
III. Muscle perfusion
  A. Muscle pH
  B. Muscle PO_2
  C. Muscle blood flow
IV. Skin blood flow
  A. Total skin blood flow
    1. Skin color
      a. Visual observation
      b. Photoplethysmography
      c. Multispectral analysis
    2. Skin temperature
      a. Palpation
      b. Thermistor thermography
      c. Liquid crystal thermography
      d. Infrared thermography
    3. Fluorescein angiography
    4. Laser Doppler flowmetry
    5. Skin flap bleeding at time of surgery
  B. Nutritional skin blood flow
    1. ^{133}Xe washout
      a. Injected
      b. Epicutaneous
    2. Hydrogen washout
V. Cutaneous oxygen delivery
  A. Intracutaneous
    1. Polarographic
    2. Mass spectrometric
  B. Transcutaneous PO_2 measurement
VI. Segmental blood pressure
  A. Skin flush
  B. Doppler technique
  C. Plethysmography
    1. Strain gauge plethysmography
    2. Volume plethysmography
    3. Photoplethysmography
    4. Impedance plethysmography
  D. ^{133}Xe clearance (distal blood pressure)
VII. Skin blood pressure
  A. Blanching of histamine-injected skin
  B. Photoelectric technique
  C. ^{133}Xe clearance
  D. ^{131}I clearance
  E. Laser Doppler flowmetry
VIII. Skin function
  A. Observation of ability to maintain skin envelope
  B. Observation of ability to produce cutaneous appendages
  C. Ability of skin to heal incisions

*From Burgess, EM and Matsen, FA, III: *Determining amputation levels in peripheral vascular disease.* J Bone Joint Surg 63A:1494, 1981, with permission.

SKIN TEMPERATURE AND TISSUE APPEARANCE

Warmth to touch and a line of demarcation have been mentioned as the most reliable signs of viability in the foot. Some surgeons consider skin temperature too nonspecific to influence the choice of amputation level. Others state that the best indices of amputation level are skin temperature and appearance at the proposed amputation site, rather than a rigid adherence to the presence of pulses or the results of oscillometry or arteriography. A demarcation line implies that the gangrene is localized and that proximal vascularity is adequate. The absence of a demarcation line usually indicates that the disease is spreading, thus precluding a local procedure. If the patient's condition permits, it is surgically advantageous to wait for a sharp line of demarcation. In general, a sharp difference in skin temperature between the proximal and distal areas suggests a recent arterial occlusion with poor collateral circulation. Delaying surgery, when possible, may allow time for the collateral circulation to develop sufficiently to permit a more distal amputation. The amputation level is usually well above the cold area. Rubor on dependency and blanching of the toes on elevation also suggest poor collateral circulation. It has been suggested that dependent rubor at the level of the proposed skin incision is an almost absolute contraindication to amputation at that level.

CONDITION OF ADJACENT AREA

Skin color should be observed. Cyanotic skin proximal to the gangrenous area which does not reverse color with elevation of the limb usually indicates advanced ischemia in the area, which is a contraindication to local surgery. Trophic changes in the area, such as thin, shiny skin with marked loss of hair and subcutaneous tissue, indicate poor vascularity. Edema in the area impedes blood flow. In the absence of venous obstruction or cardiorenal disease, the edematous limb will usually respond to elevation or pressure management.

EXTENT OF GANGRENE

The prognosis for healing after a toe amputation is more favorable if the gangrene is confined to the distal phalanx. If gangrene is present in the entire digit of one or more toes, then a transmetatarsal amputation is considered to be a safer procedure. Antibiotics, bed rest, and surgical drainage may be used preoperatively to control the degree of infection and to localize the gangrene, thereby allowing a more distal amputation.

DIABETES

The presence or absence of diabetes does not seem to be critical in the healing of a given amputation wound because the frequency of healing is as great or greater in diabetics as in patients without diabetes.

REST PAIN OR CLAUDICATION

Pain is commonly present when gangrene is spreading. Pain that radiates from the toes toward the ankle or leg is usually a contraindication for a toe or transmetatarsal amputation. Ischemic rest pain and dependent rubor are reliable signs that perfusion is inadequate for wound healing. Severe rest pain above the ankle has been reported to be an indicator of a poor prognosis for a below-knee amputation.

The degree of claudication is sometimes difficult to accurately assess from history or even physical examination. Pain is often neurologic and musculoskeletal in origin, rather than vascular. Cardiopulmonary problems can limit the exercise-testing performance of elderly patients. Intermittent claudication often has a benign course. The patient may at first experience increasing disability owing to rest pain and an inability to walk; then collateral circulation may develop, with relief of the claudication and recovery of functional capacities.

PREOPERATIVE SYMPATHECTOMY

Sympathectomy is a procedure designed to reduce vascular spasm and improve collateral circulation by cutting the sympathetic trunk. Nevertheless, lumbar sympathectomies that are performed prior to the amputation do not increase the incidence of healing of lower extremity amputations.

ARTERIAL RECONSTRUCTION

Major arterial reconstruction prior to the amputation does not have a discernible effect upon the healing rates of lower extremity amputations.

MEASUREMENT OF PERIPHERAL CIRCULATION

PERIPHERAL PULSES

The absence of palpable pulsations in major vessels of the lower extremity does not necessarily indicate severe ischemia. A collateral blood supply develops if these vessels are occluded gradually. The below-knee amputation heals as successfully with or without a popliteal pulse and usually heals in the absence of the femoral pulse. In the case of transmetatarsal or digital amputations, healing is more likely if a pedal pulse is present.

Transmetatarsal or digital amputations will heal satisfactorily in almost half of the cases if a femoral pulse is the most distal palpable pulse. Peripheral pulses must be viewed in conjunction with other factors. No correlation has been found between measurements of skin blood flow and the level of the most distal palpable pulse. These results suggest that pulse palpation is a poor predictor of blood flow and should not be used in the selection of the amputation level.

ARTERIOGRAPHY

A contrast medium is injected into the femoral artery and the vascular outline is observed roentgenographically to detect evidence of collateral circulation. Controversy exists over the utility of arteriography as a prognosticator of healing ability. William Dwyer established precise criteria for predicting safe healing in the below-knee amputation:

1. A below-knee amputation can be performed safely if the popliteal bifurcation is patent and good collateral vessels at the knee and upper third of the leg are seen on the first film.
2. If these findings are seen on the second film, taken 10 seconds later, but not on the first film, then it is a borderline case. The decision is then based on the extensiveness of the collateral network.
3. If a femoral blockage is present with absence of collateral circulation, then a below-knee amputation is contraindicated; some form of above-knee amputation is recommended.

4. An above-knee amputation, rather than a below-knee amputation, is also advised if the posterior tibial artery alone is patent without collaterals.

Other people state that arteriography is of no value in level selection.

Arteriography is an invasive, expensive, painful, risky, and relatively time-consuming procedure and therefore is not suitable for repetitive measurements.

CAPILLARY SKIN BLOOD FLOW AS MEASURED BY RADIOACTIVE XENON 133 (^{133}Xe) CLEARANCE

The most widely used technique for measuring skin blood flow at the potential amputation site is the determination of the clearance rate of intracutaneously injected ^{133}Xe. For below-knee amputations, the critical level on the anterior skin is a flow rate of 2.7 ml per 100 g tissue per minute (or greater), which will allow adequate circulation for healing at 100 percent. A trial amputation at the below-knee level is recommended for a flow rate in the range of 2.3 to 2.7 ml per 100 g tissue per minute. However, less definitive results, with healing in cases where blood flow is as low as 0.01 ml per 100 g per minute and revisions being required in cases with flows as high as 7.5 ml per 100 g per minute, have been reported. At least one repeated measurement is advised to rule out measurement error.

This technique depends on the assumption that the measurement's validity is not adversely affected by the trauma of injecting ^{133}Xe. By using the laser Doppler velocimetry technique, it was demonstrated in 1980 that the skin blood flow is increased by as much as sevenfold for at least 20 minutes when a 30-gauge needle is inserted into the skin. Thus, the technique appears to alter what it is intended to measure.

DIRECTIONAL DOPPLER FLOW DETECTION

The Doppler ultrasound velocity detector is used to perform a simple, noninvasive technique for assessing arterial velocity and extremity systolic blood pressure. Systolic pressures in excess of 70 mm Hg found below the knee are generally consistent with either primary or secondary healing of a below-knee amputation. If there is no measurable pressure or Doppler arterial sound below the popliteal level, then a below-knee amputation will not heal. If below-knee pressures are less than 70 mm Hg, then an above-knee amputation may be indicated as an initial procedure. If the thigh pressure is at least 45 percent of brachial pressure, or at least 50 mm Hg in the nondiabetic patient or 70 mm Hg in the diabetic patient, then a below-knee amputation rather than an above-knee amputation is recommended. Below-knee amputations with detectable thigh pressures of less than 50 mm Hg will heal, and thus they should not be contraindicated if other clinical signs are favorable.

Single toe amputations heal with ankle arterial pressures as low as 35 mm Hg, but forefoot amputations usually do not heal with ankle pressures of less than 55 to 60 mm Hg. In general, an ankle systolic pressure of greater than 70 mm Hg is used to predict primary healing of toe, transmetatarsal, or Syme amputations.

Diabetic patients, however, frequently have artificially elevated systolic pressures at all levels of the lower extremity, which makes Doppler assessment inaccurate. Segmental systolic pressure readings may be falsely elevated in over half of the patients undergoing a foot amputation and over a third of those having a below-knee amputation. Segmental pulse volume recordings (PVRs) give correct predictions in only half of the total cases. Systolic pressures cannot be measured at all in 5 percent to 10 percent of diabetic patients because the vessels are stiff and noncompressible. The absence of Doppler arterial signals in the popliteal space or more distally is generally agreed to predict wound failure in over 85 percent of below-knee amputations.

The noninvasive measurement of cutaneous blood flow velocity by laser Doppler has been described. This system utilizes the Doppler frequency shift in monochromatic laser light that is backscattered from moving red blood cells. This technique measures flow velocity through the superficial microvascular system; it differs from plethysmography, which is a measure of total flow. Regional or microcirculatory flow can be measured using radioactive tracers, but these techniques are invasive and require exposure to radioactivity.

PLETHYSMOGRAPHY

The best method of measuring total arterial inflow into a segment is plethysmography. It provides a picture of the sympathetic response in the limb. Venous occlusion plethysmography is performed with the extremity in an air or watertight chamber. The volume change in the receptacle after the venous return is occluded corresponds to the arterial inflow of blood. The room must be kept at a constant temperature. If venous return is not completely arrested, an erroneous reading will be made. Minimal satisfactory sympathetic response of the circulation with indirect heating is twice the control value in the calf and three times the control value in the foot. Pulse volume recordings can be taken by placing PVR cuffs around the thighs, calves, and ankles.

The pulse volume recorder can also be used to measure segmental systolic pressures. In this technique, the PVR cuff is placed distal to the occlusion cuff.

Digital photoplethysmography (PPG) is very reliable for assessing foot circulation. By using special toe cuffs, digital systolic pressures of less than 10 mm Hg can be measured. It has been reported that nondiabetic patients with a digital pressure above 10 mm Hg can be expected to heal after digit or foot amputation. Diabetics should evidence a minimal digital pressure of 25 mm Hg for healing. More recent investigations using PPG indicate the failure of forefoot amputations with toe pressures of less than 45 mm Hg (failure in all limbs with a pressure of less than 20 mm Hg) and primary healing with toe pressures greater than 55 mm Hg. Ankle pressures were not a valid estimate of forefoot perfusion and, thus, healing of forefoot amputations.

OSCILLOMETRY

The oscillometer measures the pulsatile change in volume of all of the tissues under the cuff with each heart beat. Oscillometric indices are based on the resting state. Although oscillometry is not yet viewed as a stable diagnostic tool, an oscillometric index below "trace" in the instep following indirect heating is considered to be inadequate for wound healing in the foot.

INTRA-ARTERIAL INJECTION OF RADIOACTIVE (^{99m}Tc) MICROSPHERES

The injection can be made through a translumbar aortic catheter or via a needle in the femoral artery. The degree of perfusion as related to amputation level selection is being investigated.

SKIN BLOOD PRESSURE

Skin pressures can be determined by the counterpressure necessary to stop the clearance of intradermally injected isotopes such as ^{133}Xe or ^{131}I. They can also be determined by measuring the pressure at which blushing occurs (blanching disappears) in histamine-injected skin as the inflated transparent sphygmomanometer cuff is gradually deflated. Wound healing is unlikely with skin blood pressures below 20 mm Hg; healing is variable if pressures are between 20 and 40 mm Hg; and complete healing is probable if the pressures are greater than 40 mm Hg.

TRANSCUTANEOUS Po₂

The circulatory status of the extremity can be reflected by a transcutaneous Po_2 measurement. To measure the transcutaneous oxygen tension, the skin is locally warmed to 44°C. A Clark electrode applied to the skin measures the oxygen emanating from the skin. Initial data indicate that below-knee amputations heal if the Po_2 level is greater than 40 mm Hg and fail to heal with below-knee transcutaneous Po_2 values of 26 mm Hg or less. There is variable healing if values are between 26 and 40 mm Hg.

MUSCLE PERFUSION

Measurements of the muscle pH of the clean-cut proximal surfaces of the gastrocnemius, soleus, and anterior tibial muscles do not show a relationship to the healing of below-knee amputations if the pH is above 7.0. However, when the pH is below 7.0, healing does not occur.

ONSET OF ARTERIAL OCCLUSION

A slow onset of vascular disease without sudden arterial occlusion is compatible with amputation below the knee. If the occlusion is gradual, there will usually be sufficient time for collateral circulation to develop. Sudden arterial occlusion (especially if combined with weakness or absence of the femoral pulse, coolness of the skin above mid-leg, prolonged venous filling, or evidence of extreme ischemia by elevation-dependency tests) is supporting evidence for an above-knee amputation.

OPERATIVE RISK

Some patients may have conditions such as disabling arthritis, myocardial infarction, cerebrovascular accidents, severe renal disease, or marked pulmonary disease that will make them poor risks for survival of the operation and for rehabilitation, especially if the amputation is above the knee joint. If it is felt that the patient may be able to survive only one amputation, then an above-knee amputation is required although the chance of successful rehabilitation is much greater with a distal amputation.

WOUND BLEEDING

Some surgeons believe that the presence of skin bleeding should determine the amputation level rather than a palpable pulse or bleeding from the major vessels. Mid-leg amputations heal by primary intention, however, even with poor bleeding at the intended site of amputation. Little or no bleeding from the wound edge usually mandates a more proximal amputation when considered with other factors.

PRESENCE OF ISCHEMIC MUSCLE AT THE TIME OF SURGERY

The presence of ischemic muscle at the time of surgery is not an absolute indication for an above-knee amputation. Healing can occur if the skin is viable and the necrotic muscle is resected.

AMPUTATION TECHNIQUE

No preoperative assessment method will ever predict the outcome of an amputation with certainty because the healing process depends upon postoperative—not preoperative—blood supply. The preoperative criteria used to select the amputation level may be entirely sound, and yet the amputation may fail because of intraoperative or postoperative factors.

Successful wound healing depends on the operative technique. In cases of peripheral vascular disease, surgery must be meticulous, with delicate handling of tissue and without vigorous skin retraction.

Tension on tissue occludes small blood vessels and thus must be avoided. The length, shape, and source of the flap are factors that affect the healing potential. Flaps should have adequate length to close without tension. Tissue distal to a ligature dies and thus should be minimized and should not include tissue adjacent to a vessel. The skin should be closed in a manner that will hold yet will not occlude the skin blood vessels.

POSTOPERATIVE FACTORS

INFECTION

Wound infection can ruin all prior efforts. Using the open-flap method when there is evidence of serious infection and ischemia will probably result in a lower rate of wound complication without eventual reamputation at a higher level. In the presence of local infection, antibiotics given preoperatively and postoperatively also enhance the results.

EDEMA

A major cause of failure of wound healing is edema. Edema can worsen vascularity in the residual limb not only through pressure on vessels, but also by creating tension at the suture line. Therefore, skin flaps should be long enough to accommodate some postoperative tissue swelling. This is the rationale for the use of pressure bandages or rigid support postoperatively.

TYPE OF POSTOPERATIVE DRESSING

The failure rate of below-knee amputations with immediate postoperative fittings (rigid dressings) and soft dressings is nearly identical.

SUMMARY

Although a higher primary healing rate may be achieved following above-knee amputation for peripheral vascular disease, this must be weighed against the significantly lower mortality following below-knee amputation. Also, the chance for successful prosthetic ambulation is considerably greater for below-knee amputees. Because many people who receive an amputation because of vascular insufficiency may eventually have the remaining leg amputated, every inch of the limb that is saved is valuable. As Kerstein and associates so aptly stated in 1974: "It is necessary to find a common meeting ground for what a patient will tolerate physiologically and what he needs psychologically."

AMPUTATION FOR TRAUMA

In cases of trauma, all viable tissue should be saved during the initial surgery. Revisions, such as bone shaping or skin grafting, are usually performed in a subsequent procedure.

AMPUTATION FOR TUMOR

The site of amputation for tumor depends upon the nature of the tumor and the presence or absence of metastasis. It is usually desirable to have a joint between the tumor and the amputation site.

AMPUTATION FOR DEFORMITY

Because amputation for deformity is not a life-saving procedure, primary consideration can be given to appearance and function. The patient's sex and occupation, as well as the fashions worn by the patient, are factors that may influence the decision.

CONGENITAL LIMB DEFICIENCY REVISION

Revision of congenital limb deficiencies requires a special knowledge of the effect of the growth process on various abnormalities and a thorough knowledge of prosthetic replacements. In general, epiphyses are retained to allow maximal longitudinal growth. In some situations, there may be general professional agreement to amputate. Since a young child has no say in the decision, marginal cases may best be delayed until the child is old enough to participate in the decision-making process.

SURGICAL EXPERTISE

Leg amputations are sometimes performed by surgeons who have little knowledge of human gait or the functional characteristics of various prostheses. The surgeon might select from only certain levels of amputation based on prior experience or the list of sites of election based on outmoded prosthetic considerations. The surgeon should be in close communication with the prosthetist and other members of the rehabilitation team. Decisions regarding whether to amputate, where to amputate, and the objectives of the amputation are serious and should not be undertaken in ignorance. The pathology is not the only factor under consideration. Depending on the clinical situation, anatomic, surgical, prosthetic, and personal factors should also be considered to varying degrees.

BIBLIOGRAPHY

BADDELEY, RM: *A trial of conservative amputations for lesions of the feet in diabetes mellitus.* Am Surg 30:431–433, 1964.

BADDELEY, RM AND FULFORD, JC: *The use of arteriography in conservative amputations for lesions of the feet in diabetes mellitus.* Br J Surg 51:658–663, 1964.

BAKER, WH AND BARNES, RW: *Minor forefoot amputation in patients with low ankle pressure.* Am J Surg 133:331–332, 1977.

BARNES, RW, SHANIK, GD, AND SLAYMAKER, EE: *An index of healing in below-knee amputation: Leg blood pressure by Doppler ultrasound.* Surgery 79:13–20, 1976.

BARNES, RW AND SLAYMAKER, EE: *Postoperative deep vein thrombosis in the lower extremity amputee: A prospective study with Doppler ultrasound.* Ann Surg 183:429–432, 1976.

BARNES, RW, ET AL: *Prediction of amputation wound healing: Roles of Doppler ultrasound and digit photoplethysmography.* Arch Surg 116:80–83, 1981.

BAUMGARTNER, R: *Failures in through-knee amputation.* Prosthet Orthot Int 7:116–118, 1983.

BERGTHOLDT, HT AND BRAND, PW: *Thermography: An aid in the management of insensitive feet and stumps.* Arch Phys Med Rehabil 56:205–209, 1975.

BICKEL, WH: *Amputations below the knee in occlusive arterial disease.* Surg Clin North Am 23:982–994, 1943.

BICKEL, WH AND GHORMLEY, MD: *Amputations below the knee in occlusive arterial disease.* Proc Mayo Clinic 18:361–367, 1943.

BONE, GE AND POMAJZL, MJ: *Toe blood pressure by photoplethysmography: An index of healing in forefoot amputation.* Surgery 89:569–574, 1981.

BRADHAM, RR AND SMOAK, RD: *Amputations of the lower extremity: Used for arteriosclerosis obliterans.* Arch Surg 90:60–64, 1965.

BROWSE, NL: *Choice of level of amputation in ischaemic arterial disease.* Scand J Clin Invest 31:249–252, 1973.

BURGESS, EM: *Sites of amputation election according to modern practice.* Clin Orthop 37:17–22, 1964.

BURGESS, EM: *The below-knee amputation.* Inter-Clinic Info Bull 8:1–22, 1969.

BURGESS, EM AND MATSEN, FA, III: *Determining amputation levels in peripheral vascular disease.* J Bone Joint Surg 63A:1493–1497, 1981.

BURGESS, EM, ET AL: *Segmental transcutaneous measurements of PO_2 in patients requiring below-the-knee amputation for peripheral vascular insufficiency.* J Bone Joint Surg 64A:378–382, 1982.

CAMERON, HC, LENNARD-JONES, JE, AND ROBINSON, MP: *Amputations in the diabetic: Outcome and survival.* Lancet 2:605–607, 1964.

CANTY, TJ: *Amputations and recent developments in artificial limbs.* US Armed Forces Med J 3:1147–1152, 1952.

CARTER, SA: *The relationship of distal systolic pressures to healing of skin lesions in limbs with arterio-occlusive disease: With special reference to diabetes mellitus.* Scand J Lab Invest (Suppl) 31:239–243, 1973.

CHAVATZAS, D, BUDAK, D, AND JAMIESON, CW: *An assessment of value of long posterior flaps in below-knee amputation by skin blood pressure.* J Cardiovasc Surg 16:594–596, 1975.

CRANLEY, JJ, ET AL: *Below-the-knee amputation for arteriosclerosis obliterans: With and without diabetes mellitus.* Arch Surg 98:77–80, 1969.

DALE, WA AND CAPPS, W, JR: *Major leg and thigh amputations: Ten-year survey of results.* Surgery 46:333–342, 1959.

DALE, WA AND JACOBS, JK: *Lower extremity amputation: Results in Nashville, 1956-1960.* Ann Surg 155:1011–1021, 1962.

DEAN, RH, ET AL: *Prognostic indicators in femoropopliteal reconstructions.* Arch Surg 110:1287–1293, 1975.

DEAN, RH, ET AL: *Predictive value of ultrasonically derived arterial pressure in determination of amputation level.* Am Surg 41:731–737, 1975.

DWYER, WA, JR: *Arteriography in localizing the amputation level in arteriosclerosis obliterans.* J Med Soc NJ 59:464–467, 1962.

DWYER, WA, JR: *Arteriographic determination of a safe amputation level.* J Med Soc New Jersey 66:8–12, 1969.

ECKER, ML AND JACOBS, BS: *Lower extremity amputation in diabetic patients.* Diabetes 19:189–195, 1970.

EFFENEY, DJ, LIM, RC, AND SCHECTER, WP: *Transmetatarsal amputation.* Arch Surg 112:1366–1370, 1977.

ERAKLIS, A AND WHEELER, HB: *Below-knee amputations in patients with severe arterial insufficiency.* N Engl J Med 269:938–943, 1963.

FEE, HJ, FRIEDMAN, BH, AND SIEGEL, ME: *The selection of an amputation level with radioactive microspheres.* Surg Gynecol Obstet 143:88–90, 1977.

FLEURANT, FW AND ALEXANDER, J: *Below knee amputation and rehabilitation of amputees.* Surg Gynecol Obstet 151:41–44, 1980.

FURSTÉ, W AND HERRMANN, LG: *Value of transmetatarsal amputations in the management of gangrene of toes.* Arch Surg 57:497–512, 1948.

GIBBONS, GW, ET AL: *Predicting success of forefoot amputations in diabetes by noninvasive testing.* Arch Surg 114:1034–1036, 1979.

GIBBONS, GW, ET AL: *Noninvasive prediction of amputation level in diabetic patients.* Arch Surg 114:1253–1257, 1979.

HAIMOVICI, H: *Criteria for and results of transmetatarsal amputation for ischemic gangrene.* Arch Surg 70:45–51, 1955.

HARRIS, PD, SCHWARTZ, SI, AND DeWEESE, JA: *Midcalf amputation for peripheral vascular disease.* Arch Surg 82:381–383, 1961.

HOLLOWAY, GA, JR: *Cutaneous blood flow responses to injection trauma measured by laser Doppler velocimetry.* J Invest Dermatol 74:1–4, 1980.

HOLLOWAY, GA, JR AND BURGESS, EM: *Cutaneous blood flow and its relation to healing of below-knee amputation.* Surg Gynecol Obstet 146:750–756, 1978.

HOLLOWAY, GA, JR AND WATKINS, DW: *Laser Doppler measurement of cutaneous blood flow.* J Invest Dermatol 69:306–309, 1977.

HOLSTEIN, P: *Distal blood pressure as guidance in choice of amputation level.* Scand J Clin Lab Invest 31:245–248, 1973.

HOLSTEIN, P, DOVEY, H, AND LASSEN, NA: *Wound healing in above-knee amputations in relation to skin perfusion pressure.* Acta Orthop Scand 50:59–66, 1979.

HOLSTEIN, P, SAGER, P, AND LASSEN, NA: *Wound healing in below-knee amputations in relation to skin perfusion pressure.* Acta Orthop Scand 50:49–58, 1979.

KANE, WJ: *Lower limb amputations in peripheral vascular disease: Factors influencing the level.* Minn Med 51:179–182, 1968.

KELLY, PJ, AND JANES, JM: *Criteria for determining proper level of amputation in occlusive vascular disease: A review of 323 amputations.* J Bone Joint Surg 39A:883–891, 1957.

KELLY, PJ AND JANES, JM: *Criteria for determining the proper level of amputation in occlusive vascular disease.* J Bone Joint Surg 52A:1685–1688, 1970.

KENDRICK, RR: *Below-knee amputations in arteriosclerotic gangrene.* Br J Surg 44:13–17, 1956.

KERSTEIN, MD, ET AL: *Amputation of the lower extremity: A study of 194 cases.* Arch Phys Med Rehabil 55:454–459, 1974.

KOLIND-SØRENSEN, V AND MARQVERSEN, J: *Distal blood pressure measurement in lower-limb amputees.* Acta Orthop Scand 50:571–572, 1979.

KRITTER, AE: *A technique for salvage of the infected diabetic gangrenous foot.* Orthop Clin North Am 4:21–30, 1973.

LEBEDEV, NE: *Choice of the level and method of amputation in gangrenous stages of endarteritis and atherosclerosis of vessels in extremities.* Khirurgiia (Moscow) 40:45–46, 1964.

LeCONTE, RG: *New war methods in amputations: Stumps and prosthesis of the lower limbs.* US Nav M Bull 13:244–254, 1919.

LEE, BY: *Hemodynamic evaluation in selection of amputation level.* Bull Prosthet Res 10–22:85–104, 1974.

LEE, BY, ET AL: *Noninvasive hemodynamic evaluation in selection of amputation level.* Surg Gynecol Obstet 149:241–244, 1979.

LITTLE, JM, ET AL: *A trial of flapless below-knee amputations for arterial insufficiency.* Med J Aust 1:883–887, 1970.

MALONE, JM, ET AL: *Therapeutic and economic impact of a modern amputation program.* Ann Surg 189:798–802, 1979.

MALONE, JM, ET AL: *Therapeutic and economic impact of a modern amputation program.* Bull Prosthet Res 10–32:7–17, 1979.

McCOLLOUGH, NC, III: *The dysvascular amputee.* Orthop Clin North Am 3:303–321, 1972.

MEHTA, K, ET AL: *Fallibility of Doppler ankle pressure in predicting healing of transmetatarsal amputation.* J Surg Res 28:466–470, 1980.

MILLER, MB: *Advanced occlusive arterial disease (gangrene) in the aged: And decision-making for amputation.* J Am Geriatr Soc 22:321–328, Jul 1974.

MOORE, WS: *Determination of amputation level: Measurement of skin blood flow with Xenon Xe 133.* Arch Surg 107:798–802, 1973.

MOORE, WS: Letter to the Editor. *Determination of amputation level by measurement of skin blood flow.* Arch Surg 109:124, 1974.

MOORE, WS: *Skin blood flow and healing.* Bull Prosthet Res 10–22:105–108, 1974.

MURDOCH, G: *Levels of amputation and limiting factors.* Ann R Coll Surg Engl 40:204–216, 1967.

MURDOCH, G: *Amputation surgery in the lower extremity.* Prosthet Orthot Int 1:72–83, 1977.

MURDOCH, G: *The surgery of the below-knee amputation.* In MURDOCH, G (ED): *Prosthetic and Orthotic Practice.* Edward Arnold & Co, London, 1970, pp 45–60.

MURRAY, DG: *Below-knee amputations in the aged: Evaluation and prognosis.* Geriatrics 20:1033–1038, 1965.

PALOSCHI, GB AND LYNN, RB: *Major amputations for obliterative peripheral vascular disease with particular reference to the role of below-knee amputation.* Can J Surg 10:168–171, 1967.

PEDERSEN, HE, LaMONT, RL, AND RAMSEY, RH: *Below-knee amputation for gangrene.* South Med J 57:820–825, 1964.

PERSSON, BM: *Sagittal incision for below-knee amputation in ischaemic gangrene.* J Bone Joint Surg 56B:110–114, 1974.

POLLOCK, SB, JR AND ERNST, CB: *Use of Doppler pressure measurements in predicting success in amputation of the leg.* Am J Surg 139:303–306, 1980.

RAINES, JK, ET AL: *Vascular laboratory criteria for the management of peripheral vascular disease of the lower extremities.* Surgery 79:21–29, 1976.

RECORD, EE: *Surgical amputation in the geriatric patient.* J Bone Joint Surg 45A:1742–1749, 1963.

ROMANO, RL AND BURGESS, EM: *Level selection in lower extremity amputations.* Clin Orthop 74:177–184, 1971.

ROON, AJ, MOORE, WS, AND GOLDSTONE, J: *Below-knee amputation: A modern approach.* Am J Surg 134:153–158, 1977.

ROSENDAHL, S: *Transmetatarsal amputation in diabetic gangrene.* Acta Orthop Scand 43:78–83, 1972.

SCHWARTZ, JA, ET AL: *Predictive value of distal perfusion pressure in the healing of amputation of the digits and the forefoot.* Surg Gynecol Obstet 154:865–869, 1982.

SCHWINDT, CD, LULLOFF, RS, AND ROGERS, SC: *Transmetatarsal amputations.* Orthop Clin North Am 4:31–42, 1973.

SILBERT, S AND HAIMOVICI, H: *Criteria for the selection of the level of amputation for ischemic gangrene.* JAMA 155:1554–1558, 1954.

SIZER, JS AND WHEELOCK, FC, JR: *Digital amputations in diabetic patients.* Surgery 72:980–989, 1972.

SKVERSKY, N AND ZISLIS, JM: *Peripheral-vascular disorders and the aged amputee.* Geriatrics 25:142–149, 1970.

STAHLGREN, LH AND OTTEMAN, M: *Review of criteria for the selection of the level for lower extremity amputation for arteriosclerosis.* Ann Surg 162:886–892, 1965.

STILL, JM, JR, WRAY, CH, AND MORETZ, WH: *Selective physiologic amputation: A valuable adjunct in preparation for surgical operation.* Ann Surg 171:143–151, 1970.

Suzak, Z, Gaspar, A, and Najenson, T: *Arterial occlusive disease in amputee patients: Assessment with the Doppler ultrasound flowmeter and correlation with rehabilitation.* Arch Phys Med Rehabil 61:269–272, 1980.

Thompson, RG, et al: *Amputation and rehabilitation for severe foot ischemia.* Surg Clin North Am 54:137–154, 1974.

Tolstedt, GE and Bell, JW: *Failure of below-knee amputation in peripheral arterial disease: Use of arteriography in determining site of election.* Arch Surg 83:934–936, 1961.

Vankka, E: *Study on arteriosclerotics undergoing amputations.* Acta Orthop Scand 104:1–98, 1967.

Verta, MJ, Jr, et al: *Forefoot perfusion pressure and minor amputation for gangrene.* Surgery 80:729–734, 1976.

Warren, R, et al: *The transmetatarsal amputation in arterial deficiency of the lower extremity.* Surgery 31:132–140, 1952.

Warren, R and Kihn, RB: *A survey of lower extremity amputations for ischemia.* Surgery 63:107–120, 1968.

Wessman, HC: *The amputation site in the lower extremity: Regard for the vascular efficiency.* Minn Med 40:905–908, 1966.

Young, AE, Henderson, BA, and Couch, NP: *Muscle perfusion and the healing of below knee amputations.* Surg Gynecol Obstet 146:533–534, 1978.

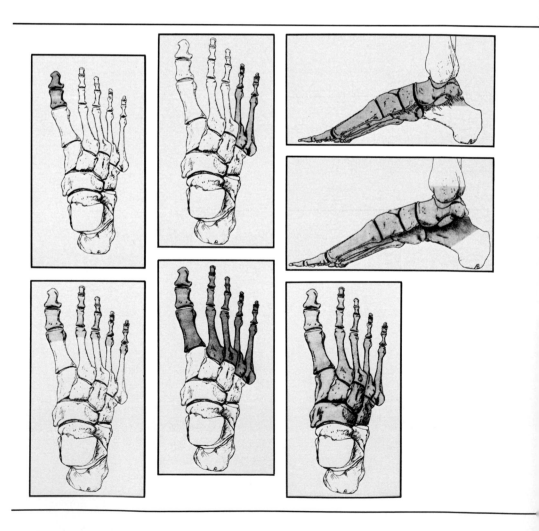

PARTIAL FOOT AMPUTATIONS

RIGID PLATE
STEEL SPRING
WITH HEEL CUP

TARSAL (Ta), PARTIAL (CHOPART, MIDTARSAL DISARTICULATION, PIROGOFF, BOYD)

CHOPART AMPUTATION

TECHNIQUE
PROBLEMS
PROSTHESES
   BOOT WITH TOE FILLER
   BOOT WITH SEMIRIGID
   METAL SOLE AND TOE FILLER
   ANKLE/FOOT ORTHOSIS

CHOPART PROSTHESIS
VARIATION

PIROGOFF AMPUTATION

TECHNIQUE
ADVANTAGES
PROBLEMS
PROSTHESES
   SHOE FILLER
   THICK SHOE SOLE
   WITH SOFT PADDING
   POSTERIOR LEAF SPRING
   AFO

BOYD AMPUTATION

TECHNIQUE
PROSTHESES

PHALANGEAL (Ph), PARTIAL (SYME TERMINAL AMPUTATION, TOE)

SYME TERMINAL AMPUTATION

The Syme terminal amputation is performed for toenails that are markedly hypertrophied, ingrown, or incurved causing pressure on the subungual tissue, or for toenails that have a chronic mycotic infection. A closed procedure is usually performed when the surgery is prophylactic. The wound is packed open when infection is present.

TOE AMPUTATION (TRANSPHALANGEAL, DIGITAL AMPUTATION)

Toe amputations are generally indicated for localized gangrene of the distal end of the toe and infection that is demarcated. The conditions that are necessary for success include freedom from pain, no dependent rubor, a venous filling time of no more than 20 to 25 seconds, no gangrene proximal to the proximal interphalangeal joint, and no discoloration extending over the metatarsal region. Amputation of a single toe can be performed through the toe, at the base of the proximal phalanx, or disarticulated at the metatarsophalangeal joint.

AMPUTATION THROUGH THE TOE

The dorsal incision is made at the level of intended bone section. The plantar incision is made farther distally to allow for a long plantar flap. The flexor and extensor tendons are sectioned and are allowed to retract. Digital vessels are ligated and sectioned. Digital nerves are also sectioned. After division at the selected level, the ends of the bone are smoothed with a rasp.

AMPUTATION AT THE BASE OF THE PROXIMAL PHALANX

Skin incisions can be fashioned to yield a variety of flap designs (fishmouth, long plantar, long dorsal, side-to-side, or any combination). The flaps must be long enough to close without tension.

The position of the sesamoids beneath the first metatarsal head can be maintained by suturing the flexor and extensor tendons together over the end of the bone. In all other toes, the tendons are drawn distally, divided, and allowed to retract. Digital nerves are divided proximal to the end of the bone. Digital vessels are ligated and sectioned. This level is preferred to disarticulation at the metatarsophalangeal joint by some surgeons who claim that the small button of bone protects the metatarsal head.

PROSTHESIS

A prosthesis is not necessary for toe amputation.

PHALANGEAL (Ph), COMPLETE (DISARTICULATION AT THE METATARSOPHALANGEAL JOINT, TOE, DIGITAL AMPUTATION)

If the great toe is being amputated (Fig. 6-1), every effort is made to retain the base of the proximal phalanx, which serves as the insertion of important intrinsic muscles. If the flexor hallucis brevis has no insertion it retracts, pulling the sesamoids proximally to the middle of the metatarsal shaft. With the lesser toes, amputation is sometimes performed at the metatarsophalangeal joint rather than through the proximal phalanx, which would leave a functionless little stump subject to friction and pressure when the patient walks. Argument has been given against amputation by disarticulation because the cartilage covering the metatarsal head has a poor blood supply and is thus susceptible to infection and healing failure. If clear synovial fluid drainage is present, then joint and cartilaginous involvement is inevitable and satisfactory healing will be unlikely.

TECHNIQUE

With the toe held in acute flexion, a dorsal incision through the capsule is made first. With the toe held straight, the remainder of the capsule is incised. Medial and lateral or dorsal and ventral flaps may be used. Scars are placed to avoid weight-bearing surfaces.

Amputation of the great toe or fifth toe is sometimes accompanied by removal of the metatarsal head as well. This allows for easier skin closure. The dorsal incision is placed toward the midline to avoid lateral pressures.

PROBLEMS

Great toe amputation does not noticeably affect standing or walking at a slow or moderate pace. Since the push-off that is normally provided by the great toe is lost, a limp is apparent during running or fast walking. Also, the lack of a great toe increases the

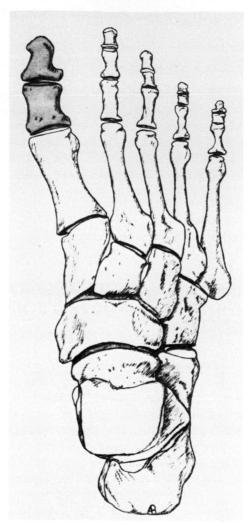

FIGURE 6-1. Phalangeal, complete.

vulnerability of the remaining toes, and plantar calluses may form. Therefore, the great toe should not be amputated unless it is absolutely necessary.

Amputation of the second toe results in severe hallux valgus.

PROSTHESES

For amputation of the toes, lamb's wool, sponge rubber, or foam is usually inserted into the tip of the shoe. If the great toe is amputated, a long steel spring shank can be used in the sole of the shoe to assist push-off and prevent deformity of the shoe. Weight is usually redistributed to the lateral aspect of the foot after loss of the great toe. A wedge (metatarsal bar) placed behind the metatarsal heads aids in the even distribution of pressure. When the second toe is amputated, a firm but pliable material is placed between the great toe and the third toe to function as a spacer to prevent hallux valgus.

AMPUTATION OF ALL TOES

Amputation of all toes is sometimes recommended in cases of multiple painful metatarsophalangeal dislocations, clawing of the toes, and severe hallux valgus. It is most applicable in cases of gross deformity when the toes are rigid, functionless, and painful. If the lateral four toes require amputation, then the great toe is usually not left because it will become grossly displaced and create problems.

TECHNIQUE

A dorsal incision is made beginning at the first metatarsal head and crossing the proximal phalanx of each toe while dipping down into the intervening web spaces. After a similar incision is made on the plantar aspect of the foot, the flexor and extensor tendons are divided and each toe is disarticulated. The suture line is dorsal to the weight-bearing areas.

PROSTHESES

An insole is used that has a metatarsal support to relieve weight from the metatarsal heads and a cavus support for the high arch that often results. A cork or foam toe block is attached distally as a filler (Fig. 6-2). Normal-length shoes with toe blocks make walking essentially normal by compensating for the amputated toes. A rocker sole may be necessary to replace the action of rocking forward on the foot. The sole can be stiffened with a long steel spring or sole plate to prevent the front part of the shoe from turning up. For patients who have amputations as a result of Hansen's disease (leprosy) or diabetes, the rest of the foot will probably have a loss of sensation and a tendency toward skin breakdown. In these cases, it is important to obtain an even distribution of pressure and to avoid high local pressures, which will cause ulcerations. An insole molded to the shape of the foot and lined with a soft material may serve this purpose. If a custom insole is used, then a larger-than-usual shoe will be needed.

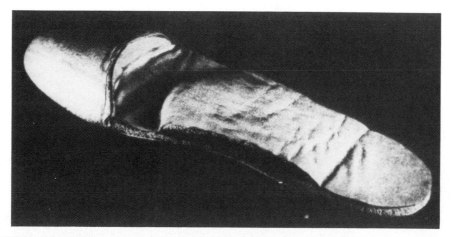

FIGURE 6-2. Sponge rubber insole with metatarsal padding and a cork toe block. (From Flint, M and Sweetnam, R: *Amputation of all toes: A review of forty-seven amputations.* J Bone Joint Surg 42B:93, 1960, with permission.)

METATARSAL (MT), PARTIAL (METATARSAL RAY RESECTION, TRANSMETATARSAL)

METATARSAL RAY RESECTION

This procedure involves removal of an entire ray (toes plus metatarsals) (Fig. 6-3). Transmetatarsal amputations are usually better because the ray amputation leaves such a narrow foot and walking surface that they interfere with balance on uneven ground.

    The metatarsal ray resection is indicated in some cases of congenital anomalies, gangrene secondary to frostbite, neoplasms, severe chronic infections of a single metatarsal, or a deep subaponeurotic foot abscess. For a congenital deformity involving supernumerary rays, a ray resection is most often done on the fifth ray. If six complete

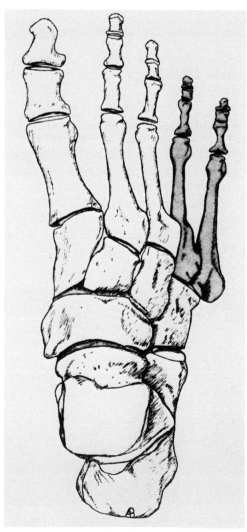

FIGURE 6-3. Metatarsal ray resection.

rays are present, the fifth ray is usually resected so that the surgical scar will not be located on the lateral aspect of the foot. Better success has been reported with amputation of the fourth and fifth rays rather than the first and second metatarsal rays, which would affect push-off during walking. Cases have been reported of removal of several lateral toes and the third metatarsal for giantism or congenital hypertrophy limited to several rays of the foot. Because simple toe disarticulations are prone to failure, some surgeons suggest that it is necessary to remove the metatarsal head along with the involved toe to obtain adequate débridement and eradicate the infected tissue.

TRANSMETATARSAL AMPUTATION

Transmetatarsal amputation (Fig. 6-4) was first described by C. Bernard and C. Heute in 1855. This procedure had limited success and was performed infrequently before the advent of antibiotics. Since that time, transmetatarsal amputations have proven to be

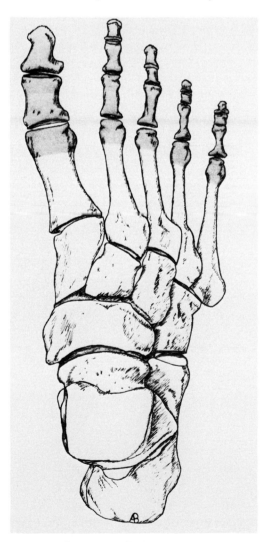

FIGURE 6-4. Transmetatarsal amputation.

successful for patients with atherosclerotic occlusive vascular disease as well as those with diabetic ischemia. In diabetics, the gangrene often results from slight trauma, such as cutting corns or trimming a callus or trophic nails. Transmetatarsal amputations are indicated when gangrene involves two or more toes, is limited to the toes, and does not extend proximally into the web or foot itself. The plantar skin must be intact. Other suggested criteria include: infection is controlled or stabilized, there is no pain (pain indicates the presence of infection or ischemia too marked to allow healing) other than in the affected toes, there is no dependent rubor, and venous filling in the dependent foot is less than 25 seconds. The absence of foot or popliteal pulses does not preclude successful healing; however, the presence of a pedal pulse is a favorable prognostic sign. Reasonable collateral circulation is desired. Transmetatarsal amputations are rarely successful when performed after toe amputations have failed. Some authors have reported a much lower success rate in diabetic patients as opposed to nondiabetic patients. This statistic may be reflective of diabetes management, however.

The preoperative preparation period is critically important to the success of the operation. During this time, it is important for infection to be controlled using antibiotics (based on culture and sensitivity testing), gentle foot baths, open drainage, débridement, vasodilators, and bed rest. Transmetatarsal amputation is contraindicated if infection is not controlled. At the time of surgery, the prognosis is more favorable if the diabetes is well controlled and the gangrene has demarcated.

The residual limb is highly acceptable functionally and cosmetically. Foot balance is maintained because the residual limb is symmetrical in shape and major muscle attachments are preserved. Disability is minimal, and there is no formal prosthetic requirement. The major disadvantage of transmetatarsal amputation is the risk of nonhealing, the failure rate being nearly 50 percent in many centers.

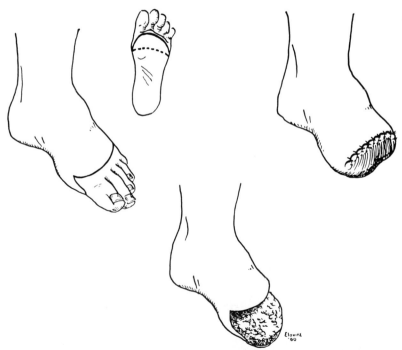

FIGURE 6-5. The incision lines of the transmetatarsal amputation. Note the long plantar flap. (From Wheelock, FC, Jr: *Transmetatarsal amputations and arterial surgery in diabetic patients.* N Engl J Med 264:316, 1961, with permission.)

TECHNIQUE

The dorsal incision is made from side to side at the level of intended bone section. The plantar incision is made distal to the metatarsal heads and is extended transversely at the level of the interdigital clefts (Fig. 6-5). The incisions are sharp and go directly down to the bone. The plantar flap containing subcutaneous fat and a layer of plantar muscles is reflected to the level of intended bone section. The dorsal and plantar incisions are carried down to the bone without dissection of any tissue planes. The metatarsals are sectioned transversely, usually just proximal to the metatarsal heads. The first and fifth metatarsals are beveled on the medial and lateral sides. All metatarsals are beveled inferiorly. Any sesamoid bones are removed. Nerves are identified and divided so that they fall proximal to the distal end of the bone. Tendons are allowed to retract. The plantar flap is brought over the distal end of the bone and sutured to the shorter dorsal flap without tension. A plantar flap is used to cover the ends of the bones (because the circulation is better than on the dorsum of the foot) and to avoid locating the scar in a weight-bearing area. Postoperative gangrene following transmetatarsal amputation in peripheral vascular disease is almost always confined to the dorsal aspect of the foot.

If the end of the stump is covered by abnormal skin—either a scar or skin graft (even a pedicle graft)—it is rarely able to withstand the stresses of weight-bearing and will ultimately result in painful callosities or ulcers. The surgical procedure should be as untraumatic as possible by not using forceps on the skin margins, avoiding dog-ears on the corners upon closure, achieving closure without tension, and allowing adequate drainage.

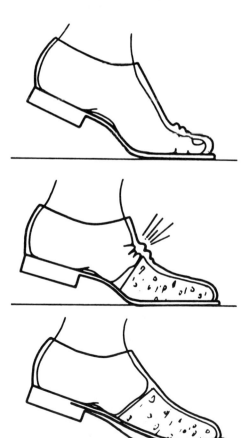

FIGURE 6-6. (*Top*) The normal toe break is at the metatarsophalangeal joints. (*Middle*) Irritation resulting from an abnormally proximal "toe break." (*Bottom*) Correction of the shoe's irritating effect by the addition of a steel shank between the inner and outer sole and the rocker bottom. (From Harris, WR and Silverstein, EA: *Partial amputations of the foot: A follow-up study.* Can J Surg 7:9, 1964, with permission.)

PROSTHESES

The break in an ordinary shoe is at the metatarsophalangeal joints, which corresponds roughly to the end of the long transmetatarsal stump (Fig. 6-6, *top*). A shoe with stuffing or foam in the toe is thus all that may be necessary. If the stump is shorter, as in the short transmetatarsal, Lisfranc, and Chopart amputations, the shoe will break at a more proximal point, giving an uncosmetic appearance. Also, the vamp of the shoe may irritate the top of the stump, resulting in sores (Fig. 6-6, *middle*). Adding a long steel spring between the inner and outer sole, along with modifying the shape to a rocker bottom, can prevent these problems (Fig. 6-6, *bottom*). Without support in the front of the shoe, the patient will display a limp (early drop-off) as the walking speed increases.

METATARSAL (MT), COMPLETE (LISFRANC, MIDFOOT AMPUTATION, TARSOMETATARSAL DISARTICULATION)

LISFRANC AMPUTATION

In 1798, William Hey from Leeds described a tarsometatarsal ablation. Jacques Lisfranc, in 1815, described a similar disarticulation (Fig. 6-7). Lisfranc and midtarsal Chopart amputations are considered in the growing child where it is desirable not to interfere with the distal tibial epiphysis and yet to allow end-bearing. Another indication for the Lisfranc or Chopart amputation is when a prosthesis is unobtainable. In individuals who do heavy labor or farm work, the Lisfranc or Chopart amputation may be desirable because each offers full limb length and total end weight-bearing and the prosthetic replacement is simple. They are sometimes performed following crush injuries of the forefoot or frostbite.

TECHNIQUE

The incision begins at the base of the fifth metatarsal and goes distally along the lateral edge of the metatarsal shaft to the neck of the metatarsal. The incision is then made down and across the sole of the foot, parallel and just proximal to the metatarsal heads. On the medial side of the foot, the incision is made proximal to the space between the medial cuneiform and the base of the first metatarsal. The dorsal incision is curved, with a distal convexity just distal and parallel to the line of the tarsometatarsal joints. The flaps are elevated to expose the tarsometatarsal joints. The lateral three metatarsals are separated from the cuboid and lateral cuneiform. The first metatarsal is separated from the medial cuneiform. The second metatarsal is then separated from the middle cuneiform (this is sometimes difficult and may require one of several modified procedures). Vessels are ligated and the flaps sutured. A rigid dressing is usually worn for several weeks to prevent equinus deformity.

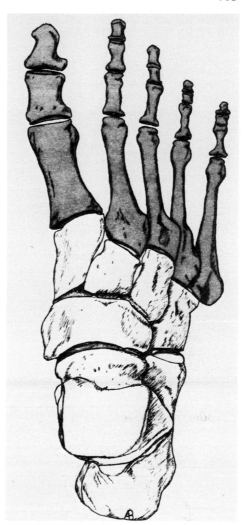

FIGURE 6-7. Lisfranc amputation.

PROBLEM

A fixed equinus deformity may result from a loss of the distal attachment of the dorsi-flexors, as with the Chopart midtarsal amputation. This results in excessive anterior weight-bearing across an area of scar tissue and adherent, tender skin that is unaccustomed to weight-bearing, thus causing pain, skin ulcerations, and infection. Therefore, many surgeons state that the Lisfranc amputation should never be done, and it has largely been discarded as an elective amputation in the English-speaking parts of the world. There are reported cases, however, of amputees who have a tarsometatarsal amputation with a contralateral Syme amputation who find the midfoot amputation superior. Prevention or correction of the ankle equinus would make this a desirable amputation level (Table 6-1). For this reason, some surgeons implant the extensor tendons into the dorsum of the foot to restore balance. If the surgeon rejects midfoot amputations and goes from the transmetatarsal amputation to the Syme amputation, then all undamaged tissue may not be saved and the leg will be shortened. A subtalar wedge osteotomy with arthrodesis will correct the equinus displacement and result in a

TABLE 6-1. RECONSTRUCTIVE PROCEDURES USED TO PREVENT OR CORRECT ANKLE EQUINUS

1. Subtalar wedge osteotomy with arthrodesis
2. Use of the peroneal and posterior tibial tendons as an anterior sling
3. Anterior tibial tendon tenodesis with or without the toe extensor tendons
4. Removal of the talus
5. Lengthening of the Achilles tendon may be combined with these procedures

residual limb that uses the plantar surface of the foot for weight-bearing. This procedure preserves talocrural movement, leaves the healthy talus, and does not shorten the limb.

PROSTHESES

SHOE FILLER

If the equinus deformity has been corrected surgically, a forefoot shoe filler may be used. Weight-bearing will be on the plantar heel skin, but push-off will be lost. If only a shoe filler is used, the "toe" break is located more proximal than in the normal foot; this is usually regarded as cosmetically unsatisfactory.

RIGID PLATE

If an equinus deformity that can be passively corrected is present, then prosthetic stabilization is necessary. This has been attempted by a plate that supports the residual foot and is rigidly attached to the shank piece that goes above the calf (Fig 6-8).

STEEL SPRING WITH HEEL CUP

A more cosmetic version is a prosthesis with an arch of spring steel that is thin enough to be flexible. The steel extends out to the toe and posteriorly to form a heel cup. The toe area is filled with soft silicone to provide the elastic compression necessary to hold the back of the foot against the heel cup.

TARSAL (Ta), PARTIAL (CHOPART, MIDTARSAL DISARTICULATION, PIROGOFF, BOYD)

CHOPART AMPUTATION

Disarticulation at the midtarsal joint (through the talonavicular and calcaneocuboid joints)
Long plantar flap

A disarticulation through the midtarsal joint, which was developed by François Chopart while he was working at the Charitable Hospital in Paris where he was Professor of Surgery, was first described in 1792 (Fig. 6-9).

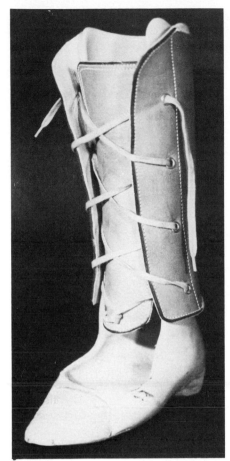
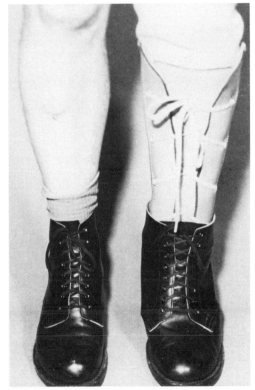

FIGURE 6-8. A prosthesis for the Lisfranc or Chopart amputation. *(Left)* The sole plate is rigidly attached to the shank, which is fitted with a laced leather corset. *(Right)* A large boot is needed because the prosthesis is bulky. (From Harris, WR and Silverstein, EA: *Partial amputations of the foot: A follow-up study.* Can J Surg 7:10, 1964, with permission.)

A Chopart amputation is recommended in the growing child for fibular amelia. This would allow end-bearing without interfering with the nutrition to the distal tibial epiphysis. A Syme revision can be performed later if needed.

Because the midtarsal amputation is more likely to heal than the transmetatarsal amputation, it has been used for neuropathic lesions with extensive destruction of the foot, as well as ischemic gangrene and traumatic injuries. The anterior tibialis and other ankle dorsiflexors are attached to the plantar fibrous tissue or to the talar neck (the insertion of the anterior tibialis is detached and passed through a hole that is drilled in the neck of the talus) in order to partially counterbalance the triceps surae.

TECHNIQUE

The incision goes from just behind the tubercle of the navicular bone distally along the medial border of the foot toward the head of the first metatarsal. Midway on the shaft of the metatarsal, the incision is carried down across the sole to fashion the plantar flap. On the lateral side of the foot, the incision is made proximally along the shaft of the fifth

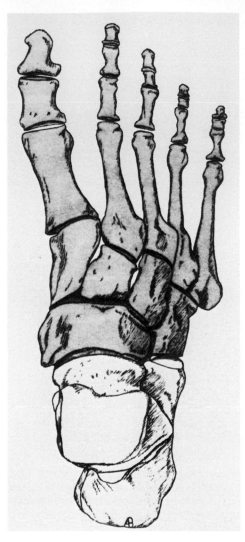

FIGURE 6-9. Chopart amputation.

metatarsal to a point midway between the lateral malleolus and the base of the fifth metatarsal. The dorsal incision is curved with a distal convexity to parallel the line of the metatarsal heads. The plantar flap is carefully elevated with as little damage to the subcutaneous tissue as possible. The ligaments holding the talonavicular joint are divided. The anterior tibialis muscle is firmly attached to the neck of the talus (usually by a hole drilled in the bone). Division of the ligaments between the calcaneus and cuboid completes the disarticulation. Vessels are tied and flaps are opposed. A rigid dressing to prevent equinus deformity is usually applied and is worn for several weeks.

PROBLEMS

The remaining foot is usually drawn into equinovarus by the triceps surae, causing a poor weight-bearing surface that results in ulceration and necrosis of the skin (Table 6-2). As the calcaneus migrates downward, weight-bearing occurs on the anterior surface of the talus and anterior and inferior portions of the calcaneus. The skin over the antero-inferior aspect of the residual foot tends to develop calluses. This painful and deformed limb is not effective for weight-bearing. James Syme, who claimed to have introduced

TABLE 6-2. FEATURES OF VARIOUS PARTIAL FOOT AMPUTATIONS

| | Technique | | | |
Features	Lisfranc	Chopart	Pirogoff	Boyd
arthrodesis	–	–	+	+
weight-bearing through tissue normally used for such	– (if equinus develops)	– (if equinus develops)	–	+
equinus deformity is a problem	+	+	–	–
ulceration of skin and necrosis are common problems	+	+	+	–
abnormal joint is created	–	–	–	–

(–) absent
(+) present

Chopart's amputation in Edinburgh in 1929, reported satisfactory results. He explained that the cut tendons acquired new attachments, thus counteracting the extensor muscles of the ankle acting through the Achilles tendon. Releasing the Achilles tendon or using residual muscles to suspend the anterior part of the foot is often ineffective or of only temporary benefit. Cases have been reported, however, of amputees who preferred the Chopart amputation, which they described as being more comfortable, to a contralateral Syme amputation.

PROSTHESES

BOOT WITH TOE FILLER

A simple boot with stuffing in the toe is an easy way to manage the foot, but it does nothing to improve the gait over walking barefooted. Also, the filler acts with the shoe to rub the end of the stump, causing pressure or ulceration. With use, the toe of the shoe points up and becomes uncosmetic.

BOOT WITH SEMIRIGID METAL SOLE AND TOE FILLER

A leather lacer (bootee) with a steel shank that fits inside the shoe or a long steel spring shank inserted from heel to toe between the outer and inner sole of a custom-made orthopedic shoe gives the patient added support while walking. From mid-stance until toe-off, the long steel spring shank assists push-off by resisting the forces acting to dorsiflex the forefoot. A long, high-reinforced counter or a toe filler, usually made of foam or silicone rubber, may also be used. A reverse Thomas heel or lateral heel wedge may be used when a varus hindfoot is present. The high-laced anklet with steel arch support is heavy and bulky and requires a special shoe. The steel cracks or bends, requiring frequent replacement. The long steel spring inserted between the insole and outsole does not touch the patient's foot and is very light in weight.

ANKLE/FOOT ORTHOSIS (AFO)

A posterior leaf spring AFO made of high thermal plastic may be used inside the shoe. The AFO will give resistance to plantarflexion at heel-strike, allowing a slow descent of the foot. It will also resist dorsiflexion and assist push-off from mid-stance to toe-off.

CHOPART PROSTHESIS

The Chopart prosthesis is almost identical to the Syme prosthesis in fabrication. Unlike the Syme amputation, there is no distance between the end of the residual limb and the floor with the Chopart amputation. To compensate, a small lift may be used on the sound side. In addition, less reinforcement is used under the heel pad on the prosthetic side to minimize thickness of the socket under the remaining limb.

Variation

To counteract the equinus tendency, the socket can be designed to comfortably grip the concavities on each side of the calcaneus posteriorly and hold it downward, restraining plantarflexion. The prosthesis, made of plastic or stainless steel, fits into a ready-made shoe.

PIROGOFF AMPUTATION

> Calcaneal fragment–tibial arthrodesis
> End-bearing stump

In 1854, Nicolai Ivanovitch Pirogoff, the greatest Russian surgeon of his day (Fig. 6-10), published a new surgical procedure at the ankle joint that sought to improve upon the Syme amputation (Fig. 6-11). Pirogoff considered the separation of the heel flap from the bone the most difficult part of the Syme amputation. Because this skin was so adherent, it was easy to injure the flap during dissection or to make the flap too thin. Another characteristic of Syme's operation that Pirogoff attempted to improve or eliminate was formation of a depression in the heel flap when the calcaneus was removed.

TECHNIQUE

The skin incision (Fig. 6-12), which resembles the Syme amputation, begins below the malleoli and passes anteriorly across the ankle joint to the opposite malleoli. Division of soft tissue and tendons is carried down to the bone. The ankle joint capsule is divided anteriorly. The lateral ligaments are detached from the malleoli, and the talus is displaced to expose the superior surface of the calcaneus. The calcaneus is divided obliquely from a point behind the body of the talus and in front of the Achilles tendon superiorly to a point between the middle and posterior third of the bone inferiorly (Fig. 6-13). The posterior third forms an undetached part of the heel flap. The malleoli are removed at the level of the inferior articular end of the tibia (Fig. 6-14). After vessel ligation and division, the heel flap is brought up and sutured. Arthrodesis of the calcaneal fragment to the tibia forms an end-bearing limb that is longer than the Syme limb (Fig. 6-15) and is fixed firmly in place.

ADVANTAGES

If the calcaneal fragment fuses to the tibia without difficulty, a long end-bearing limb results. If no prosthesis is available, the amputee is able to walk with less limp than following a Syme amputation. The heel flap does not wobble as it may do on the Syme limb.

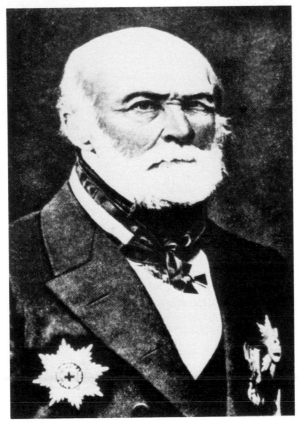

FIGURE 6-10. Nicolai Ivanovitch Pirogoff (1810–1881), who devised an amputation at the ankle to improve certain features of Syme's amputation that he regarded as detrimental. (From Harris, RI: *History and development of Syme's amputation*. Artificial Limbs 6:14, 1961, with permission.)

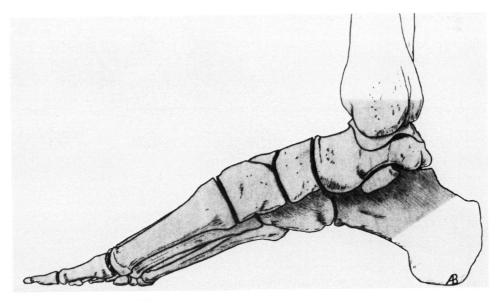

FIGURE 6-11. Pirogoff amputation.

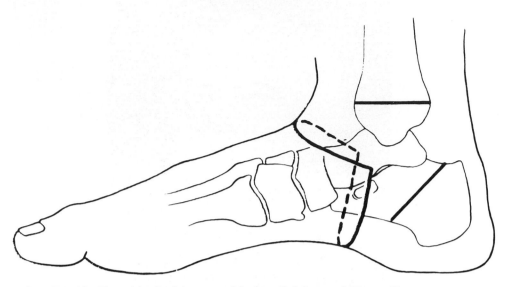

FIGURE 6-12. The skin incisions and bone divisions of Pirogoff's amputation. (From Harris, RI: *History and development of Syme's amputation.* Artificial Limbs 6:15, 1961, with permission.)

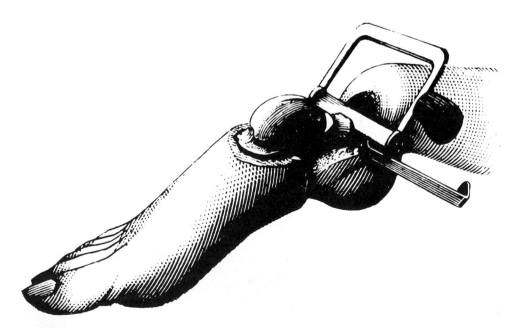

FIGURE 6-13. Calcaneal division in Pirogoff's amputation. (From Harris, RI: *History and development of Syme's amputation.* Artificial Limbs 6:15, 1961, with permission.)

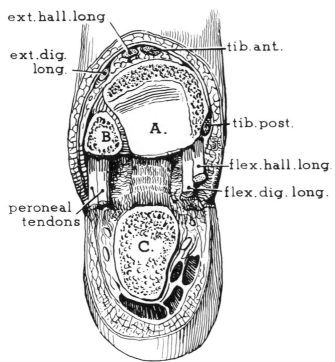

FIGURE 6-14. The residual limb after removal of the foot. (*A*) Tibia. (*B*) Fibula. (*C*) Calcaneus. (From Harris, RI: *History and development of Syme's amputation.* Artificial Limbs 6:15, 1961, with permission.)

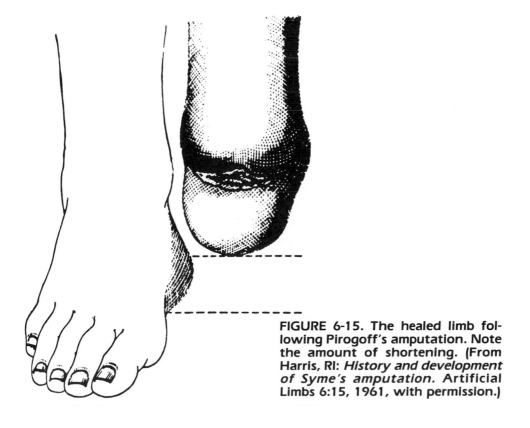

FIGURE 6-15. The healed limb following Pirogoff's amputation. Note the amount of shortening. (From Harris, RI: *History and development of Syme's amputation.* Artificial Limbs 6:15, 1961, with permission.)

PROBLEMS

If the calcaneal fragment and tibia fail to unite, a painful, unstable limb results. Chronic osteomyelitis of the calcaneal fragment or distal tibia is likely to result if the wound becomes infected. The skin over the back of the heel (where the Achilles tendon inserts) is not as well suited for weight-bearing as the plantar surface of the foot. Recurrent bursitis, ulcerations, and osteophytes may develop in this region. Another major problem is the difficulty in providing an adequate ankle/foot mechanism in the small distance between the end of the residual limb and the floor.

PROSTHESES

SHOE FILLER

With only a shoe filler, push-off is lost, which impairs walking.

THICK SHOE SOLE WITH SOFT PADDING

Again, there is no push-off.

POSTERIOR LEAF SPRING AFO

A flexible plastic ankle/foot orthosis (AFO) can be used. It provides dorsiflexion assistance during swing phase, plantarflexion assistance during the last part of stance phase, and resistance to plantarflexion from heel-strike to mid-stance.

BOYD AMPUTATION

> Calcaneotibial arthrodesis
> No posterior migration of heel pad
> End-bearing stump

TECHNIQUE

The incision is made from just below the lateral malleolus across the dorsum of the foot at the talonavicular joint to just below the medial malleolus. The plantar incision is made across the base of the metatarsals. A talectomy is performed, as well as excision of all tarsals except the calcaneus. Articular cartilage is removed from the entire ankle joint mortise and the superior surface of the calcaneus. After removal of a portion of the sustentaculum tali, the calcaneus is brought forward until the weight-bearing surface of the heel is under the long axis of the leg. The calcaneus is fitted into the ankle mortise. Steinmann pins or Kirschner wires may be used for internal fixation of the arthrodesis. The long plantar skin flap is brought forward to cover the anterior portion of the calcaneus. The scar is located at the anterior joint and goes just below the lateral malleolus (Fig. 6-16). Weight-bearing is through tissue that is normally used for weight-bearing.

PROSTHESES

The same prostheses used for the Syme amputation can be used for the Boyd amputation. Since the Boyd amputation results in a slightly longer limb than the Syme amputa-

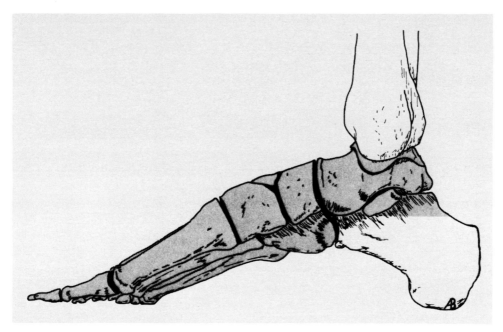

FIGURE 6-16. Boyd amputation.

tion, it may be necessary to put a small lift on the shoe of the sound foot to obtain adequate clearance for installation of the Syme foot under the socket.

BIBLIOGRAPHY

BADDELEY, RM: *A trial of conservative amputations for lesions of the feet in diabetes mellitus.* Am Surg 30:431–433, 1964.

BADDELEY, RM AND FULFORD, JC: *A trial of conservative amputations for lesions of the feet in diabetes mellitus.* Br J Surg 52:38–43, 1965.

BAKER, WH AND BARNES, RW: *Minor forefoot amputation in patients with low ankle pressure.* Am J Surg 133:331–332, 1977.

BARNES, R: *Rehabilitation of a partial forefoot amputee: A case report.* J Am Podiatry Assoc 54:333–334, 1964.

BINGHAM, J: *The surgery of partial foot amputations.* In MURDOCH, G (ED): *Prosthetic and Orthotic Practice.* Edward Arnold & Co., London, 1970, pp 141–147.

BOYD, HB: *Amputation of the foot with calcaneotibial arthrodesis.* J Bone Joint Surg 21:997–1000, 1939.

BRADHAM, GB, LEE, WH, AND STALLWORTH, JM: *Transmetatarsal amputation.* Angiology, 11:495–498, 1960.

BRADHAM, RR AND SMOAK, RD: *Amputations of the lower extremity: Used for arteriosclerosis obliterans.* Arch Surg 90:60–64, 1965.

BRYANT, RC: *Forefoot amputation.* Letter to the Editor. Arch Surg 115:889, 1980.

BURGESS, EM: *Prevention and correction of fixed equinus deformity in midfoot amputations*. Bull Prosthet Res 10–5:45–47, 1966.

BURGESS, EM: *Prevention and correction of fixed equinus deformity in midfoot amputations*. Inter-Clinic Info Bull 6:20–22, 1966.

CARNES, EH: *Amputations, stumps and prostheses*. War Med 1:656–663, 1941.

CARNEY, WI AND GOLDOWSKY, SJ: *Amputation in peripheral vascular disease*. Am J Surg 93:795–797, 1957.

CHAPMAN, MW: *Amputations*. In INMAN, VT (ED): *DuVries' Surgery of the Foot*. CV Mosby, St. Louis, 1973.

CHRISTIE, J, CLOWES, CB, AND LAMB, DW: *Amputations through the middle part of the foot*. J Bone Joint Surg 62B:473–474, 1980.

CLAUGUS, CE, ET AL: *Amputations of the lower extremity for arteriosclerosis*. Arch Surg 76:992–996, 1958.

CONDIE, DN: *Biomechanics of the partial-foot amputation*. In MURDOCH, G (ED): *Prosthetic and Orthotic Practice*. Edward Arnold & Co, London, 1970, pp 149–160.

EFFENEY, DJ, LIM, RC, AND SCHECTER, WP: *Transmetatarsal amputation*. Arch Surg 112:1366–1370, 1977.

FLINT, M AND SWEETNAM, R: *Amputation of all toes: A review of forty-seven amputations*. J Bone Joint Surg 42B:90–96, 1960.

FRIEDMANN, LW: *The Surgical Rehabilitation of the Amputee*. Charles C Thomas, Springfield, Illinois, 1978.

FURSTÉ, W AND HERRMANN, LG: *Value of transmetatarsal amputations in management of gangrene of toes*. Arch Surg 57:497–512, 1948.

GAZELEY, WE AND HOLMBLAD, JE: *Congenital foot deformities requiring surgery and prosthesis in Lisfranc's amputations*. Inter-Clinic Info Bull 6:14–20, 1967.

HAIMOVICI, H: *Criteria for and results of transmetatarsal amputation for ischemic gangrene*. Arch Surg 70:45–51, 1955.

HANGER, HB: *The Syme and Chopart Prostheses: A Manual for Prosthetists*. Northwestern University Medical School, Chicago, 1961.

HARRIS, RI: *The history and development of Syme's amputation*. Artificial Limbs 6:4–43, 1961.

HARRIS, WR AND SILVERSTEIN, EA: *Partial amputations of the foot: A follow-up study*. Can J Surg 7:6–11, 1964.

HASLAM, ET: *Surgical treatment of segmental giantism of the foot*. Inter-Clinic Info Bull 5:1–6, 1966.

HERMAN, BE: *Transmetatarsal amputation in arteriosclerotic diabetic gangrene*. NY State J Med 62:1432–1434, 1962.

HUNTER, GA: *Results of minor foot amputations for ischemia of the lower extremity in diabetes and nondiabetics*. Can J Surg 18:273–276, 1975.

JONES, RF: *Amputee rehabilitation: Basic principles in prosthetic assessment and fitting*. Med J Aust 2:290–293, 1977.

KRITTER, AE: *A technique for salvage of the infected diabetic gangrenous foot*. Orthop Clin North Am 4:21–30, 1973.

LATEGAN, LR: *Hemiamputation of the left foot*. Proc Mine Med Off Assoc 48:28–29, 1968.

LEVY, SE: *Total contact restoration prosthesis for partial foot amputations*. J Am Podiatry Assoc 50:887–896, 1960.

LINDQVIST, C AND RISKA, EB: *Results after amputation of Chopart, Pirogoff and Syme*. Acta Orthop Scand 36:344–345, 1965.

LINDQVIST, C AND RISKA, EB: *Chopart, Pirogoff and Syme amputations: A survey of 21 cases*. Acta Orthop Scand 37:110–116, 1966.

LISFRANC, J: *Nouvelle methode operatoire pour l'amputation partielle due pied dans sons articulation tarso-metatarsienne: Methode precedes des nombreuse modifications qu'a subies celle de Chopart.* Gabon, Paris, 1815.

MACDONALD, A: *Chopart's amputation: The advantages of a modified prosthesis.* J Bone Joint Surg 37B:468–470, 1955.

McCOLLOUGH, NC, III: *The dysvascular amputee.* Orthop Clin North Am 3:303–321, 1972.

McKITTRICK, LJ, McKITTRICK, JB, AND RISLEY, TS: *Transmetatarsal amputation for infection and gangrene in patients with diabetes mellitus.* Ann Surg 130:826–842, 1949.

McKITTRICK, LS: *Recent advances in the care of the surgical complications of diabetes mellitus.* N Engl J Med 235:929–932, 1946.

MURDOCH, G: *Amputation surgery in the lower extremity.* Prosthet Orthot Int 1:72–83, 1977.

NAKHGEVANY, KB AND RHOADS, JE, JR: *Ankle-level amputation.* Surgery 95:549–552, 1984.

NISSEN, KI: *The place of amputation of all toes.* J Bone Joint Surg 35B:488–489, 1953.

NORTON, WL: *Tarsal amputation.* J Korea Med Assoc 6:1174–1177, 1963.

OMER, GE, JR AND POMERANTZ, GM: *Initial management of severe open injuries and traumatic amputations of the foot.* Arch Surg 105:696–698, 1972.

PEDERSON, HE AND DAY, AJ: *The transmetatarsal amputation in peripheral vascular disease.* J Bone Joint Surg 36A:1190–1199, 1954.

POTTER, JW AND SOCKWELL, JE: *Custom-foamed toe filler for amputation of the forefoot.* Orthot Pros 28:57–60, 1974.

PRIOROV, NN: *Amputation of the extremities and prosthesis in the U.S.S.R.* J Internat Coll Surgeons 8:13–19, 1945.

RECORD, EE: *Surgical amputation in the geriatric patient.* J Bone Joint Surg 45A:1742–1749, 1963.

REVENKO, TA AND PARSHCHIKOVA, LS: *Reconstructive surgery for faulty short amputation stumps of foot.* Acta Chir Plast 16:42–47, 1974.

ROOT, HP: *Factors favoring successful transmetatarsal amputation in diabetes.* N Engl J Med 239:453–458, 1948

ROSENDAHL, S: *Transmetatarsal amputation in diabetic gangrene.* Acta Orthop Scand 43:78–83, 1972.

SCHWINDT, CD, LULLOFF, RS, AND ROGERS, SC: *Transmetatarsal amputations.* Orthop Clin North Am 4:31–42, 1973.

SILBERT, S AND HAIMOVICI, H: *Criteria for the selection of the level of amputation for ischemic gangrene.* JAMA 115:1554–1558, 1954.

SILBERT, S AND HAIMOVICI, H: *Results of midleg amputations for gangrene in diabetics.* JAMA 144:454–458, 1980.

SIZER, JS AND WHEELOCK, FC, JR: *Digital amputations in diabetic patients.* Surgery 72:980–989, 1972.

STAROS, A AND PEIZER, E: *Orthopaedic shoes for bilateral partial foot amputations.* Artificial Limbs 9:27–34, 1965.

SYME, J: *Amputation at the ankle joint.* Lon and Edin Mon J Med Sci 2 (No. XXVI):93–96, 1843.

TAURISANO, MR: *Sock suited for foot amputations.* Phys Ther 54:749, 1974.

THOMPSON, RG: *Amputation in the lower extremity.* J Bone Joint Surg 45A:1723–1734, 1963.

THOMPSON, RG, ET AL: *Amputation and rehabilitation for severe foot ischemia.* Surg Clin North Am 54:137–154, 1974.

TOOMS, RE: *Amputations.* In CRENSHAW, AH (ED): *Campbell's Operative Orthopaedics.* CV Mosby, St. Louis, 1971.

TUCK, WH: *Partial foot prosthesis.* In MURDOCH, G (ED): *Prosthetic and Orthotic Practice.* Edward

Arnold & Co, London, 1970, pp 161–167.

VERTA, MJ, JR, ET AL: *Forefoot perfusion pressure and minor amputation for gangrene.* Surgery 80:729–734, 1976.

WAGNER, FW, JR: *Amputations of the foot and ankle.* Clin Orthop 122:62–69, 1977.

WARREN, R, ET AL: *The transmetatarsal amputation in arterial deficiency of the lower extremity.* Surgery 31:132–140, 1952.

WARREN, R AND KIHN, RB: *A survey of lower extremity amputations for ischemia.* Surgery 63:107–120, 1968.

WHEELOCK, FC, JR: *Transmetatarsal amputations and arterial surgery in diabetic patients.* N Engl J Med 264:316–320, 1961.

WHEELOCK, FC, JR, MCKITTRICK, JB, AND ROOT, HF: *Evaluation of transmetatarsal amputation in patients with diabetes mellitus.* Surgery 41:184–189, 1957.

WHITE, RW: *Guillotine amputation of the foot followed by skin graft for distal gangrene.* S Afr J Surg 10:149–151, 1972.

WIGNEY, WA: *A prosthesis to restore balance and prevent pressure ulcers after partial amputation of the foot.* Med J Aust 1:852–853, 1965.

WILSON, ABK: *Hand and foot prostheses.* Practitioner 201:759–766, 1968.

YOUNG, AE: *Transmetatarsal amputation in the management of peripheral ischemia.* Am J Surg 134:604–607, 1977.

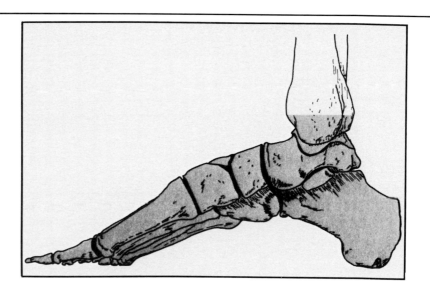

CHAPTER 7

ANKLE DISARTICULATION AND SYME (TARSAL [Ta], COMPLETE)

END-BEARING LIMBS

Amputation limbs in the lower extremity must be designed to perform the essential functions of the normal lower extremity: weight-bearing and locomotion. Weight-bearing is best accomplished through the end of the limb. To provide weight-bearing through the end of the residual limb, the bone must be sectioned where the cross-sectional area is great and the whole area of transected bone is capable of weight-bearing. These criteria can be met if the section is through the strong cancellous bone rather than through the shaft of the bone. Also, the skin that is used to cover the end of the bone must be free of hair follicles, have a thick epidermis, and be tolerant of weight-bearing. The lower ends of the femur or tibia meet these requirements.

Locomotion is best accomplished when the amputated limb has the greatest residual length and normally functioning joints, nerves, muscles, and vessels. The Syme amputation, as well as supracondylar amputations through the femur, adheres to these principles.

SURGICAL PROCEDURES

ANKLE DISARTICULATION

See Stage One under the Two-Stage Syme Amputation.

SYME AMPUTATION

James Syme (1799–1870) was known in his day as the most eminent surgeon in the English-speaking world. During his occupancy of the Chair of Clinical Surgery at the University of Edinburgh (1833–1869), he developed a new surgical procedure that has survived until now. This procedure, first performed in 1842 and described in 1843, was a disarticulation amputation through the ankle joint with end weight-bearing on the preserved heel flap. A similar procedure had already been described by Jean-Baptiste-Lucien Baudens of the Hôtel des Invalides, Paris, in 1842, and later by Philibert-Joseph Roux in 1845. Baudens' method of tibiotarsal disarticulation failed because the flap was from the dorsum of the foot, which was not tolerant of weight-bearing pressure. Roux's supramalleolar amputation used a large medial flap for assured blood supply from the posterior tibial artery. However, the flap was too thin for weight-bearing, and the area of the transected tibia and fibula was too small.

While studying in Europe, Syme learned the Chopart amputation (midtarsal joint disarticulation with a long plantar flap) and was the first to employ it in Great Britain. Syme noted that Chopart's amputation had fewer complications than amputations through the leg, although he did not understand why. Syme began performing Chopart's amputation prior to Pasteur's work on fermentation in 1856, which first revealed the world of microorganisms. It was later realized that in the presence of sepsis, disarticulation is a safer—and thus more successful—procedure than amputation through muscle masses and medullary canals of long bones. Articular cartilage, when left on the end of the bone, provides a natural barrier to the spread of infection.

Since the mortality for below-knee amputations, in which the tissue spaces and medullary cavity were widely opened, was as high as 50 percent at the time, Syme worked on developing a surgical procedure at the ankle joint that utilized the merits of Chopart's amputation, namely, joint disarticulation and an end weight-bearing limb. Although rated by Syme as the most valuable partial amputation, Chopart's amputation was inadequate for caries or compound injury involving the talus or calcaneus. Syme strove to make disarticulation at the ankle a success by creating a comfortable end-bearing limb and decreasing mortality.

Syme's amputation is indicated for many destructive and infective lesions of the foot that cannot be treated with a more distal, usually transmetatarsal, amputation. These include severe injuries of the foot, intractable infections of bones and joints of the foot (Syme first performed the operation for tuberculous infection of the talus and calcaneus), deformities of the foot, and frostbite. Syme's amputation has been performed in selected cases of obliterative vascular disease, neuropathic joints in the foot, diabetes, malignant disease, ulceration of the forefoot from irreparable injury to the sciatic nerve or spina bifida, and the insensitive foot of the leprosy patient. Its use in the neuropathic limb, however, is very limited because weight-bearing on an anesthetic limb usually results in ulceration. In cases of obliterative vascular disease, claudication is eliminated because the calf muscles no longer function. Syme recommended the amputation even in cases where the joint itself was diseased. The procedure is sometimes performed for congenital deformities of the foot. In children, it is indicated in some cases of fibular hemimelia, proximal femoral focal deficiency, and congenital foot amputations.

It is preferable to below-knee amputations for the bilateral amputee, for children because the distal growth is not disturbed, and in underdeveloped countries where no prosthetic services are available. The Syme amputation is preferred to partial foot amputations if good lower limb function cannot be reasonably assured with a more distal amputation. It is often preferred over the Boyd amputation because failure of bony union is not an issue and a greater distance exists between the distal end of the limb and the floor for fitting a prosthetic foot.

The classic Syme amputation is not recommended as a primary procedure where open, infected wounds of the foot are present. The heel pad, with good nerve and blood supply, must be large enough to provide a weight-bearing cover for the cut ends of the tibia and fibula.

TECHNIQUE AS DESCRIBED BY SYME

With the foot at a right angle to the leg, the plantar skin incision is made from the center of one malleolus directly across the sole of the foot to the other malleolus. The anterior incision is made from one malleolus to the other at a 45-degree angle to the sole of the foot and the long axis of the leg. The periosteum and plantar aponeurosis, which form the superior attachment of the septa that enclose the fat cells, are removed with the heel flap to preserve the specialized subcutaneous tissue. Great care must be taken in the technique of separating the heel flap from the calcaneus. If a cut is made into the subcutaneous layer, between the periosteum and plantar aponeurosis above and the dermis below, the septa will open, decompressing the heel pad. The stress-resistant properties of the elastic adipose tissue will be lost, and it will no longer be able to function as a hydraulic buffer. Syme stated that this amputation can be disastrous if performed incorrectly.

After separation of the heel flap, the Achilles tendon is divided and the foot is disarticulated. The malleolar projections are removed if the ankle joint is sound. A thin slice of tibia connecting the malleoli is also removed if the articulating surfaces are diseased. To ensure adequate circulation to the flap, the posterior tibial artery must not be divided above where it branches into the medial and lateral plantar arteries. Also, the heel flap must attach firmly to the cut end of the tibia.

MORE RECENT VARIATION

Today, the plantar incision is tilted slightly forward to give a larger heel flap than the one described by Syme. Syme advocated the smaller heel flap so as not to impair circulation. The larger heel flap has the advantage of providing more protection to the anterior margin of the lower end of the tibia. The ankle joint is entered through an incision that runs from the malleoli at a 45-degree angle with the line of the tibia and the plantar surface of the foot (Fig. 7-1A and B). The tibial and fibular collateral ligaments are divided from within the joint (Fig. 7-1C). The posterior tibial artery is avoided medially. The talus is dislocated downward from the ankle joint mortise (Fig. 7-1D). The Achilles tendon is carefully divided, avoiding damage to the skin flap behind it (Fig. 7-2). The talus, calcaneus, and foot are removed, avoiding damage to the posterior tibial artery.

The malleoli and a thin slice of the lower end of the tibia are removed, maintaining a broad weight-bearing surface. The tibia and malleoli should be removed in a plane that is parallel to the ground when the patient stands. This is determined individually and is not necessarily in the same plane as the articular surface of the tibia. The subcutaneous layer and skin of the heel flap are sutured to the margin of the anterior incision across the front of the ankle. The suture line should be slightly above the anterior margin of the distal end of the tibia. The dog-ears of skin are not trimmed but are allowed to shrink. Either a Penrose drain or a Hemovac is used to drain the dead space (Fig. 7-3). The heel flap is held in place by adhesive strips (Fig. 7-4), transfixion pins, or a plaster cast over a tension sock. Transfixion pins prevent early postoperative weight-bearing and can get lost in the wound. The periosteum readily adheres to the cut ends of the tibia and fibula. The position of the heel flap should be inspected frequently in the postoperative period. Stitches are removed at about 2 weeks postoperatively. Weight-bearing usually begins at about 4 weeks postoperatively but may begin earlier if a cast is applied in the immediate postoperative period.

TWO-STAGE SYME AMPUTATION

The two-stage Syme amputation was first proposed by Alvin Hulnick and colleagues in 1949 and was later supported by August W. Spittler and colleagues in 1954. It is advocated for involvement of the plantar skin or overt infections of the foot for which the original Syme amputation is not indicated. A success rate of nearly 95 percent has been claimed when this procedure is used on patients with diabetes, arteriosclerosis, or other dysvascular conditions, as long as the following indications are met:

1. The patient is a potential prosthetic user.
2. The heel pad is free of open lesions.
3. Doppler systolic pressure at the ankle is 70 mm Hg or greater.

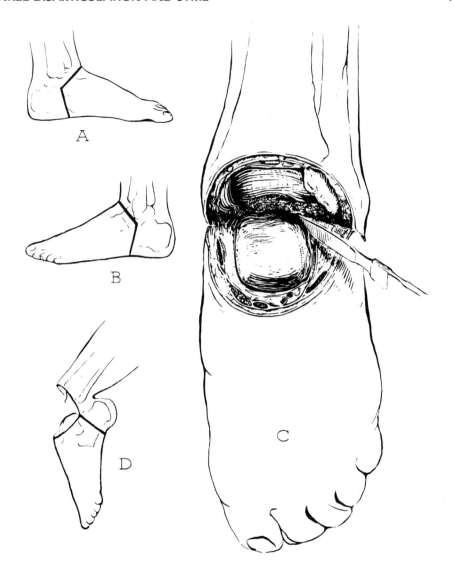

FIGURE 7-1. Techniques for the Syme amputation. *(A)* Skin incision from the medial side. *(B)* Skin incision from the lateral side. *(C)* Division of the collateral ligaments. *(D)* Dislocation of the talus downward from the ankle joint mortise. (From Harris, RI: *History and development of Syme's amputation.* Artificial Limbs 6:28, 1961, with permission.)

4. The ratio of ankle to arm systolic pressure is over 0.45.
5. There is no gross pus at the amputation site or ascending lymphangitis.
6. There is no gas in the tissue proximal to the amputation site, as evaluated by palpation or roentgenogram.
7. Bleeding occurs in the skin flaps within 3 minutes after release of the tourniquet.

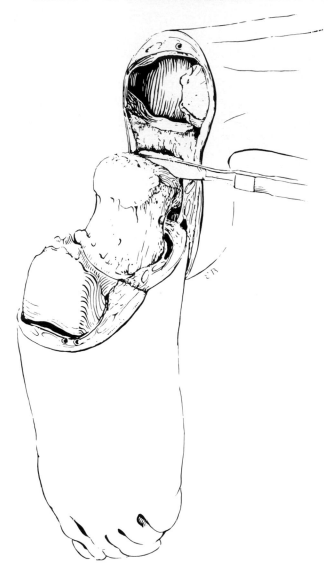

FIGURE 7-2. The calcaneus is subperiosteally dissected from the heel flap. The Achilles tendon is divided at its insertion. (From Harris, RI: *History and development of Syme's amputation.* Artificial Limbs 6:29, 1961, with permission.)

STAGE 1: DISARTICULATION AT THE ANKLE

In Stage 1, a disarticulation at the ankle is performed. The incision is parallel and 2.5 to 4 cm (1 to 1½ in) more distal to the classic Syme amputation. This allows for the size of the malleoli. Anterior and posterior skin flaps are preserved. These are closed loosely to allow adequate drainage and to avoid constricting the skin flap circulation. A wound drain connected to a bottle that contains an antibiotic solution is often placed into the cavity of the ankle joint. Usually, the infection will not spread into the distal end of the tibia and fibula because the articular cartilage acts as a natural barrier. Hematoma formation from bone bleeding is also avoided. A compression dressing that maintains

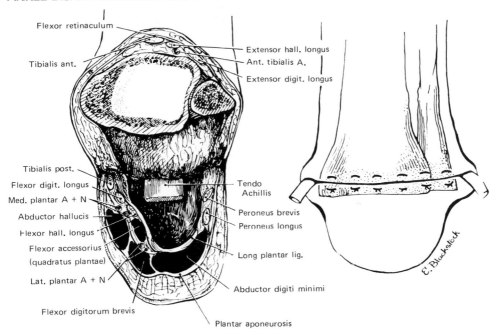

Flexor retinaculum

Tibialis ant.

Extensor hall. longus
Ant. tibialis A.
Extensor digit. longus

Tibialis post.
Flexor digit. longus
Med. plantar A + N
Abductor hallucis
Flexor hall. longus
Flexor accessorius
(quadratus plantae)
Lat. plantar A + N

Tendo
Achillis

Peroneus brevis
Peroneus longus

Long plantar lig.

Flexor digitorum brevis

Abductor digiti minimi

Plantar aponeurosis

E. Blackstock

FIGURE 7-3. *(Left)* Anatomy of the operative field just prior to closure. *(Right)* Wound closure with drainage. (From Harris, RI: *History and development of Syme's amputation.* Artificial Limbs 6:30, 1961, with permission.)

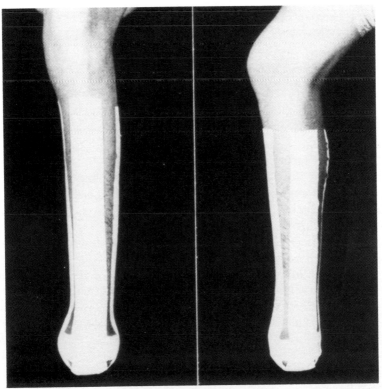

FIGURE 7-4. Method of adhesive strapping of the heel flap to the leg to ensure proper positioning in relation to the cut ends of the tibia and fibula. (From Harris, RI: *History and development of Syme's amputation.* Artificial Limbs 6:30, 1961, with permission.)

the position of the heel pad is applied. The drain is removed within 2 to 7 days post-operatively. At 7 to 10 days, a nonwalking cast is applied. Walking casts are occasionally applied if the malleoli are not prominent and the pad is tough.

STAGE 2: CONVERSION OF THE ANKLE DISARTICULATION TO THE SYME AMPUTATION

Once the wound is healed and infection is controlled (usually by 6 weeks), then the malleoli are removed. Medial and lateral incisions are made over the dog-ears, and the malleoli are removed flush with the ankle joint surface. The articular cartilage is left undisturbed. Next, the flares of the tibia and fibula are removed parallel to the tibial shaft, which leaves the distal limb relatively square. This allows for better control of the prosthesis. At approximately 7 to 10 days postoperatively, the patient is placed into a walking cast.

TECHNIQUE AS DESCRIBED BY SARMIENTO

This surgical procedure was designed to cosmetically improve the bulbous residual limb necessitating a bulbous-ended prosthesis and yet retain the end-bearing feature of the limb. In this procedure, the circumference of the bulbous end is reduced by about one-third by removing the metaphyseal flare of the distal tibia and beveling the distal fibula. This results in a distal bony end that is only slightly wider than the diaphyseal portion of the lower leg. Tibial length (Sarmiento later described removal of a half inch of the tibia and fibula) and end weight-bearing are maintained. A cast is applied at surgery. The attachment of a SACH foot and ambulation usually begin in the first post-operative week. This rigid plaster prosthesis seems to control excessive edema and enhance adherence of the heel flap to the cut distal end of the tibia.

ADVANTAGES OF THE SYME AMPUTATION

Syme noted that the advantages of his amputation over below-knee amputations were less mutilation, decreased risk of serious hemorrhage, decreased mortality, a more comfortable limb, and a more useful limb for weight-bearing. Since weight-bearing is the main function of the legs, residual limbs that allow weight-bearing on the end offer the best possibility of good function. Syme emphasized the importance of end-bearing, although in his day its merits were secondary to the lower operative mortality. Function is also enhanced by limb length. The Syme amputation offers comfortable end weight-bearing and long length.

The Syme amputee may walk about the house without using a prosthesis or crutches. This is especially useful when the amputee gets up at night to go to the bathroom or needs to move quickly in an emergency. Also, the amputee is afforded a means of adequate ambulation even if a prosthesis cannot be procured. If the Syme amputee is fitted with a prosthesis, adjustments are usually fewer than those needed by the best-fitted below-knee amputee. Bilateral Syme amputees walk with a better gait and can stand longer than bilateral below-knee amputees. Since the calf muscles are no longer functioning, the vascular insufficiency symptom of claudication is eliminated. Phantom pain is rare after a Syme amputation.

The Syme limb rarely needs surgical revision. The few problems that occur are most often the result of imperfections in the surgeon's technique. The Syme amputation requires more skill on the part of the surgeon than many other amputations. A satisfactory limb can be obtained only by rigid adherence to a precise surgical technique. The major objection to the Syme limb has been the uncosmetic bulbous distal end. For that reason, for many years the Syme amputation was not recommended for women. With the current surgical modifications and prosthetic improvements, this objection is no longer justified.

PROBLEMS WITH THE SYME AMPUTATION

SURGICAL DAMAGE TO THE WEIGHT-BEARING STRUCTURE OF THE HEEL FLAP

This is usually due to faulty surgical technique. If attention is given to subperiosteal separation of the heel flap from the calcaneus instead of attempting to trim the flap by removing origins of small muscles, this problem is avoided. Once the weight-bearing qualities of the flap are impaired, there is no subsequent procedure to restore them.

MISPLACED HEEL FLAP

The heel flap should be located beneath the center of the cut end of the tibia. The flap will become misplaced if it is not secured in this position until sound healing has occurred. Frequent careful postoperative inspection and painstaking care are important because the flap fits loosely over the lower end of the tibia. If the flap becomes misplaced, impairment of the limb's end-bearing capability results. This can sometimes be surgically corrected.

SLOPING SURFACE OF THE LOWER END OF THE TIBIA

The plane of transection of the tibia must be parallel to the ground when the patient is standing, not necessarily at a right angle to the long axis of the shaft of the tibia. Failure to do this will result in displacement of the heel flap toward the high side of the slope during weight-bearing. The oblique weight-bearing surface is prone to ulceration.

WOBBLY OR UNSTABLE HEEL FLAP

A flaccid, loose heel flap is usually due to dissection through the subcutaneous elastic adipose tissue (buttonholing) rather than to subperiosteal dissection. This disrupts the septa of the flap, opens fat loculi, and allows fat to escape. A loose heel flap can be avoided by proper operative technique; but once present, it cannot be surgically corrected.

NEUROMA ON THE POSTERIOR TIBIAL NERVE

A neuroma inevitably develops on any cut nerve, but in this case, the nerve is rarely sensitive. In cases where the nerve is painful, it should not be divided at a higher level because of potential damage to the posterior tibial artery. The nerve can be cut well above the ankle joint without removal of the distal segment of the nerve.

MARGINAL GANGRENE OF THE HEEL FLAP

Gangrene can be caused by injury to the posterior tibial artery, division above its bifurcation, a postoperative dressing applied too tightly, swelling beneath unloosened adhesive strips, or infection. If infection is present preoperatively, a two-stage procedure should be performed.

TENDER HEEL FLAP WITH CALLUSES

Tenderness is usually due to surgical damage to the fibroelastic adipose tissue of the heel flap, which is accentuated if the area of tibia and fibula transection is small or spurs are present. Bony spurs can be removed, but a damaged heel flap or an inadequate tibia and fibula support area cannot be corrected by subsequent surgery.

IMPERFECT SKIN COVERING OF THE DISTAL LIMB

If the skin covering the distal limb is ill adapted to weight-bearing, little can be done by surgery. Prosthetic socket modification can distribute weight-bearing between the end of the amputated limb and the proximal end of the socket, as with the below-knee prosthesis.

HEEL PAD CLASSIFICATION

An arbitrary classification of the mobility of the heel pad was developed by George Murdoch of Dundee, Scotland (Fig. 7-5).

Class I   The heel pad is securely fixed to the end of the bone but permits enough movement to accommodate shifts of a surface in contact (Fig. 7-6A).

Class II   The heel pad as a whole cannot be displaced, but the substance of the pad can be moved beyond the diameters of the cut bone.

Class III   The whole heel pad can be displaced in any direction about the end of the bones.

Class IV   The heel pad is grossly mobile and permanently displaced so that it cannot be reposed over the bone ends (Fig. 7-6B).

Heel pads in Classes I and II are satisfactory within the criteria described by Syme.

Attempts to improve upon Syme's amputation by sectioning at the supramalleolar level have been unsuccessful. Although the residual limb is no longer bulbous, the area of support is too small and the poorly padded end of the limb does not tolerate continued end weight-bearing. The satisfactory results of the Syme amputation depend upon a wide area of bony support covered by a large, thick heel pad.

REAMPUTATION

Reamputation of Syme limbs is indicated when transection of the tibia is so high that the area of support for the heel flap is too small, the weight-bearing structures of the heel flap are damaged, the heel flap is uncontrollably unstable, or there is nutritional impairment of the heel flap. A bursa may develop between the tibia and the heel pad if the flap is excessively mobile. Often, a satisfactory result can be obtained by removal of the bursa and freshening of the tibial surface. New bone formation in the pad usually does not cause discomfort; however, sometimes it warrants surgical exploration, especially in the case of spurs. Postoperative sepsis and vascular insufficiency are the most frequent causes of failure requiring reamputation at a higher level.

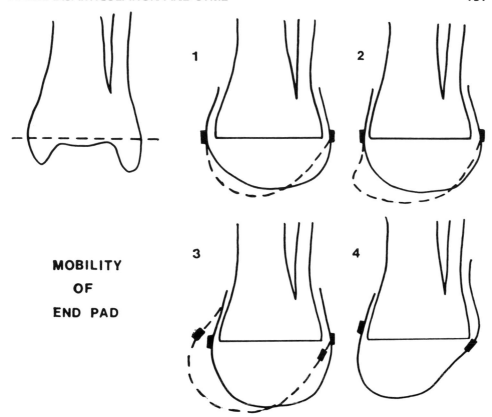

FIGURE 7-5. Classification of the mobility of Syme's stump end pads. (From Murdock, G: *Syme's amputation.* J R Coll Surg Edinb 21:22, 1976, with permission.)

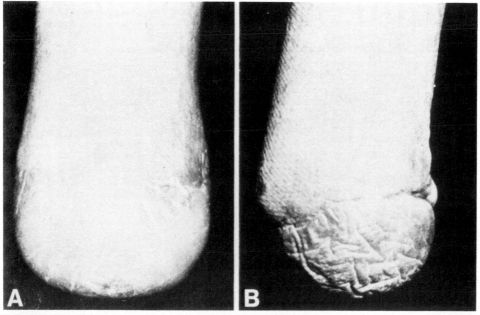

FIGURE 7-6. Syme's amputation stumps. *(A)* Class I end pad. *(B)* Class IV end pad. (From Murdock, G: *Syme's amputation.* J R Coll Surg Edinb 21:23, 1976, with permission.)

PROSTHESES

The Syme amputation has had only limited popularity until recently, at least in part because of the difficulty of providing a suitable prosthesis. The prosthesis should provide satisfactory ankle function in the limited space between the end of the limb and the floor, should have structural durability, especially in the ankle region, and should improve the appearance of the leg.

HISTORIC SYME PROSTHESIS

This prosthesis (Fig. 7-7) consists of a front-lacing leather socket (bucket) that is molded to the limb. A strong steel frame forms medial and lateral uprights that reinforce the leather. A full-length anterior opening allows entry. The tightness of the thigh-lacer provides a means of adjusting the relative distribution of weight-bearing between the proximal and distal aspects of the limb. Such a prosthesis can be adjusted to reduce end weight-bearing to as little as 40 percent of the body weight. The prosthesis is bulky to

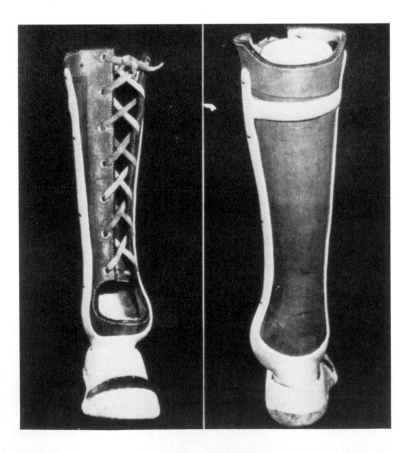

FIGURE 7-7. A standard Syme prosthesis: anterior and posterior views. (From Harris, RI: *Syme's amputation: The technical details essential for success.* J Bone Joint Surg 38B:628, 1956, with permission.)

accommodate the bulbous limb and heavy to withstand the stresses that are transmitted through it. A single-axis joint located below the socket provides the ankle motion.

This prosthesis is uncosmetic because of the large ankle circumference, which does not match the other leg. The leather absorbs perspiration, which results in hygiene problems in warm climates. The prosthesis is heavy because of the metal components, and it sometimes requires auxiliary suspension. The laces cause uneven pressure along the tibial crest. Obtaining proper leg-length equality is difficult because of the space required by the single-axis foot. The sidebars are also subject to mechanical failure. This prosthesis is rarely used now except in countries where plastic laminates are unavailable.

CANADIAN SYME PROSTHESIS

In 1955, The Canadian Department of Veteran Affairs Center sponsored the development of a plastic Syme prosthesis (Fig. 7-8). A posterior door that extends to the brim of the socket allows insertion of the limb and then is buckled into place for closure. Because the entire socket is constructed of polyester laminate, socket reliefs can be made simply by modifying the plaster model of the patient's limb or by grinding or sanding areas of pressure concentration. The socket is also perspiration-resistant. The

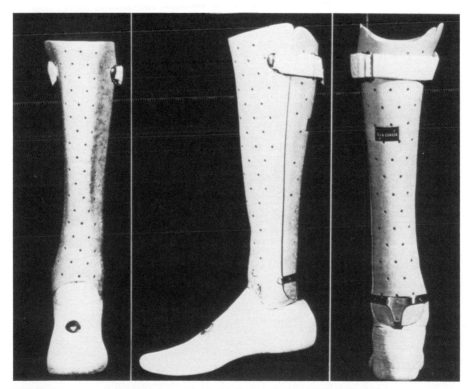

FIGURE 7-8. Laminated synthetic resin bonded Canadian Syme prosthesis: anterior, lateral, and posterior views. (From Harris, RI: *Syme's amputation: The technical details essential for success.* J Bone Joint Surg 38B:629, 1956, with permission.)

foot used is a modified solid-ankle–cushion-heel (SACH) type, which allows for more accurate height adjustment and eliminates the necessity of elevating the shoe on the sound side. Although the ankle circumference is less than the historic Syme prosthesis, the Canadian prosthesis has a bulky ankle area and an unattractive posterior opening with conspicuous straps. The prosthesis is more durable, lighter, and less expensive than the historic prosthesis, and auxiliary suspension is unnecessary. Shock at heel-strike is reduced for more comfort during walking than with the historic prosthesis.

VETERANS ADMINISTRATION SYME PROSTHESIS (MEDIAL OPENING PLASTIC SYME PROSTHESIS)

The Veterans Administration Prosthetics Center (VAPC) in New York developed a prosthesis (Fig. 7-9) that differs from the Canadian Syme prosthesis. A removable medial panel, which does not extend to the proximal brim, replaced the posterior window.

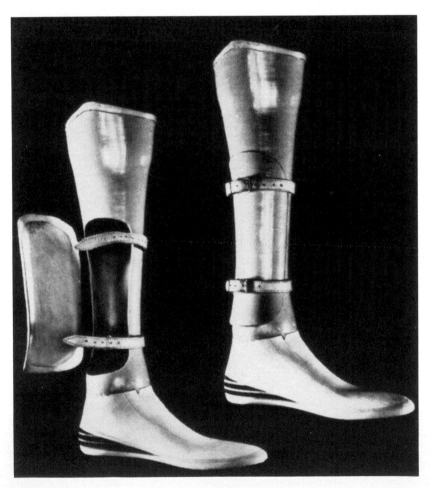

FIGURE 7-9. The Syme prosthesis developed at the Veterans Administration Prosthetics Center, New York. An opening in the medial wall allows donning of the prosthesis. Weight-bearing can be divided between the proximal and distal portions of the socket, as desired. (From Wilson, AB, Jr: *Prostheses for Syme's amputation*. Artificial Limbs 6:57, 1961, with permission.)

This modification enhances the mechanical strength of the prosthesis over the Canadian Syme prosthesis, although either type of opening weakens the structure. Because the medial opening does not extend to the proximal brim, the prosthesis can be designed so that some weight-bearing occurs along the proximal portions of the socket (which is similar to the patellar-tendon-bearing [PTB] socket), with pressure over the patellar tendon, medial tibial flare, and shaft of the fibula. The amount of proximal weight-bearing depends on the extent of the proximal trim lines during fabrication. Posteriorly there are reliefs for the hamstrings. The socket flares posteriorly at the proximal margin behind the knee. Adequate relief is made for the peroneal nerve just below the fibular head. The patient's knee is flexed about 10 degrees during casting, which is less than for a PTB socket. Thus, the Syme prosthesis is designed to enhance end weight-bearing rather than proximal weight-bearing. The socket extends slightly above the tibial plateau. Additional reliefs are made over the tibial tubercle and the entire tibial crest. Both posterior-opening and medial-opening prostheses can have sockets that extend proximally to include the tibial condyles. Shorter sockets would result in intolerable pressure along the tibia because of less surface area and less mediolateral stability because of a shorter lever arm.

SUSPENSION

The decrease in limb circumference proximal to the bulbous end makes suspension possible by virtue of the irregular contours of the socket itself. Other natural suspension can be obtained by the gastrocnemius muscle because the posterior part of the socket curves into the popliteal space. In exceptional cases, a femoral condyle strap may be used for auxiliary suspension.

FOOT

A prefabricated Syme foot is usually used.

ELASTIC-LINER SYME PROSTHESIS (CLOSED, EXPANDABLE-SOCKET SYME PROSTHESIS; MIAMI SYME PROSTHESIS; WINDOWLESS PROSTHESIS)

This prosthesis was developed at the University of Miami Prosthetic-Orthotic Laboratory in 1965. The elastic-liner Syme prosthesis (Fig. 7-10) is more cosmetic (without windows or straps) and stronger (without window openings) than the Canadian or VAPC Syme prostheses. The inner liner (socket), which is made of Silastic elastomer or pelite, extends proximally to a point where the diameter of the proximal leg equals the bulbous end of the leg distally. A space is created between the inner socket and the outer laminated polyester resin socket by using a wax buildup during fabrication (Fig. 7-11). Silastic elastomer foam is usually used to fill this space. This foam is compressed as the limb is pushed into the prosthesis during donning. The distal end of the liner is attached to the outer shell to prevent it from separating when the limb is withdrawn. Because of the cylindrical construction, it does not need an excessively thick laminate for requisite strength. It cannot be used when the bulbous end of the limb is larger than the proximal brim or is too large for a satisfactory cosmetic appearance of the cylindrical portion of the socket. This prosthesis was designed to accommodate the modified Syme limb, which is narrower distally because the malleoli have been trimmed. When

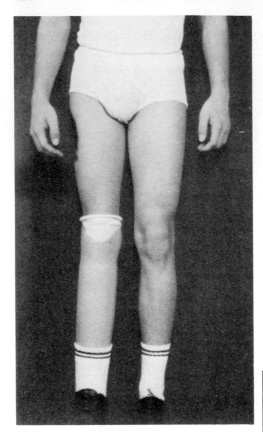

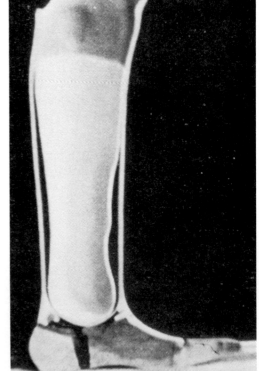

FIGURE 7-10. An elastic-liner Syme prosthesis. (From LeBlanc, MA: *Elastic-liner type of Syme prosthesis: Basic procedure and variations.* Artificial Limbs 15:22, 1971, with permission.)

FIGURE 7-11. A cutaway lateral view of an elastic-liner Syme prosthesis. The space between the inner elastomer socket and the outer shell of the socket allows entry of the stump without a window. (From LeBlanc, MA: *Elastic-liner type of Syme prosthesis: Basic procedure and variations.* Artificial Limbs 15:23, 1971, with permission.)

inserted into the prosthesis, the limb compresses the soft silicone foam rubber of the inner wall in the distal half of the prosthesis. Expansion of the silicone rubber after donning helps maintain total contact and suspension. This prosthesis, like the medial opening type, is easily modified for proximal weight-bearing.

SOCKET-FOOT JUNCTION FAILURE

Failure at the junction of the socket and the foot sometimes occurs in Syme prostheses. This is the weakest point in the prosthesis. A shearing force is created at push-off as the anterior section is compressed and the posterior section is tensioned. Reinforcement of the mechanical bond may be necessary to maintain socket-foot attachment in prostheses for Syme as well as Chopart or long below-knee amputations.

BIBLIOGRAPHY

ALLDREDGE, RH: *Indications for the Syme's amputation.* Surg Clin North Am 26:422–431, 1946.

ALLDREDGE, RH AND THOMPSON, TC: *Technique of Syme amputation.* J Bone Joint Surg 28:415–426, 1946.

BAKER, GCW AND STABLEFORTH, PG: *Syme's amputation: A review of sixty-seven cases.* J Bone Joint Surg 51B:482–487, 1969.

BOCCIUS, CS: *Standard Syme's prosthesis.* In *Syme's Amputations and Prosthesis.* Prosthetic Service, Department of Veterans Affairs, Canada, 1954, pp 14–18.

BOCCIUS, CS: *The plastic Syme prosthesis in Canada.* Artificial Limbs 6:86–89, 1961.

CANTY, TJ: *Amputations and recent developments in artificial limbs.* US Armed Forces Med J 3:1147–1152, 1952.

CARNES, EH: *Amputations, stumps and prostheses.* War Med 1:656–663, 1941.

CATTERALL, RCF: *Syme's amputation by Joseph Lister after sixty-six years.* J Bone Joint Surg 49B:144, 1967.

DALE, GM: *The Syme's amputation.* In *Syme's Amputation and Prosthesis.* Prosthetic Service, Department of Veterans Affairs, Canada, 1954, pp 6–13.

DALE, GM: *Syme's amputation for gangrene from peripheral vascular disease.* Artificial Limbs 6:44–51, 1961.

DANKMEYER, CH, JR, DOSHI, R, AND ALBAN, CR: *Adding strength to the Syme prosthesis.* Orthot Pros 28:3–7, 1974.

DANKMEYER, CH, JR, DOSHI, R, AND ALBAN, CR: *Adding strength to the Syme prostheses.* In *Selected Readings: A Review of Orthotics and Prosthetics.* The American Orthotic and Prosthetic Association, Washington, DC, 1980, pp 90–94.

DIVELEY, RL AND KIENE, RH: *An improved prosthesis for a Syme's amputation.* J Bone Joint Surg 38A:219–221, 1956.

EASTON, AL, REICHELT, AE, AND ITOH, M: *A modified Canadian type Syme's pylon.* J Am Phys Ther Assoc 43:452–453, 1963.

ECKHARDT, AL AND ENNEBERG, H: *The use of a Silastic liner in the Syme's prosthesis.* Inter-Clinic Info Bull 9:1–4, 1970.

FOORT, J: *The Canadian type Syme prosthesis (Series II, Issue 30)*. Lower-Extremity Amputee Research Project, Institute of Engineering Research, University of California, Berkeley, 1956.

GARDNER, HF: *A report of the checkout of the UC-Berkeley Syme prosthesis and fabrication manual*. Veterans Administration Prosthetics Center, New York, 1958.

GLADSTONE, H AND IULIUCCI, L: *Some American experiences with Syme prostheses*. Artificial Limbs 6:90–101, 1961.

GORDON, EJ AND ARDIZZONE, J: *Clinical experiences with the S.A.C.H. foot prosthesis*. J Bone Joint Surg 42A:226–234, 1960.

GRAHAM, WP, III, ET AL: *Transarticular joint amputations: The value of preserving articular cartilage*. J Surg Res 14:524–537, 1973.

HAIG, G: *Syme's amputation*. Injury 4:164, 1972.

HAMPTON, F: *Recent developments in the fitting and fabrication of the Syme's prosthesis*. Orthot Pros Appl J 14:45–57, 1960.

HAMPTON, F: *Suspension casting for below-knee, above-knee, and Syme's amputation*. Artificial Limbs 10:5–26, 1966.

HAMPTON, FL: *Prosthetic principles in the lower extremity amputee*. Orthop Clin North Am 3:339–347, 1972.

HANGER, HB: *The Syme and Chopart prostheses: A manual for prosthetists*. Northwestern University Medical School, Chicago.

HARDING, HE: *Knee disarticulation and Syme's amputation*. Ann R Coll Surg Engl 40:235–237, 1967.

HARRIS, RI: *Introduction*. In *Syme's Amputation and Prosthesis*. Prosthetic Service, Department of Veterans Affairs, Canada, 1954, pp 1–5.

HARRIS, RI: *Syme's amputation: Technical details essential for success*. J Bone Joint Surg 38B:614–632, 1956.

HARRIS, RI: *The history and development of Syme's amputation*. Artificial Limbs 6:4–43, 1961.

HARRIS, RI: *Syme's amputation: The technique essential to secure a satisfactory end-bearing stump, Part I*. Can J Surg, 6:456–469, 1963.

HARRIS, RI: *Syme's amputation: The technique essential to secure a satisfactory end-bearing stump, Part II*. Can J Surg, 7:53–63, 1964.

HINTERBUCHNER, C, SAKUMA, J, AND SATUREN, P: *Syme's amputation and prosthetic rehabilitation in focal scleroderma*. Arch Phys Med Rehabil 53:78–84, 1972.

HORNBY, R AND HARRIS, WR: *Syme's amputation: Follow-up study of weight-bearing in sixty-eight patients*. J Bone Joint Surg 57A:346–349, 1975.

HULNICK, A, HIGHSMITH, C, AND BOUTIN, FJ: *Amputations for failure in reconstructive surgery*. J Bone Joint Surg 31A:639–649, 1949.

IULIUCCI, L AND DEGAETANO, R: *VAPC technique for fabricating a plastic Syme prosthesis with medial opening*. Veterans Administration Prosthetics Center, New York, 1969.

JONES, RF: *Amputee rehabilitation: Basic principles in prosthetic assessment and fitting*. Med J Aust 2:290–293, 1977.

KAY, HW AND STAROS, A: *Plastic laminate Syme prosthesis*. Prosthetic Devices Study, New York University and Veterans Administration Prosthetic Center, New York, 1959.

LAMB, R: *Present evaluation of the Syme amputation*. Am J Surg 95:688–692, 1958.

LEBLANC, MA: *Elastic-liner type of Syme's prosthesis: Basic procedure and variations*. Artificial Limbs 15:22–26, 1971.

LEVY, SJ: *A case of Syme's amputation*. Proc Mine Med Off Assoc 46:57–58, 1966.

LINDQVIST, C AND RISKA, EB: *Results after amputations of Chopart, Pirogoff and Syme*. Acta Orthop Scand 36:344–345, 1965.

LINDQVIST, C AND RISKA, E: *Chopart, Pirogoff and Syme amputations: A survey of twenty-one cases.* Acta Orthop Scand 37:110–116, 1966.

MARX, HW: *An innovation in Syme's prosthetics.* Orthot Pros 23:131–138, 1969.

MAUCH, HA: *The development of artificial limbs for lower limbs.* Bull Prosthet Res 10–22:158–166, 1974.

MAZET, R, JR: *Syme's amputation: A follow-up study of fifty-one adults and thirty-two children.* J Bone Joint Surg 50A:1549–1563, 1968.

McCOLLOUGH, NC, III: *The dysvascular amputee.* Orthop Clin North Am 3:303–321, 1972.

McLAURIN, CA: *The Syme type prosthesis.* In MURDOCH, G (ED): *Prosthetic and Orthotic Practice.* Edward Arnold & Co, London, 1970, pp 125–137.

MERCER, W: *Syme's amputation.* J Bone Joint Surg 38B:611–612, 1956.

MEYER, LC, BAILEY, HL, AND FRIDDLE, D, JR: *An improved prosthesis for fitting the ankle-disarticulation amputee.* Inter-Clinic Info Bull 9:11–15, 1970.

MURDOCH, G: *Levels of amputation and limiting factors.* Ann R Coll Surg Engl 40:204–216, 1967.

MURDOCH, G: *Syme's amputation.* J R Coll Surg Edinb 21:15–30, 1976.

MURDOCH, G: *Amputation surgery in the lower extremity.* Prosthet Orthot Int 1:72–83, 1977.

OMER, GE AND POMERANTZ, GM: *Initial management of severe open injuries and traumatic amputations of the foot.* Arch Surg 105:696–698, 1972.

PAVOT, AP: *Ankle-disarticulation: A definitive type of amputation in adults.* Arch Phys Med Rehabil 54:307–310, 1973.

PHELPS, ME AND STANFORD, JW: *Fabricating an expandable inner-socket prosthesis.* Inter-Clinic Info Bull 11:7–10, 1971.

RADCLIFFE, CW: *The biomechanics of the Syme prosthesis.* Artificial Limbs 6:76–85, 1961.

RATLIFF, AHC: *Syme's amputation: Result after forty-four years—report of a case.* J Bone Joint Surg 49B:142–143, 1967.

RENTOUL, WW: *Syme's amputation.* J Bone Joint Surg 36B:672–673, 1954.

ROSENMAN, LD: *Syme amputation for ischemic disease in the foot.* Am J Surg 118:194–199, 1969.

SARMIENTO, A: *A modified surgical-prosthetic approach to the Syme's amputation: A follow-up report.* Clin Orthop 85:11–15, 1972.

SARMIENTO, A, GILMER, RE, JR, AND FINNIESTON, A: *A new surgical-prosthetic approach to the Syme's amputation: A preliminary report.* Artificial Limbs 10:52–55, 1966.

SHELSWELL, JH: *Syme's amputation.* J Bone Joint Surg 36B:507, 1954.

SHELSWELL, JH: *Syme's amputation.* Lancet 2:1296–1299, 1954.

SHEPLAN, L, LIEBERMAN, B, AND SARMIENTO, A: *Patellar tendon bearing prostheses: Value of routine x-ray studies.* South Med J 62:1223–1226, 1969.

SINCLAIR, WF: *Below the knee and Syme's amputation prosthesis.* Orthop Clin North Am 3:349–357, 1972.

SPITTLER, AW, BRENNAN, JJ, AND PAYNE, JW: *Syme amputation performed in two stages.* J Bone Joint Surg 36A:37–42, 1954.

SRINIVASAN, H: *Syme's amputation in insensitive feet: A review of twenty cases.* J Bone Joint Surg 55A:558–562, 1973.

STAROS, A: *The SACH (solid-ankle cushion-heel) foot.* Orth Pros Appl J 11:23–32, 1957.

SYME, J: *Amputation at the ankle joint.* Lon and Edin Mon J Med Sci 2:93–96, 1843.

SYME, J: *Amputation at the ankle joint.* Lon and Edin Mon J Med Sci 3:274, 1843.

SYME, J: *Amputation at the ankle joint.* Lon and Edin Mon J Med Sci 4:647–653, 1844.

SYME, J: *Amputation at the ankle joint*. Lon and Edin Mon J Med Sci 5:337–344, 1845.

SYME, J: *Amputation at the ankle*. Lon and Edin Mon J Med Sci 6:81–84, 1846.

SYME, J: *Mr. Syme on amputation at the ankle-joint*. Lancet 2:480–481, 1857.

THOMPSON, RG: *Amputation in the lower extremity*. J Bone Joint Surg 45A:1723–1734, 1963.

WAGNER, FW, JR: *Amputations of the foot and ankle*. Clin Orthop 122:62–69, 1977.

WARREN, R, ET AL: *The Syme amputation in peripheral arterial disease: A report of six cases*. Surgery 37:156–164, 1955.

WEIR, EA AND FOORT, J: *Plastic Syme's prosthesis*. In *Syme's Amputations and Prosthesis*. Prosthetic Service, Department of Veterans Affairs, Canada, 1954, pp 19–27.

WHITEFIELD, GA: *Syme's amputation*. In MURDOCH, G (ED): *Prosthetic and Orthotic Practice*. Edward Arnold & Co, London, 1970, pp 119–124.

WILDER, MJ: *Modified Syme Amputation*. Inter-Clinic Info Bull 4:6–15, 1965.

WILSON, AB, JR: *Prostheses for Syme's amputation*. Artificial Limbs 6:52–75, 1961.

WILSON, AB, JR: *Limb prosthetics: 1970*. Artificial Limbs 14:1–52, 1970.

WILSON, ABK: *Hand and foot prostheses*. Practitioner 201:759–766, 1968.

WILSON, PD: *The Syme amputation*. Surg Clin North Am 1:711–728, 1921.

WOOD, WL, ZLOTSKY, N, AND WESTIN, GW: *Congenital absence of the fibula: Treatment by Syme amputation—indications and techniques*. J Bone Joint Surg 47A:1159–1169, 1965.

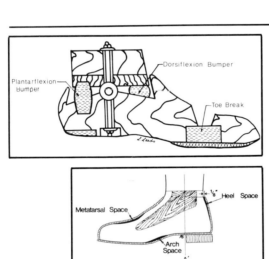

Dorsiflexion Bumper

Plantarflexion Bumper

Toe Break

Metatarsal Space

⅛" Heel Space

Arch Space

A′

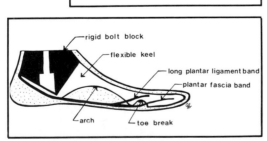

rigid bolt block

flexible keel

long plantar ligament band

plantar fascia band

arch

toe break

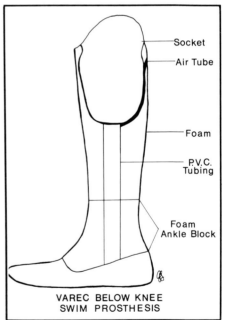

Socket

Air Tube

Foam

P.V.C. Tubing

Foam Ankle Block

VAREC BELOW KNEE
SWIM PROSTHESIS

ANKLE/FOOT MECHANISMS

The prosthetic foot is important for determining the forces that are transmitted to the socket-limb interface. The foot should be designed to absorb the plantarflexion and dorsiflexion forces at the ankle, the subtalar inversion and eversion forces, transverse rotation, and torque. All of these features are especially important if the amputee will be walking over uneven surfaces. The ankle/foot assembly should be durable and relatively simple in construction to minimize repairs and replacement. It should be comfortable, lightweight, and cosmetically acceptable.

Many different prosthetic ankle/foot assemblies have been designed. The nonarticulated, multiaxial solid-ankle–cushion-heel (SACH) foot is by far the most common prosthetic foot used in the world today. Variations of the SACH foot are being used primarily for cosmetic versatility. The single-axis wooden foot and the multiple-axis cable ankle are becoming obsolete; the hydraulic ankles are still largely experimental; the Greissinger foot is increasing in popularity; and the SAFE foot has yet to withstand the test of time.

SINGLE-AXIS ANKLE

The single-axis ankle joint allows no mediolateral or transverse movement (Fig. 8-1). Dorsiflexion (5 to 7 degrees) and plantarflexion (about 15 degrees) are limited by bumpers made of hard felt or rubber. During plantarflexion, the plantarflexion bumper, which is located behind the ankle axis, is compressed and hence offers resistance to the movement. The dorsiflexion bumper, which is slightly firmer than the plantarflexion bumper, resists dorsiflexion. Resistance to dorsiflexion or plantarflexion can be varied by using rubber bumpers of different densities. The good excursion permitted in plantarflexion provides increased knee stability. If properly "tuned," the single-axis foot offers as much function as the multiple-axis foot in ordinary activities.

ADVANTAGES

1. Allows foot-flat without much force on the heel to ensure knee stability (permits a greater range of plantarflexion and dorsiflexion than the SACH foot).
2. Can adjust plantarflexion and dorsiflexion.
3. Simpler to maintain than multiple-axis articulated assemblies.
4. More economical than multiple-axis articulated assemblies.

DISADVANTAGES

1. No mediolateral or transverse rotary motion of the foot; thus, torque forces are transmitted through the socket to the residual limb.
2. Moving parts wear and may become noisy.
3. Rubber bumpers wear, thus offering varying resistance and requiring adjustments and more maintenance than nonarticulated feet. If the rubber bumpers harden or wear, gait is affected.
4. Heavier than the SACH foot.
5. Less cosmetic than the SACH foot.

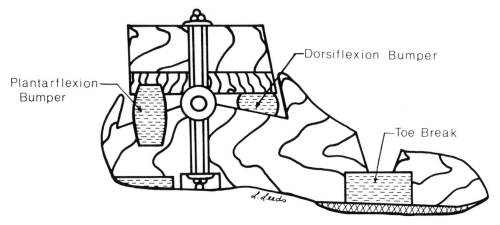

FIGURE 8-1. The historic wooden foot with a single-axis ankle and a toe break.

WOODEN FOOT (THE HISTORIC FOOT)

The wooden foot (see Fig. 8-1) usually has some type of flexible sole such as belting or felt. Recesses for bumpers are located at the toe break and at the ankle joint. The location and angle of the toe break varies. The toe break should be far enough forward for stability during stance, but far enough back to allow a smooth transition from stance to swing phase. This corresponds to the metatarsophalangeal joints of the normal foot. The toe break should be at right angles to the line of progression. The standard wooden foot usually has a single-axis ankle.

ADVANTAGES

1. Durable.
2. Easily installed and repaired.

DISADVANTAGES

1. Little shock absorption at heel-strike.
2. The toe break is in one plane, allowing little variation in gait.
3. Socks sometimes catch in the toe break and tear.

VARIATIONS OF THE WOODEN FOOT (COMPRESSIBLE HEELS AND TOES)

One variation of the wooden foot is the replacement of the wooden toe from the toe break forward with a compressible material such as rubber or felt (Fig. 8-2). The bottom of the foot from the toe break back may also be replaced with a compressible material (Fig. 8-3).

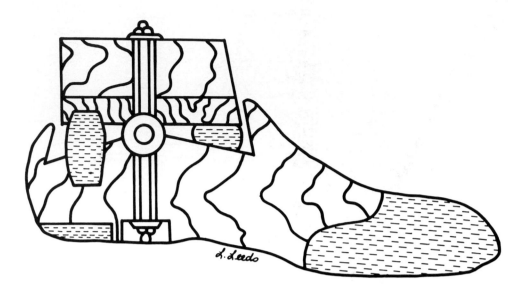

FIGURE 8-2. A variation of the wooden foot with a toe section of compressible rubber. The dorsiflexion rubber bumper is located anterior to the single-axis ankle. The plantarflexion bumper is located posterior to the single-axis ankle.

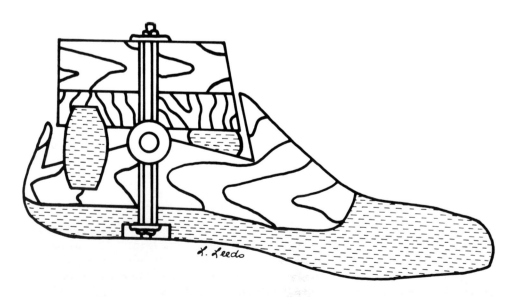

FIGURE 8-3. A variation of the wooden foot with compressible material along the entire bottom of the foot.

ADVANTAGES

1. It bends more naturally than a foot with a toe break because the amputee can roll onto the toe from various angles.
2. There is more shock absorption at heel-strike than with the wooden foot, which increases the comfort and durability of other parts of the prosthesis.

DISADVANTAGES

1. The rubber tends to increase the weight of the foot.
2. Felt tends to swell if it gets wet, which can damage the shoe.
3. Felt tends to curl.

MULTIPLE-AXIS (FUNCTIONAL) ANKLE

ARTICULATED ASSEMBLIES

ADVANTAGES

1. Mediolateral and torsional forces on the limb are reduced because some rotation is absorbed during walking.
2. Accommodates well to uneven ground.

DISADVANTAGES

1. Bulky.
2. Maintenance and adjustment are frequent; cable breakage is not unusual.
3. Noisy.
4. Heavier than single-axis or SACH foot.
5. Less cosmetic than single-axis or SACH foot.
6. Expensive.

CABLE

This ankle has a flexible cable that runs between the foot and shank through a large rubber block. Since there is no set axis of motion, movement occurs in any direction of plantarflexion and dorsiflexion, inversion, eversion, and some transverse rotation.

OTTO BOCK UNIVERSALLY MOVABLE GREISSINGER FOOT

The universally movable Greissinger foot (Fig. 8-4) offers lateral and rotary movements, which absorb the unevenness of the ground. A separate plantarflexion bumper allows the adjustment of plantarflexion resistance. The foot is made of light wood with a flexible, shock absorbent sole, and a toe and heel made of Pedilan, a permanently elastic plastic material. This foot can be used for above-knee or below-knee amputees. It is more cosmetic and lighter in weight, and it requires less maintenance than the cable ankle.

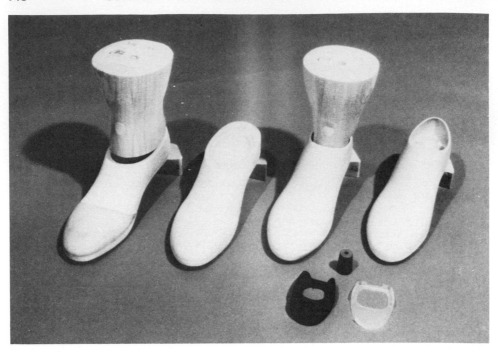

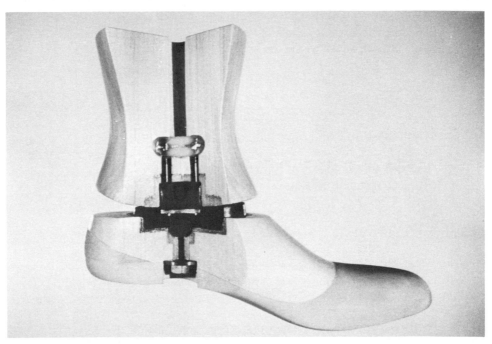

FIGURE 8-4. *(Top)* On the left is the Greissinger 1A6 foot, which has a full rocking rubber that comes in soft, medium, or hard density. It offers more range of motion and flexibility than the 1A12. On the right side is the Greissinger 1A12, which is more cosmetic than the 1A6 and comes in medium or hard rocking rubber used in conjunction with a hard or normal plantarflexion bumper. The Greissinger 1A12 can be used with the endoskeletal system in combination with the 2R11 modular ankle joint. *(Bottom)* A cutaway view of the Greissinger 1A6. (From Otto Bock Orthopedic Industry, Minneapolis, with permission.)

NONARTICULATED ASSEMBLIES

SOLID-ANKLE–CUSHION-HEEL (SACH) FOOT

The idea of a solid rubber foot is not new. The first rubber foot was patented in 1863. In 1952, a prosthetic foot with a neoprene crepe sole was developed at the Prosthetic Services Center of the Canadian Department of Veterans' Affairs for a Syme prosthesis. The first prototypes of the present version of the SACH foot were developed by James Foort and Charles W. Radcliffe at the University of California at Berkeley in the mid-1950s. It was released as a SACH foot in 1956. The SACH foot is used for most amputees, especially children and women.

The SACH foot (Fig. 8-5) does not have an articulated ankle joint; the ankle and foot are combined into one component. Shock absorption and ankle motion, like the normal ankle, are provided by the material and structure. The SACH foot differs from earlier attempts at a rubber foot in that it has a combination of a keel and an external cushioning material. The keel, made of hardwood or aluminum, is rigidly bolted to the shank.

At heel-strike, the molded heel wedge compresses to cushion the impact and simulate normal plantarflexion. From mid-stance to push-off, the shape and length of the wooden keel provide the smooth rocker motion and support. The flexible, high-density foam rubber sole and forefoot deform under pressure to provide resistance to toe extension during late stance phase and an overall cushion throughout stance phase. The toe section may be reinforced with nylon belting.

The SACH foot may have either an external or internal keel. The internal keel is covered by the high density foam on the dorsum of the foot and thus cannot be seen

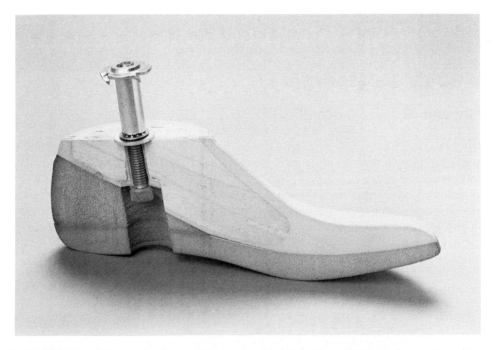

FIGURE 8-5. Cutaway of a solid-ankle–cushion-heel (SACH) foot. Note the molded heel wedge, wooden keel, and nylon belting extending into the anterior aspect of the keel.

from the outside. An external keel extends to the dorsum of the foot and is visible. The wooden external keel can be trimmed so that the lamination over the shank can be brought over the ankle onto the foot. This improves the appearance; however, the foot cannot be removed. The external keel is wider than the internal keel, which adds to the mediolateral stability.

With a conventional foot that has a soft plantarflexion bumper and a firm dorsiflexion bumper, the patient may experience a sudden change in resistance during the stance phase. This will not be true with the SACH foot.

FITTING

The amount of heel stiffness (soft, medium, or firm) selected for a particular amputee depends on the amputation level and the amputee's weight and activity level. The SACH foot allows some motion in all directions by compression of various parts of the foot.

A properly sized SACH foot should be selected to fit the shoe. If shaping the foot is necessary, material should be removed from the toe section rather than from the heel section. A minimal amount of rubber should be removed from the toe section because the resulting foot will have a disproportionately long keel and thus push-off will be hindered.

The final shape of the SACH foot and its fit in the shoe determine foot function. The foot should fit the shoe in both the uncompressed and the compressed states. The entire sole, except for the arch, should fit the shoe closely (Figs. 8-6, 8-7). The arch should provide at least 0.3 cm (⅛ in) clearance between the foot and the shoe's inner sole. If adequate clearance is not provided, motion will be restricted, resulting in shoe damage. There should also be a slight space above the metatarsal area of the foot to allow for material expansion during roll-over in the weight-bearing phase. A gap of at least 0.3 cm (⅛ in) should be present between the upper posterior part of the heel section of the foot and the top of the shoe. This space tapers posteriorly and inferiorly and terminates at the lower third of the heel to allow for heel wedge expansion during plantarflexion. The lower third of the SACH foot heel should fit snugly into the heel counter of the shoe. All other areas of the SACH foot should fit the shoe snugly.

ADVANTAGES

The SACH foot has no moving parts and thus requires virtually no maintenance. It has a better appearance than an articulated prosthetic foot, with no gap between the shank and the foot. It operates quietly even after long use and is light in weight. The SACH foot offers good cushioning of the shock at heel-strike and a smooth transition of weight from heel-strike to toe-off. The material has a good "memory" (returns to the original shape). It is able to withstand weather changes, particularly dampness. It offers more stability than the single-axis ankle on rough or uneven terrain because of the flexible heel.

DISADVANTAGES

Since plantarflexion and dorsiflexion adjustments are limited, initial correct selection and installation are necessary for desired function. Compression of the heel makes walking up an incline unstable. SACH feet must be used with caution with high bilateral amputees because of the rocker action caused by the compressible heel. Getting a

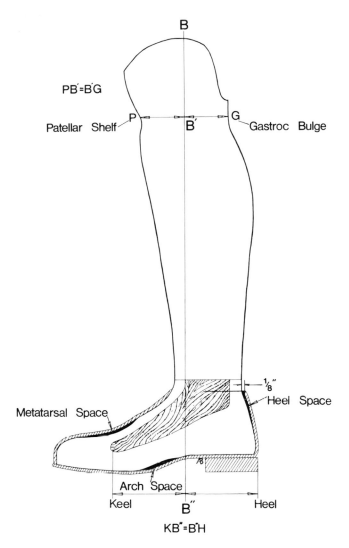

FIGURE 8-6. Alignment of a SACH foot to a patellar-tendon-bearing prosthesis. Note the fit of the SACH foot, in an uncompressed state, in the shoe.

sock over the foot is sometimes difficult, especially with an internal keel. In cases like this, a thin nylon sock may be left on the foot over which a second sock can be applied. Shoes of different heel heights require different prosthetic feet or prostheses with appropriate alignment. Gait will be adversely affected if the amputee changes heel heights with a single SACH foot. Excessive stress at the anterior end of the wooden keel may cause the formed foot to crack and the anterior end of the keel to protrude through the belting and rubber sole. The toe will curl or turn up excessively. The metal bolt may also erode the wooden keel if the foot is attached and detached very often. The material gradually loses elasticity. The SACH foot provides little absorption of torque during locomotion. If noise or clicking occurs, it usually means that the belting beneath the keel has loosened or become detached.

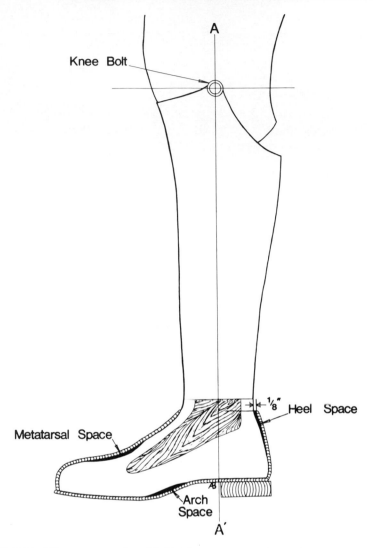

FIGURE 8-7. Alignment of a SACH foot to an above-knee prosthesis. Heel, arch, and metatarsal spaces are present between the foot and shoe in the uncompressed state.

VARIATIONS OF THE SACH FOOT

SYME FOOT

A standard SACH foot can be used for the Syme prosthesis. Because the Syme limb is about 8 cm (3 in) shorter than the contralateral intact limb, there is enough space for a modified SACH assembly. The SACH-foot keel, which is weakened by the removal of material to shorten the foot, needs to be reinforced with a hardwood base. A hole is drilled in the center of the wood to accommodate the foot attachment bolt. Fiberglass epoxy laminate running parallel to the keel is used to reinforce the keel-to-socket bond.

SACH feet made especially for Syme's prostheses are commercially available. They are designed for clearances as low as 2.5 cm (1 in). The heel wedges are thinner than on the standard SACH feet, and the keel is larger and wider for stability and durability. The stud bolt is reversed to prevent any potential irritation of the end of the long amputation limb.

SCULPTURED TOE SACH FOOT

This foot (Fig. 8-8) has a more natural appearance than the standard SACH foot and may be desirable if the amputee wears shoes in which the forefoot is exposed. It comes in various heel heights and firmnesses as well as shoe sizes.

HI-HEEL MALE MOLDED SACH FOOT

This foot was designed to be worn with high-heeled men's shoes and western boots.

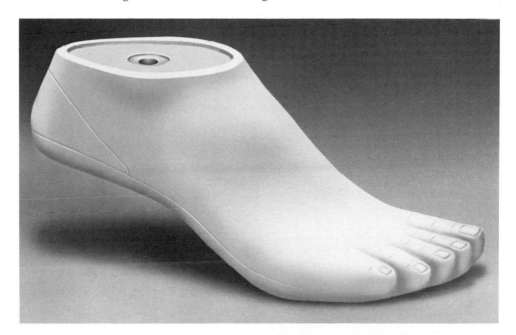

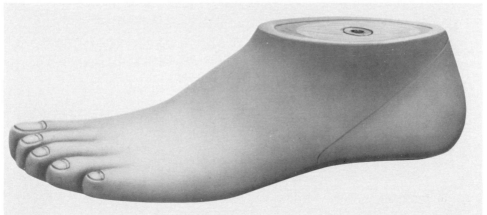

FIGURE 8-8. *(Top)* Sculptured toe ladies' SACH foot, "Fashion," for 45-mm heel shoes. *(Bottom)* "Low Profile" male SACH foot, for 18-mm heel shoes. **(From Kingsley Manufacturing, Costa Mesa, California, with permission.)**

POSTOPERATIVE FLAT-HEELED FOOT

This foot (Fig. 8-9, bottom) was originally designed for ambulation without a shoe following an immediate postoperative fitting of a prosthesis. It permits equal leg length while standing and walking without shoes or with flat-heeled shoes. The wide heel and extra-wide toe offer good lateral stability. The foot weighs about 20 percent less than a regular molded foot. Resistance to toe break is less than with the standard SACH foot. The foot is used for swimming and water skiing. It is also used with flat-heeled shoes such as tennis shoes.

LITEFOOT

This foot is lighter and softer than the regular SACH foot. It was originally designed for older amputees. It is suitable for early ambulation and for a definitive prosthesis.

VETERANS ADMINISTRATION/KINGSLEY "BEACHCOMBER" FOOT

A prosthetic foot is now commercially available for the fabrication of a swim prosthesis. The Veterans Administration Rehabilitation Engineering Center (VAREC) swim prosthesis can be fabricated for a below-knee amputee (Fig. 8-10), or for an above-knee amputee by using the Otto Bock plastic knee setup. In the below-knee prosthesis, a piece of

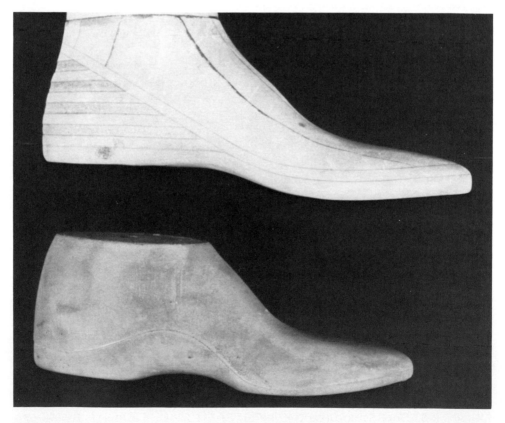

FIGURE 8-9. On the top is an old laminated-heel SACH foot, and on the bottom is a postoperative flat-heeled foot.

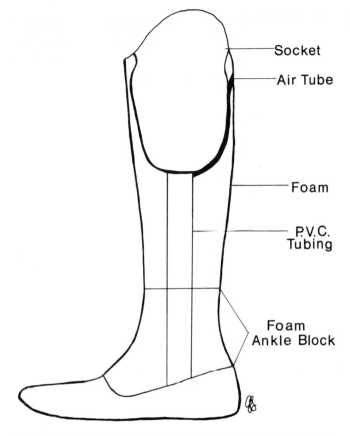

VAREC BELOW KNEE SWIM PROSTHESIS

FIGURE 8-10. The VAREC below knee swim prosthesis.

polyvinylchloride (PVC) tubing connects the socket to the foot. It is centered in the ankle block and extends proximally to the distal end of the socket. A smaller flexible tube is attached to the rigid PVC tube in the distal socket and runs proximally and posteriorly to exit at the posterior trim line of the socket. The flexible tube allows air to escape as water enters the large tube. The shank is made of foam and the prosthesis is laminated.

A two-position-lock ankle for a swim prosthesis was designed at the Veterans Administration Prosthetic Center (VAPC) and has been in use since 1978. The ankle is constructed of polypropylene and is thus waterproof and will not corrode in salt water. The Kingsley Syme foot can be attached to this ankle. The ankle locks at 90 degrees for walking and 120 degrees for swimming. The amputee is able to walk on the beach, stand with the prosthesis on to shower, and plantarflex the ankle to swim. A ring for activating the lock is located in the calf area (Fig. 8-11).

STATIONARY ATTACHMENT FLEXIBLE ENDOSKELETAL (SAFE) FOOT

The SAFE foot (Fig. 8-12) was designed to simulate the action of the human foot. It has a bolted attachment to the shin and a flexible keel. A soft foam cover encases the bolt block and the keel.

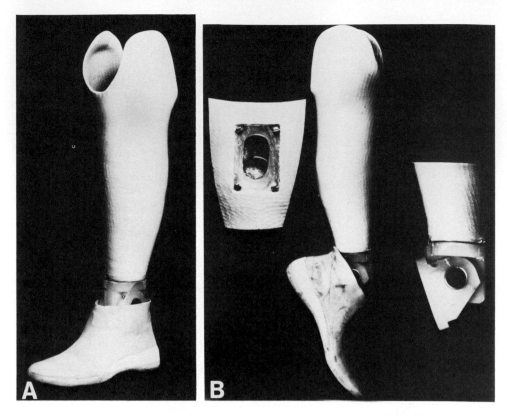

FIGURE 8-11. The VAPC swim/walk ankle. *(A)* Ankle in walk position. *(B)* On the left is the pull lever to adjust the ankle. In the center and on the right is the ankle in the swim position. (From Staros, A and Peizer, E: *Veterans Administration Prosthetics Center report.* Bull Prosthet Res 10–32:446, 1979, with permission.)

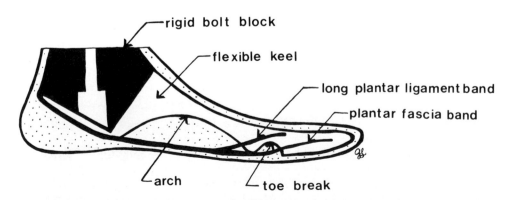

FIGURE 8-12. The stationary attachment flexible endoskeletal (SAFE) foot.

In the normal foot, flexibility is provided by ligaments, particularly the long plantar ligament and the plantar aponeurosis (plantar fascia). The arches are triangular shaped with the calcaneus proximally and the five metatarsal heads distally. If the feet are placed together, the arches form a geometrical dome. When separated, each foot is half of a dome. The half-dome provides the basic geometry for the SAFE foot.

In the normal foot, the plantar fascia, which attaches distal to the metatarsophalangeal joints, becomes tense as the foot moves from heel-rise to toe-off and the toes extend. The tension on the plantar fascia helps convert the foot into a semirigid lever. This has been called the "windlass effect" of the plantar fascia. The SAFE foot has a toe break that corresponds to that of the normal foot and a plantar fascial strap that crosses the toe break and the arch with a fixed attachment to the heel area of the foot. As the heel rises, the strap tightens to create a semirigid toe lever for a smooth transition to toe-off. The flexible keel allows the SAFE foot to adapt to irregular surfaces better than other nonarticulated prosthetic feet.

A long plantar ligament band spans the arch to stabilize the foot when the wearer stands. The toe break is carved on the plantar surface of the foot. The anterior surface of the bolt block is cut at a 50-degree angle and is rounded to provide a subtalar-like surface. The SAFE foot is made entirely of plastic and has no mechanical joints.

Plantarflexion is provided by the soft heel and by some relative motion of the bolt block to the rest of the foot. Very slight dorsiflexion can be achieved by this relative motion. Twisting of the flexible keel in the shoe permits some transverse rotation. A smooth roll-over to toe-off is provided by the gradual tightening of the plantar fascial band.

AXIAL ROTATION DEVICE

Rotation occurs at the hip, knee, and ankle during normal walking. When wearing an above-knee quadrilateral socket, the amputee actively extends the hip on the amputated side at the instant of heel contact on the amputated side to assure prosthetic knee stability. This generates an external rotation torque about the long axis of the socket. With no axial rotation device to relieve the external rotation of the socket, the residual limb tends to rotate internally within a fixed socket. Conversely, just prior to toe-off, the amputee flexes the hip to initiate knee flexion, which generates an internal rotation torque about the long axis of the socket.

Axial rotation devices (Fig. 8-13) were designed to simulate normal skeletal rotation in the lower extremity prosthesis. The rotator allows the socket to respond to the demands of the residual limb and rotate independently of the foot position through the entire stance phase from heel-strike through toe-off. The rotator functions to reduce the magnitude and abruptness of torque and shear forces at the residual limb and socket interface (Fig. 8-14), thus reducing the possibility of skin abrasions as well as reducing fatigue and improving function. This is especially necessary when prosthetic components such as side joints with a thigh-lacer or a hip joint with a pelvic band limit rotation at functioning anatomic joints. Without a means of transverse rotation either at the foot or in the shank, the amputee will need to alter gait.

A rotator can be used with above-knee and below-knee prostheses, modular systems, and conventional wood setups. It allows the amputee to perform rotational movements associated with sports such as golf or activities such as dancing. Also, kneeling is easier because the foot will rotate in relation to the floor when the rotator is located below the knee joint. Good suspension is especially necessary for the below-knee

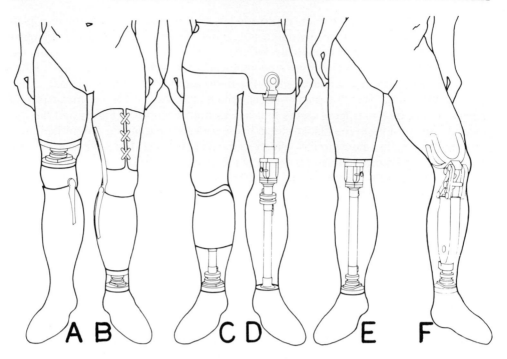

FIGURE 8-13. *(A)* Conventional above-knee prosthesis with a rotator installed above the knee. *(B)* Conventional below-knee prosthesis with a rotator installed directly on the SACH foot. *(C)* Modular below-knee system with a rotator installed directly on the SACH foot. *(D)* Hip disarticulation prosthesis with a rotator installed distal to the knee module. *(E)* Above-knee modular system with a rotator installed directly on the SACH foot. *(F)* OHC four-bar-linkage prosthesis with a rotator installed directly on the SACH foot. (From United States Manufacturing Company, Pasadena, California, with permission.)

amputee to compensate for the additional weight. Cuff suspension may allow too much movement; therefore, supracondylar brim suspension is usually preferred. A rotator that is light in weight is most desirable.

ADVANTAGES

1. Movement feels more natural and comfortable.
2. Gait appears more symmetrical and natural.
3. Less possibility of skin abrasions (reduced frequency of sebaceous cysts).
4. More rotation mobility for activities such as working at a counter or participating in sports.

DISADVANTAGES

1. Added weight.
2. May require a better suspension device to accommodate the added weight.

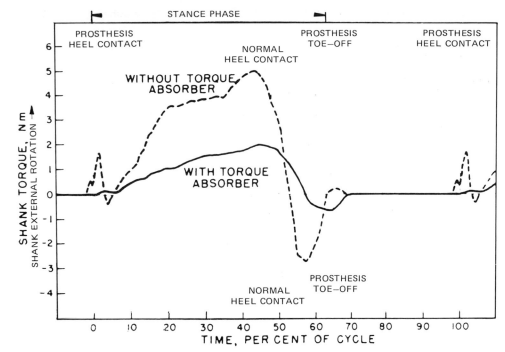

FIGURE 8-14. A comparison of axial torques occurring in an above-knee prosthesis with and without an axial rotation unit in operation. (From Racette, W and Breakey, JW: *Clinical experience and functional considerations of axial rotators for the amputee.* Orthotics and Prosthetics 31:31, 1977, with permission.)

3. Additional maintenance.
4. May compromise stability, especially in the bilateral amputee.

BIBLIOGRAPHY

BARCLAY, W: *Below-knee amputation-prosthesis.* In MURDOCH, G (ED): *Prosthetic and Orthotic Practice.* Edward Arnold & Co, London, 1970, pp 69–78.

CAMBELL, JW AND CHILDS, CW: *The S.A.F.E. foot.* Orthot Pros 34:3–16, 1980.

CONDIE, DN: *Ankle/foot mechanisms.* In MURDOCH, G (ED): *Prosthetic and Orthotic Practice.* Edward Arnold & Co, London, 1970, pp 89–103.

DOANE, NE AND HOLT, LE: *A comparison of the SACH and single axis foot in the gait of unilateral below-knee amputees.* Prosthet Orthot Int 7:33–36, 1983.

FLEER, B AND WILSON, AB, JR: *Construction of the patellar-tendon-bearing below-knee prosthesis.* Artificial Limbs 6:25–73, 1962.

GORDON, EJ AND ARDIZZONE, J: *Clinical experiences with the S.A.C.H. foot prosthesis.* J Bone Joint Surg 42A:226–234, 1969.

GORDON, E AND MUELLER, CF: *Clinical experiences with the SACH foot.* Orth Pros Appl J 13:71–74, 1959.

HAMPTON, FL: *Above-knee prostheses.* Orthop Clin North Am 3:359–372, 1972.

IULIUCCI, L AND DEGAETANO, R: *VAPC Technique for Fabricating a Plastic Syme Prosthesis with*

Medial Opening: Fabrication Manual. Veterans Administration Prosthetic Center, New York, 1969.

KAY, HW AND NEWMAN, JD: *Report of a workshop on below-knee and above-knee prosthetics.* Orthot Pros 27:9–25, 1973.

LAMOUREUX, LW AND RADCLIFFE, CW: *Functional analysis of the UC-BL shank axial rotation device.* Prosthet Orthot Int 1:114–118, 1977.

PIERCE, JN, WALKER, SW, AND MATTHEWS, JG: *The swimming prosthesis.* Inter-Clinic Info Bull 17:1–4, 1978.

RACETTE, W AND BREAKEY, JW: *Clinical experience and functional considerations of axial rotators for the amputee.* Orth Pros 31:29–33, 1977.

RADCLIFFE, CW AND FOORT, J: *The Patellar-Tendon-Bearing Below-Knee Prosthesis.* Biomechanics Laboratory, University of California, San Francisco-Berkeley, 1961.

STAROS, A AND PEIZER, E: *Veterans Administration Prosthetics Center report.* Bull Prosthet Res 10–32:444–446, 1979.

TINDALL, GA AND NITSCHKE, RO: *The ROL rotator.* Orthot Pros 33:11–15, 1979.

WILSON, AB, JR: *A report on the SACH foot.* Orth Pros Appl J 14:67–72, 1960.

WILSON, AB, JR: *Recent advances in above-knee prosthetics.* Artificial Limbs 12:1–27, 1968.

WILSON, ABK: *Hand and foot prostheses.* Practitioner 201:759–766, 1968.

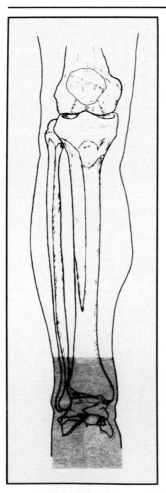
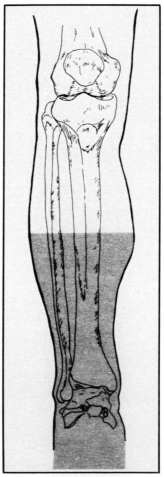
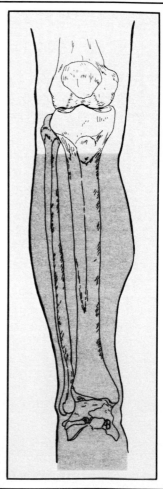

CHAPTER 9

BELOW KNEE (BK) (LEG [LEG], PARTIAL)

BRIM
WALL
MEDIAL AND LATERAL SOCKET
BRIM
WALL
NON–WEIGHT-BEARING (RELIEF) AREAS
INTERFACE: HARD (UNLINED) AND SOFT (LINED) SOCKETS
  HARD SOCKET
  SOFT INSERT SOCKET

ULTRALIGHT BELOW-KNEE PROSTHESIS
SOCKET
SHANK-FOOT SECTION
SOLE AND HEEL CUSHION
ADVANTAGES
DISADVANTAGES

BENT-KNEE PROSTHESIS

SUSPENSION MECHANISMS
THIGH-LACER (CORSET)
  ADVANTAGES
  DISADVANTAGES
  CHECK-STRAP
  CORSET WITH ISCHIAL SUPPORT
CUFF SUSPENSION STRAP, SUPRACONDYLAR CUFF

ADVANTAGES
DISADVANTAGES

FORK, JACK, OR INVERTED Y STRAP TO A WAIST BELT
ADVANTAGES
DISADVANTAGES

SOCKET BRIM SUSPENSION
SUPRACONDYLAR/SUPRA-PATELLAR (SC/SP) SUSPENSION PROSTHESIS (PTS)
  ADVANTAGES
  DISADVANTAGES
SUPRACONDYLAR (SC) WEDGE SUSPENSION
  ADVANTAGES
  DISADVANTAGES
SUPRACONDYLAR WEDGE METHODS
  LOCATION
  TYPES
    HARD OR SOFT
    INFLATABLE WEDGE
    DETACHABLE (REMOVABLE) MEDIAL BRIM

MOLDED RUBBER SLEEVE SUSPENSION
ADVANTAGE
DISADVANTAGES

SUPRAPATELLAR STRAP

AMPUTATION LEVELS

LONG BK (LEG [LEG], PARTIAL [LOWER $^1/_3$])
STANDARD BK (LEG [LEG], PARTIAL [MIDDLE $^1/_3$]
  [MID-LEG AMPUTATION])
SHORT BK (LEG [LEG], PARTIAL [UPPER $^1/_3$]
  [LESS THAN 5-CM (2-IN) RESIDUAL LIMB])

A below-knee amputation is indicated as an initial procedure for gangrene that has spread beyond the metatarsal area and shows no tendency to demarcate, that extensively involves the heel, that has spread above the ankle, or when the spreading gangrene is accompanied by an uncontrollable infection of the foot. Below-knee amputations are also performed in cases where transmetatarsal or other foot amputations have failed and the necrosis is spreading to and beyond the ankle. Successful mid-leg amputations have been done in the presence of extensive necrosis of the musculature below the knee.

SURGICAL PROCEDURES

For a long time, it was accepted that amputation through the middle third of the leg, giving a residual limb at 12.7 to 17.8 cm (5 to 7 in) below the knee joint, was the best site for a below-knee amputation. The reasons given were that short residual limbs less than 5 cm (2 in) long were prosthetically undesirable and amputations in the lower third resulted in a lower healing rate owing to relatively poor circulation. Also, since the knee is set into flexion in the prosthesis, a long residual limb would protrude posteriorly. Augusto Sarmiento and others more recently have argued that the below-knee limb should be as long as possible to achieve better prosthetic control during walking and less "popping out" of the prosthesis while sitting. This does not mean that the other levels are never indicated. Short below-knee limbs are preferable to the above-knee level if the insertion of the patellar tendon can be retained or re-established. Long below-knee limbs are preferred and indicated if circulation and soft tissue are adequate.

ANTERIOR-POSTERIOR FLAP TECHNIQUE

Because the skin over the posterior leg has a better blood supply than that over the anterior leg, a long posterior flap is usually used. The anterior skin flap is cut at approximately the level of anticipated section of the tibia. The posterior flap is 13 to 15 cm (5 to 6 in) longer to ensure adequate coverage without undue tension (Fig. 9-1). Dissection is carried down through the deep fascia to the bone. The periosteum is incised and stripped on the tibia proximally for 2.5 cm (1 in). The muscles are divided. Blood vessels are ligated and divided. Nerves are severed high with a sharp scalpel. Large nerves may be ligated. The tibia and fibula are sectioned. The tibia is beveled at 45 degrees to 60 degrees over the anterodistal aspect. Care is taken to avoid rough bony areas or a long bevel. The posterior muscle mass is beveled to allow the flap to come forward (Fig. 9-2). The posterior muscle mass is sutured anteriorly to the deep fascia of the anterolateral muscle group and to the periosteum that is reflected over the anterior aspect of the tibia. The skin is brought forward and sutured. The resulting anterior scar usually presents no problem to limb fitting.

MEDIAL-LATERAL FLAP TECHNIQUE

A sagittal technique for below-knee amputation that utilizes large equal medial and lateral musculocutaneous flaps was described by Herbert Robb, Lyle Jacobson, and Prescott Jordan in 1965, and by G.D. Tracy in 1966. The tibia is tapered at a 45-degree angle anteriorly. Muscle and intermuscular septa are sutured over the end of the bone.

The potential advantages of the medial-lateral flap technique over the more commonly used posterior flap technique include: (1) with two symmetrical flaps, the skin can be cut at a level more proximal to the area of ischemia or infection for a given bone length; (2) the ratio of flap length to width is less, and thus the risk of flap necrosis should be less; (3) the skin-cut readily exposes the tibia for division; (4) spontaneous drainage without pocket formation is more likely; and (5) the amputation limb does not have wrinkles or dog-ears from the beginning. A total-contact socket can be used successfully if the scar is not adherent.

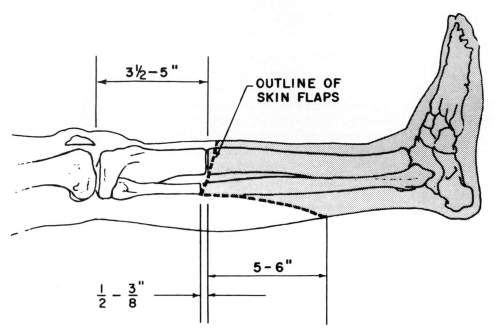

FIGURE 9-1. Below-knee amputation with a long posterior flap. The fibula has been sectioned shorter than the tibia. (From Burgess, EM: *The below-knee amputation.* Inter-Clinic Information Bulletin 8:4, 1969, with permission.)

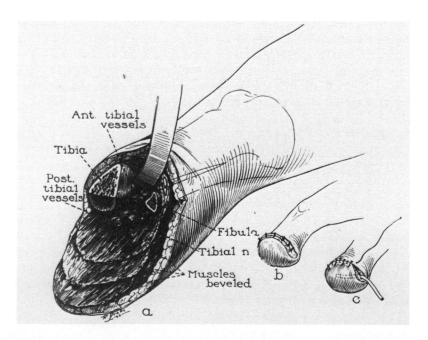

FIGURE 9-2. *(a)* The posterior muscles are beveled and ready for closure. *(b)* Closure without a drain. *(c)* Closure with a drain. (From Bickel, WH: *Amputations below the knee in occlusive arterial disease.* Surg Clin North Am 23:988, 1943, with permission.)

OPERATIVE OPTIONS

MYODESIS

Myodesis is accomplished by drilling holes in the tibia about 1 cm (³/₈ in) proximal to the distal end of the tibia. Sutures are passed through the anterior and posterior muscle groups and are fixed to the tibia by being tied within the marrow cavity. Myodesis is not usually performed in the below-knee amputation for vascular disease because the encircling sutures carry the risk of local muscle constriction and the muscle-to-bone sutures require additional operative handling of tissues.

OSTEOPLASTY

In the normal leg, the tibia and fibula are connected to one another by proximal and distal syndesmoses. After a below-knee amputation, the bones are abnormally mobile. Bier and Ertl developed procedures to stabilize the bone ends.

BIER'S OSTEOPLASTIC PROCEDURE

In 1893, August Bier recommended an osteoplastic procedure in which cortical bone with attached periosteum is used to cover the cut end of the bone to make the distal end of the limb less sensitive and capable of more weight-bearing. Weight-bearing through the long axis of the bone is necessary to avoid degenerative changes such as sclerosis and narrowing of the joint spaces. Also, changes in mineral metabolism cause osteoporosis, which can result in tenderness and spontaneous pain. The problems encountered with this procedure are lack of bony union, sclerosis of the plate, and prolonged healing time.

ERTL'S OSTEOPLASTIC PROCEDURE

The idea of covering the cut end of the bone with osteogenic material was continued by J. Ertl. His procedure, described in 1949, utilizes three periosteal flaps, two from the tibia and one from the fibula. Two small periosteal flaps (the fibular one being the shorter) with flakes of cortical bone attached are chiseled from opposite surfaces of the tibia and fibula and are sutured together (Fig. 9-3A). The larger third flap is cut from the anteromedial surface of the tibia and is brought across the distal surfaces of the tibia and fibula. It is sutured to the other flaps and the periosteum of the bones, thus forming a bridge between the tibia and fibula (Fig. 9-3B). This method eliminates the exposed cut surface of the bone, provides an insensitive surface that can bear partial weight, prevents rotation and lateral deviation of the fibula by the biceps femoris, restores the normal intramedullary pressure and deep venous return by occlusion of the tibial and fibular medullary cavities, and provides a protective wall for the cut ends of nerves and vessels in the interosseous space.

MYOPLASTY

MONDRY MYOPLASTIC PROCEDURE

When the muscles of amputated limbs no longer have their distal attachment, atrophy results. The muscle pump, which is an aid to venous return, is lost, causing stasis,

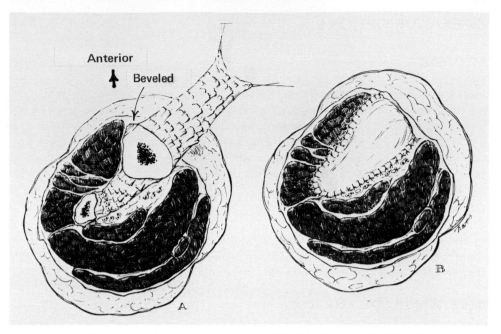

FIGURE 9-3. Ertl's osteoplastic procedure. *(A)* The shorter fibular flap and the tibial flap from the opposing surface are sutured together. The anterior crest of the tibia is beveled. The two bones are sectioned at the same level after the periosteal flaps with flakes of cortical bone have been chiseled free. *(B)* The larger tiblal flap, which is cut from the anteromedial surface, is brought across the cut ends of the bone to cover the distal surface. By suturing the third flap to the other flaps and the periosteum of the bones, a tube-like bridge is formed between the tibia and fibula. (From Loon, HE: *Below-knee amputation surgery.* Artificial Limbs 6:90, 1962, with permission.)

edema, lowered temperature, and pain in the amputation limb. Dr. Felix Mondry, in 1952, described a method of restoring the physiologic effects of muscle in the amputation limb by suturing together the flexors and extensors, including the musculature of the fibula, over the osteoperiosteal bridge and to the tibial periosteum. The residual limb is stronger due to the new attachment and better circulation. In many cases, the muscles are able to hold a total-contact prosthesis by contraction alone. The cut nerves are embedded in muscle. The end of the limb is rounded and the skin is smooth. Negative results are usually due to muscle sutures that do not hold or secondary infection.

OSTEOMYOPLASTY

Osteomyoplasty, which is a combined procedure, is recommended for elimination of hypersensitivity of the distal limb. This allows a close-fitting socket over the full length, which reduces the mechanical irritation caused by a loose-fitting socket. The best results are obtained when the two bones are transected at the same level approximately horizontal to the ground. A slant will result in vertical shearing forces.

Good circulation is maintained to deep as well as to superficial tissues. Because the bones are protected by a bone bridge and are used for axial weight-bearing through the entire length, they are not subjected to avascular necrosis of the distal end, as with the conventional amputation. Hypertrophy of the cortex with an increase in the overall diameter of the fibula (usually not a weight-bearing bone) results. Distal contact and weight-bearing result in improved proprioception, which improves prosthetic use.

LESS THAN 5-CM (2-IN) RESIDUAL LIMB

The main objections to having a residual limb shorter than 5 cm (2 in) were less area for force distribution, greater tendency to form a contracture, and difficulty in maintaining the limb in the socket. Successful prosthetic management is now possible provided that some distal weight-bearing is obtained. At high levels, the cut surface of the tibia is insensitive because the cancellous bone at this level heals with a solid bony cover. The choice of what to do with the fibular head becomes critical. If it is removed, the limb becomes conical, which results in excessive rotation inside the socket. With no treatment, the biceps pulls the fibula into abduction and rotates the head. An osteoplastic procedure can be used to anchor the fibula in a very short limb.

MANAGEMENT OF THE TIBIA AND FIBULA

Because it is close to the surface of the skin, the tibia is always beveled anteriorly. The fibula, which is normally not a weight-bearing bone, is managed in a variety of ways:

1. *Complete excision:* Complete excision is usually recommended in very short limbs because the biceps tendon tends to rotate and laterally deviate the fibula and because the protuberance of the fibular head is subjected to pressure by the prosthesis. This procedure has the advantage of exposing the lateral tibial flare to accommodate some of the weight-bearing.
2. *Section about 1 cm (³/₈ in) above the tibia:* This is usually recommended for limbs of average length.
3. *Section the same length as the tibia:* This is necessary in order to obtain the best results when using the osteoplastic procedure. It is claimed that if the fibula is amputated at the same level as the tibia, a conical limb is avoided and the rotational force is lessened, a wider area of sensory feedback is provided, and the end-bearing quality of the limb is improved.

ADVANTAGES OF BELOW-KNEE AMPUTATION AS OPPOSED TO THIGH AMPUTATION

A below-knee amputation offers several major advantages over an above-knee amputation: (1) Mortality is lower; the operative mortality with thigh amputations has decreased significantly with the advent of antibiotics, but it continues to exceed that for below-knee amputations. (2) There is a much better prospect of prosthetic rehabilitation even with bilateral below-knee amputations. (3) Persistent phantom limb and pain seem to be more common after thigh amputations.

PROSTHESES

HISTORIC BELOW-KNEE PROSTHESIS

The historic below-knee prosthesis consists of a leather thigh corset (lacer), metal side-bars with joints, and an open-ended socket (Fig. 9-4). The older sockets were usually carved out of wood. Weight-bearing is carried on the residual limb (with little or none on the anterior aspect) and through the suspension mechanism (thigh corset). The thigh

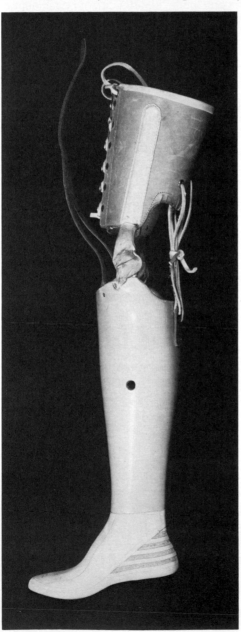

FIGURE 9-4. Historic below-knee prosthesis with leather thigh corset, metal sidebars and joints (covered with leather), a check-strap posteriorly, an inverted Y strap anteriorly, and a SACH foot.

corset transmits weight to the shank via the sidebars and knee joints, thus reducing the unit pressure on the distal limb. The mechanical knee joint has a single axis of rotation, whereas the anatomic knee joint has a polycentric axis that changes instantaneously as the knee is flexed and extended. The mechanical and anatomic axes are incongruent as the knee flexes and extends, resulting in relative motion between the amputee's limb and the socket and thigh corset. This motion is minimized if the mechanical axis is at its optimum location, which is usually above the axis of the extended knee (closer to the axis of the flexed knee). Such joint placement allows the limb to pull out of the socket somewhat during sitting.

ADVANTAGES

1. The thigh corset supports some of the weight-bearing load, thus reducing the unit pressure on the distal limb.
2. The prosthesis prevents hyperextension at the knee.
3. The prosthesis provides medial-lateral stability to the knee.
4. The socket is cooler than the PTB prosthesis because of lack of total contact.

DISADVANTAGES

1. Edema may develop easily in the distal limb because of the lack of total contact distally and the constrictive corset proximally.
2. The prosthesis is bulky and heavy.
3. It is uncosmetic.
4. The corset tends to produce atrophy of the thigh muscles.
5. Relative motion occurs between the amputee's limb and the socket/corset, causing irritation.
6. The knee hinge breaks frequently.
7. The skin tends to stretch over the end of the limb, resulting in ischemia and skin breakdown.
8. The open-ended socket accentuates weight-bearing on the thigh-lacer and proximal residual limb.
9. Normally appearing gait is not possible because of the restricting artificial knee.
10. The thigh-lacer is more expensive than cuff suspension.

SLIP SOCKET

The slip socket is an insert socket in the top portion of the shank, designed to minimize relative motion between the socket and skin, thus reducing chafing. The socket is either elastically suspended from the sidebars or is attached to the shank by a compression spring (Fig. 9-5). The socket is connected to the shank so that it can rotate and piston up and down, while at the same time allowing the amputee's own knee to activate the shank of the prosthesis. Fixed sockets are used for most amputees. The slip socket is usually used only for those people with short or tender residual limbs.

Advantages:
1. The amputee with a skin graft on the residual limb can ambulate early.
2. It preserves the knee joint.

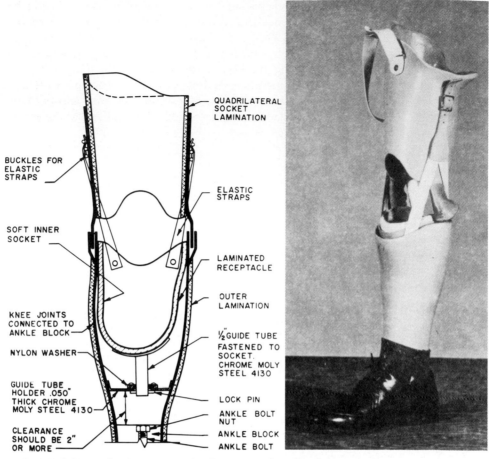

FIGURE 9-5. *(Left)* **A schematic diagram of a slip-socket below-knee prosthesis.** *(Right)* **The permanent prosthesis. (From Bochman, D and Thomson, HG:** *The slip-socket prosthesis for juveniles: A new clinical application.* **Inter-Clinic Information Bulletin 8:4–5, 1969, with permission.)**

Disadvantages:
1. The slip socket is uncosmetic.
2. It is fragile.
3. It is bulky and heavy.
4. The corset tends to produce atrophy of the thigh muscles.
5. There is excessive wear and tear of clothing.
6. Gait appearance is compromised (walk more like an above-knee amputee).

PATELLAR-TENDON-BEARING (PTB) PROSTHESIS

The PTB prosthesis was developed at the University of California and was introduced in 1959 (Figs. 9-6, 9-7). This prosthesis provides a more intimate fit and more efficient distribution of pressure than the historic below-knee prosthesis. Mediolateral knee stability is provided by the amputee's own knee. By aligning the foot more medially under

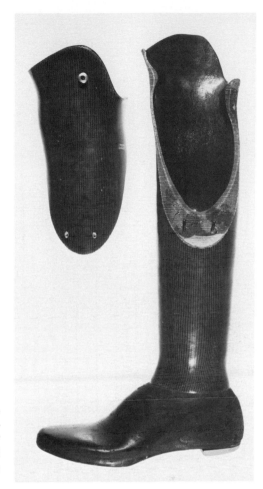

FIGURE 9-6. A patellar-tendon-bearing (PTB) prosthesis. The proximal cutaway exposes the patellar tendon bulge on the anterior socket wall and the gastroc, or popliteal, bulge on the posterior socket wall.

the socket, a narrower gait during stance phase is obtained and weight-bearing on the medial tibial flare is enhanced.

ADVANTAGES

1. The total-contact design:
   - improves circulation
   - helps prevent edema
   - provides a greater area over which to distribute the weight-bearing load
   - provides better proprioception (sensory feedback) and, hopefully, better control.
2. The prosthesis weighs less than a thigh corset (although a corset can be used with the PTB socket).
3. Allows more freedom of movement than with a thigh corset. Natural unrestricted use of the knee is possible.
4. Thigh muscles usually get larger because of the muscular activity required to control the PTB prosthesis (if a corset is not used with the PTB prosthesis).
5. Inset foot offers a more cosmetic gait than the historic below-knee prosthesis.
6. Gait looks essentially normal except for a lack of push-off.

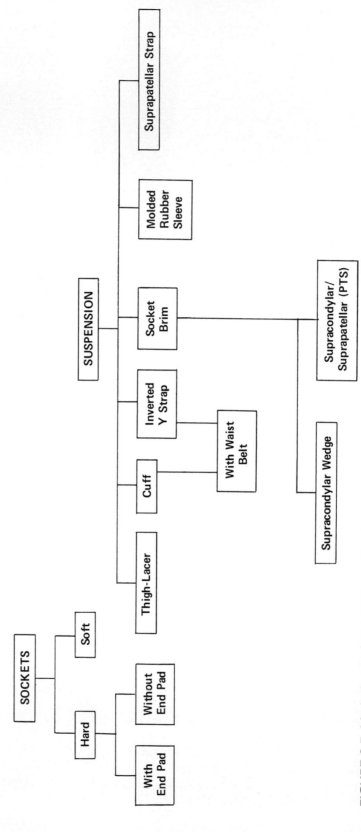

FIGURE 9-7. Variations of the PTB prosthesis.

7. More cosmetic than the historic prosthesis.
8. Easier to don and remove than the historic below-knee prosthesis if thigh-lacer is not used for suspension.
9. Requires less time for fabrication than the historic below-knee prosthesis.

DISADVANTAGES

1. Requires a more critical fit than the historic below-knee prosthesis and therefore more skill on the part of the prosthetist.
2. Excessive perspiration, especially during the summer, may result from the total-contact plastic socket but is less of a problem with a supracondylar cuff than with a thigh corset.
3. Requires stability of the anatomic knee.
4. The PTB prosthesis remodels the limb because of the intimate fit and causes shrinkage of the residual limb, thus requiring frequent observation and evaluation by the therapist during the first year.
5. Inset of foot can be a problem initially to amputees who have previously relied on the lateral stability provided by the corset and uprights.
6. There is a tendency for the amputee to hyperextend the knee and to spend too much time on the heel of the prosthesis while standing if a corset and uprights were previously worn.
7. Frequent readjustments may be necessary because of the change in shape of the residual limb.

The most common errors in the fabrication of the PTB prosthesis are not providing total contact in the distal end of the socket and making the proximal brim either too loose or too tight.

SHANK

The shank of the prosthesis connects the ankle/foot assembly with the socket in a specific alignment. The shank is usually made of wood with an exterior finish of plastic laminate that is colored appropriately. The outer surface of the shank is shaped to the contours of the sound limb. The shank may also be made with a foam center and outer plastic laminate covering or metal.

SOCKET

The socket of molded plastic laminate is aligned with the knee in a flexed position to enhance utility of the patellar tendon and tibial flares as weight-bearing surfaces. The socket, a total-contact design, offers a more intimate fit than the historic below-knee socket. The distal end of the socket is closed, providing just enough pressure to better control edema and to provide sensory feedback through a greater area of contact.

WEIGHT-BEARING AREAS

Because various areas of the residual limb tolerate pressure differently, the tissues are selectively loaded so that the most weight is borne on the pressure-tolerant areas and less weight is on the pressure-sensitive areas (Fig. 9-8). This is accomplished by reliefs over the pressure-sensitive areas and inward contours over the pressure-tolerant areas.

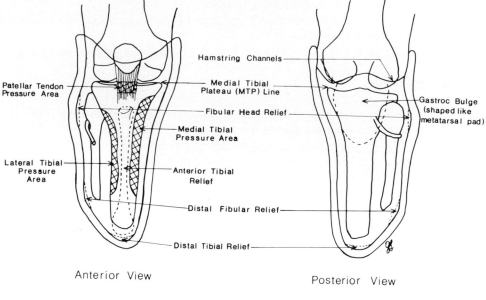

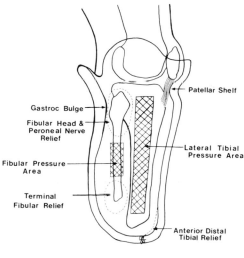

Anterior View

Posterior View

Lateral View

FIGURE 9-8. Pressure and relief areas for the PTB prosthesis.

Patellar Tendon

The socket wall has a bulge between the inferior border of the patella and the insertion of the patellar tendon on the tibial tubercle (Fig. 9-9). This places initial tension on the tendon and permits the tendon to assume a larger vertical load. The socket is set in 5-degree to 8-degree initial flexion, which enhances both the vertical aspect of load-bearing and the initial tension on the quadriceps.

Flares of the Tibia

The flares of the tibia are covered by tissue that is capable of weight-bearing. The medial flare offers more weight-bearing area because the head of the fibula blocks part of the lateral tibial flare. The proximity of the head of the fibula, the sharp tibial crest,

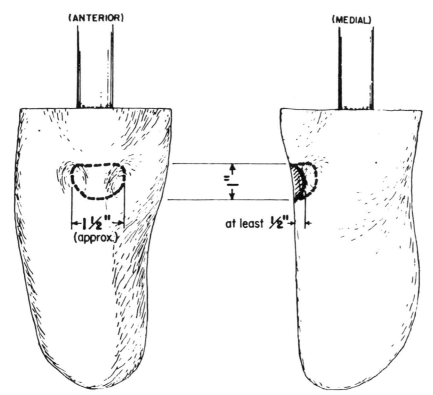

(ANTERIOR)

(MEDIAL)

←1 ½"→
(approx.)

at least ½"→

FIGURE 9-9. Modification of the positive plaster model to enhance support on the patellar tendon. (From Fleer, B and Wilson, AB, Jr: *Construction of the patellar-tendon-bearing below-knee prosthesis.* Artificial Limbs 6:29, 1962, with permission.)

and the rough tibial tubercle make fitting critical. The area over the atrophied anterior tibialis (anterolateral) can tolerate a considerable load without causing the patient discomfort.

Distal End of the Limb

Weight-bearing is possible in short residual limbs where amputation is through cancellous bone and in cases where there is a bone bridge between the distal ends of the tibia and fibula. Weight-bearing at the distal end is minimal in other below-knee limbs.

POSTERIOR SOCKET

Brim

The optimum level for the posterior brim is the popliteal crease (higher for very short limbs). It must be low enough to avoid constriction during sitting and yet high enough to prevent undue bulging of flesh over the brim. The posterior brim is generally 0.6 to 1.3 cm (¼ to ½ in) higher than the patellar tendon shelf. Grooves or cutouts are necessary for the hamstring tendons during flexion because they insert below this level. Since the semitendinosus muscle inserts more distally on the tibia than the biceps femoris on the fibula, the medial groove is deeper than the lateral. The proximal aspect of the posterior wall is flared away from the limb. For very short limbs, the posterior brim may be so high that flexion is limited to 60 degrees.

Wall

The posterior wall bulges inwardly slightly to push the limb anteriorly and maintain it on the patellar shelf (Fig. 9-10). This provides a counterforce for the patellar shelf to prevent the limb from sliding downward and backward. This counterforce must be applied over as great an area as possible because of the location of nerves and vessels in the popliteal area. When the socket is set in flexion, the need for counterpressure by the posterior wall (gastroc, or popliteal, bulge) is reduced, so there is less risk of pressure over the vessels and nerves in the popliteal area.

ANTERIOR SOCKET

Brim

The anterior brim comes to the midpatellar level.

Wall

A horizontal bulge, the patellar tendon bar or shelf, is provided at the midpoint of the patellar tendon (halfway between the inferior aspect of the patella and the tibial tuber-

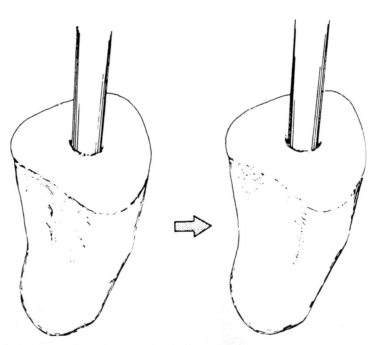

FIGURE 9-10. Modification of the positive model by shaving away plaster in the popliteal area to provide a counterpressure against anterior pressure, thus maintaining anteroposterior stability of the socket. (From Fleer, B and Wilson, AB, Jr: *Construction of the patellar-tendon-bearing below-knee prosthesis.* Artificial Limbs 6:30, 1962, with permission.)

cle) to produce tension on the patellar tendon. Weight is also borne over the medial tibial flare and, to a lesser extent, over the lateral tibial flare (Fig. 9-11). Reliefs are provided over the crest of the tibia, the anterior distal aspect of the tibia, and the lateral tibial condyle. Weight-bearing is influenced by the amount of initial flexion built into the socket. The anterior socket wall is somewhat wedge shaped, depending upon the prominence of the crest of the tibia, the tibial tubercle, and the distal end of the tibia, as well as atrophy of the pretibial muscle group (Fig. 9-12).

MEDIAL AND LATERAL SOCKET

Brim

The medial and lateral brims come to about the level of the proximal edge of the patella, which is higher than the historic below-knee prosthesis. The proximal aspects

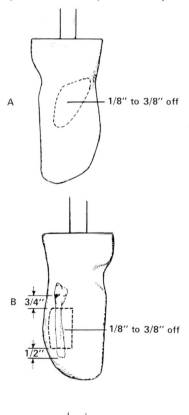

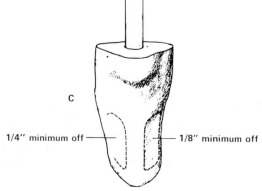

FIGURE 9-11. Modification of the positive model to enhance support on the: *(A)* medial tibial flare; *(B)* shaft of the fibula; and *(C)* antero-medial and anterolateral tibia. (From Fleer, B and Wilson, AB, Jr: *Construction of the patellar-tendon-bearing below-knee prosthesis.* Artificial Limbs 6:30, 1962, with permission.)

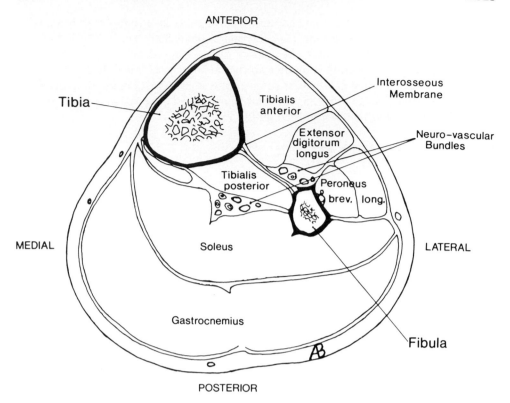

FIGURE 9-12. A cross section of a right below-knee limb. Note the wedge shape anteriorly.

of the medial and lateral walls support the femoral condyles and are usually 6.5 cm (2½ in) above the medial tibial plateau (MTP) in height. This assists in providing some mediolateral stability to the knee joint.

Wall

The lateral wall provides firm pressure over the middle and distal parts of the limb. A relief is provided over the head of the fibula and the distal end of the cut fibula (Fig. 9-13). The areas of weight-bearing are located over the mid-portion of the fibula shaft and the anterolateral aspect of the tibia. Care must be taken not to compromise the peroneal nerve. The medial wall provides a weight-bearing area over the flare of the medial tibial condyle.

NON-WEIGHT-BEARING (RELIEF) AREAS

The tibial crest, the lateral aspect of the distal end of the fibula, and the anterior aspect of the distal end of the tibia cannot tolerate much compressive stress because of the high unit pressures. The head of the fibula cannot tolerate significant pressure because of the sharp bony prominence and the location of the common peroneal nerve, which passes on the lateral side below the head. (See Figs. 9-8 and 9-13.) These concave areas of the socket are flared gently to avoid sudden pressure changes.

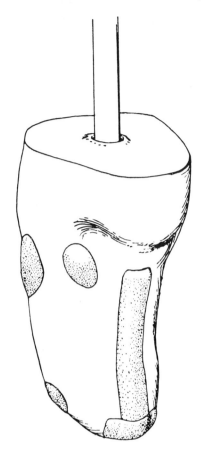

FIGURE 9-13. Buildup of the positive model to provide relief in pressure-sensitive areas. (From Fleer, B and Wilson, AB, Jr: *Construction of the patellar-tendon-bearing below-knee prosthesis.* **Artificial Limbs 6:31, 1962, with permission.)**

INTERFACE: HARD (UNLINED) AND SOFT (LINED) SOCKETS

Soft liners do not add considerably to the comfort of a properly fitting socket. They may, however, offset a fitting inaccuracy or inadequate relief over sensitive areas. The hard socket is clean and maintenance-free and thus provides a more cosmetic appearance and reduced financial costs. Hard socket is really a misnomer since the amputee wears a resilient sock with it.

Hard Socket

The hard socket may or may not have a distal pad (see Fig. 9-7). Air space should be filled with foam to ensure total contact. A soft end pad should be formed in place rather than carved after the socket has been made. A Silastic foam or silicone rubber distal pad is the type used for most amputees.

Advantages:
1. Less problem with perspiration.
2. Easy to clean.
3. Less bulk at knee than with insert type.
4. Modify by grinding or use liner insert.
5. Permits the employment of a porous socket wall when needed.

6. Fabrication time is less.
7. The soft end assures total contact temporarily.
8. The foam end is easier to make than the liner.
9. More intimate fit than with an insert.

Disadvantages:
1. More difficult to fit to bony or sensitive limbs than the lined socket.
2. Requires more skill in fabrication. All reliefs must be feathered into the mold so that there is a smooth transition from pressure-bearing to pressure-relief areas.
3. Less adjustability.

Soft Insert Socket

Soft inserts are used between the hard socket and the limb to accommodate minor incongruities between the limb and the socket or inadvertent irregularities in the socket. If a liner is to be used, it must be formed over the modified plaster positive of the limb before the socket is prepared.

The Kemblo (rubber) insert with a leather liner is made of horsehide and sponge rubber. The leather is fitted to the model with the smooth side in, for eventual contact with the skin (Fig. 9-14). A disc of sponge rubber (Kemblo) is used to form the distal end pad of the socket. Layers of Kemblo are then put along the sides of the model so that the

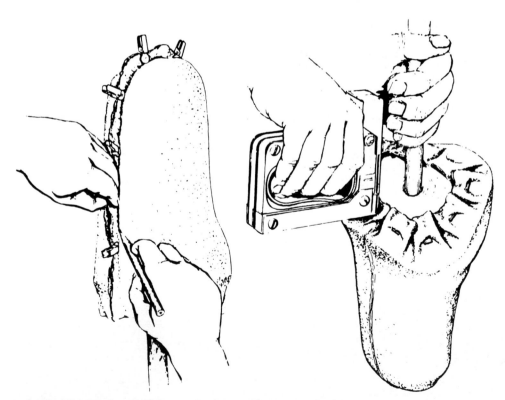

FIGURE 9-14. Preparation of the leather insert socket liner. (From Fleer, B and Wilson, AB, Jr: *Construction of the patellar-tendon-bearing below-knee prosthesis.* Artificial Limbs 6:33, 1962, with permission.)

leather will be backed through its entirety by the soft sponge rubber. Pelite is a material that has more recently been utilized for socket liners.

Advantages:
1. Less difficult to fit than a hard socket with or without a soft end pad.
2. Possible added comfort to improperly fitted socket owing to soft weight-bearing surface, which may relieve excessive unit pressure.
3. Adjustments of fit can be made more easily.
4. Can make donning easier if the residual limb is bulbous.

Disadvantages:
1. It is hot. Perspiration wets the sock, resulting in skin abrasions.
2. Perspiration causes a deterioration of the leather, especially in a humid climate. Modifications are required earlier than with a hard socket because weight is shifted to areas that cannot tolerate weight-bearing.
3. Poor hygiene owing to retention of perspiration in insert.
4. Additional bulk at the knee.
5. More weight.
6. Some sacrifice of stability.

ULTRALIGHT BELOW-KNEE PROSTHESIS

Dr. Joseph Barredo, a physicist and traumatic below-knee amputee, in cooperation with the US Naval Hospital, Philadelphia, developed a completely crustacean PTB-type prosthesis that weighs less than half of the conventional below-knee prosthesis. An ultralight prosthesis functions like the PTB prosthesis but weighs much less, which makes suspension less of a problem and thus reduces the degree of pistoning. The prosthesis is comprised of a socket, a shank-foot section, and a sole and heel cushion (Fig. 9-15). Although it may appear at first that the endoskeletal design would be lighter than the exoskeletal design, actually the exoskeletal type can be much lighter in weight while providing the same strength. The outer structure is farther from the axis and thus has a longer lever arm.

SOCKET

To make the socket, polypropylene is vacuum-formed over a positive model of the residual limb. The socket is then attached to an adjustable leg, and the prosthesis is aligned.

SHANK-FOOT SECTION

A form of the shank is made with a curved foam filler based on the alignment determined dynamically and statically. A single sheet of polypropylene is used to mold the shank-foot section over the foam filler.

SOLE AND HEEL CUSHION

A sole and heel cushion like that used with any SACH foot can be used for the ultralight prosthesis.

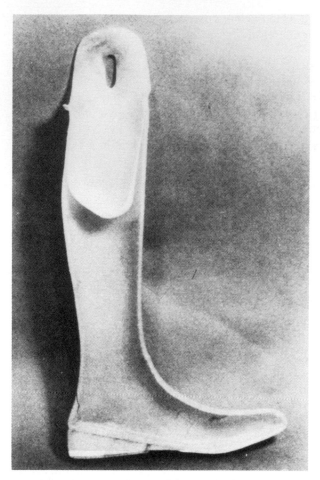

FIGURE 9-15. A cross section of the ultralight below-knee prosthesis made of polypropylene. (From Wilson, AB, Jr, Pritham, C, and Stills, M: *Manual for an Ultralight Below-Knee Prosthesis*, p. 4. Moss Rehabilitation Hospital, Temple University, Philadelphia, with permission.)

The ultralight prosthesis is difficult to modify. The use of a rigid toe section often results in structural failure at the foot. Although waterproof, the presence of buoyancy causes a problem during swimming.

ADVANTAGES

1. Requires less energy to walk.
2. Less pistoning than with conventional PTB prosthesis.
3. Can be worn in and around water.

DISADVANTAGES

1. Frequent structural failure at the foot if a rigid toe section is used (not durable).
2. Difficult to modify.
3. Jarring at heel-strike and difficulty in rolling over the foot if the foot is too rigid.

BENT-KNEE PROSTHESIS

The bent-knee prosthesis is perhaps the only prosthetic device that has remained essentially unchanged since the beginning of recorded medical history. It is indicated in cases of irreducible knee flexion contractures for which surgical revision is contraindicated.

A plaster negative is made of the entire limb from well up on the lower third of the femur with the knee joint in maximum extension. The socket is molded from a plaster positive. The lining is of horsehide with a layer of rubber between it and the firm leather socket. The socket is incorporated into the thigh corset. External knee joints connect the socket to the shank. Weight is borne through the remaining portion of the tibia, the patellar tendon, and the thigh cuff (Fig. 9-16). The prosthesis is durable and relatively cheap.

The amputee who uses the bent-knee prosthesis has no more control over or sense of position of the shank than a person with an end-bearing knee disarticulation amputation. Even if a modified below-knee prosthesis is required because of poor skin condition, limited weight-bearing capabilities, or limited knee function, it is preferable to a bent-knee prosthesis.

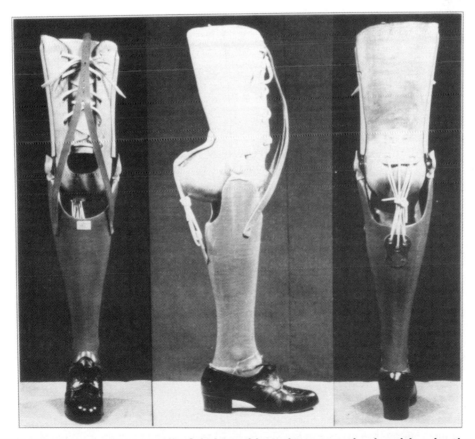

FIGURE 9-16. A commercially fabricated bent-knee prosthesis with a leather thigh cuff. (From Record, EE: *Surgical amputation in the geriatric patient.* J Bone Joint Surg 45A:1746, 1963, with permission.)

SUSPENSION MECHANISMS

THIGH-LACER (CORSET)

The leather thigh-lacer is attached by sidebars, with hinged joints at the knee, to the socket and shank (see Figs. 9-4 and 9-7). This is the usual suspension method of the historic below-knee prosthesis, but it may be used with the PTB prosthesis if there is either extreme mediolateral ligamentous instability about the amputee's knee or muscular weakness. In addition to prosthesis suspension during the swing phase, the thigh corset supports part of the body weight during the stance phase. Since the human knee joint is not a simple, single-axis joint like the prosthetic knee joint, relative motion takes place between the residual limb and the prosthesis. This may cause skin chaffing or irritation as well as popliteal pressure while sitting. The residual limb is forced out of the socket to some extent during sitting because the prosthetic joints are located proximal to the anatomic knee axis.

ADVANTAGES

1. The thigh corset provides mediolateral stability at the knee.
2. Supports part of the body weight during the stance phase.
3. Prevents hyperextension at the knee.
4. Easy to adjust.

DISADVANTAGES

1. The thigh corset is uncosmetic.
2. Relative motion takes place between the residual limb and the prosthesis owing to knee axis location.
3. The thigh corset can constrict, causing edema and retarded healing.
4. The thigh corset can cause atrophy of the thigh muscles.
5. Heat dissipation is difficult during hot weather.
6. The knee hinge is subject to breakage.
7. The leather absorbs perspiration, which eventually results in an odor.
8. The leather becomes deformed under load.
9. Donning and removal of the prosthesis are slow.
10. It is heavier than other suspension methods.
11. It limits knee rotation.
12. It is bulky, causing excessive wear on clothing.

CHECK-STRAP

A check-strap, usually a continuous thong of leather or nylon, extends from the posterior aspect of the thigh corset to the shank. Its purpose is to check the motion of extension at the knee as the shank moves forward, thus preventing abrupt and noisy contact by the metal hinge joints. It is not used with the PTB prosthesis.

CORSET WITH ISCHIAL SUPPORT

Sidebars and a corset with ischial support may be indicated when there are impairments of the bone or joint that will not permit full weight-bearing loads or when the skin cannot tolerate weight-bearing. The ischial support can be either an ischial ring or the usually more successful quadrilateral ischial weight-bearing thigh socket.

CUFF SUSPENSION STRAP, SUPRACONDYLAR CUFF

The supracondylar cuff or strap is attached via studs to the proximal part of the socket in the posteromedial and posterolateral areas (Fig. 9-17). It encircles the thigh just above the femoral condyles and patella. It suspends the prosthesis during swing phase and checks against hyperextension of the knee joint during stance phase. When properly fitted, it holds the prosthesis on over the patella, and not circumferentially around the supracondylar aspect of the thigh. This method is adequate for most amputees. On occasion, a waist strap may be attached to the supracondylar strap for auxiliary suspension.

ADVANTAGES

1. Allows full use of the thigh muscles so atrophy does not occur.
2. Does not have an artificial knee axis and thus does not create relative motion between the residual limb and the socket.

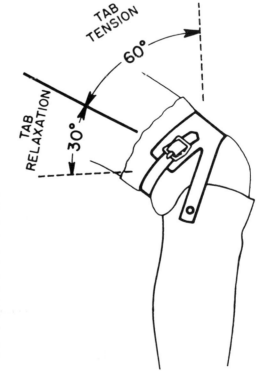

FIGURE 9-17. The side-tabs of the cuff suspension strap are positioned so that tension is provided in complete extension and through 60 degrees of flexion in the swing phase, while comfort is provided by relaxation of the tabs through an additional 30 degrees to give comfortable sitting at 90 degrees. (From Fleer, B and Wilson, AB, Jr: Construction of the patellar-tendon-bearing below-knee prosthesis. Artificial Limbs 6:45, 1962, with permission.)

3. Makes donning and removal of the prosthesis easier than with the thigh-lacer.
4. Adjustable to variations in thigh circumference.
5. Helps check hyperextension at the knee joint.
6. Lightweight; not as bulky as the thigh-lacer.
7. More cosmetic than the thigh-lacer.

DISADVANTAGES

1. Does not give mediolateral knee stability.
2. May be contraindicated for obese or extremely muscular patients because it is more restrictive than the supracondylar suspension sockets when the knee is flexed, which can cause pinching between the posterior superior socket and cuff.
3. The leather absorbs perspiration, which eventually results in odor.
4. Positioning of studs is critical.
5. Uncosmetic when sitting (the cuff's contours show through clothing).

FORK, JACK, OR INVERTED Y STRAP TO A WAIST BELT

This type of suspension is sometimes used to suspend the PTB prosthesis of a dysvascular amputee when circumferential constriction by the cuff supracondylar strap needs to be avoided. It may also be used along with a thigh corset or cuff for extra suspension. The fork strap attaches to the shank of the prosthesis (see Fig. 9-4). An elastic strap connects the fork strap to the light web waist belt. When the hip is extended and the knee is flexed during walking, the fork strap is under tension and acts to extend the knee and bring the shank forward. The fork strap slips over the knee during sitting to prevent excessive extension forces.

A variation of the inverted Y strap is the "D" ring suspension, which attaches to four points on the medial and lateral aspects of the socket via two straps that pass through a D ring. The straps slide on the D ring during walking, which reduces movement at the limb/socket interface.

ADVANTAGES

1. Can loosen or remove supracondylar strap.
2. Good auxiliary suspension aid when other types are inadequate.

DISADVANTAGES

1. Difficult to don under clothing.
2. Belt can be uncomfortable.
3. Uneven suspension through swing phase.
4. Uncosmetic.
5. Difficult to keep clean.
6. Needs frequent repair.

SOCKET BRIM SUSPENSION

SUPRACONDYLAR/SUPRAPATELLAR (SC/SP) SUSPENSION PROSTHESIS (PTS*)

The name PTS was derived from the initials of the original name, prosthèse-tibiale-supracondylienne, given by Guy Fajal of France, who developed it about 1963. The proximal brim of the PTS provides suspension by extending over the patella and a major portion of the femoral condyles (Fig. 9-18). It provides better medial-lateral stability than the PTB prosthesis. The patellar tendon shelf is less pronounced in the PTS than in the PTB, and the posterior brim is slightly higher. The supracondylar/suprapatellar prosthesis was developed in the United States for two groups of below-knee amputees who were not candidates for the PTB prosthesis: those with short limbs (<7.5 cm

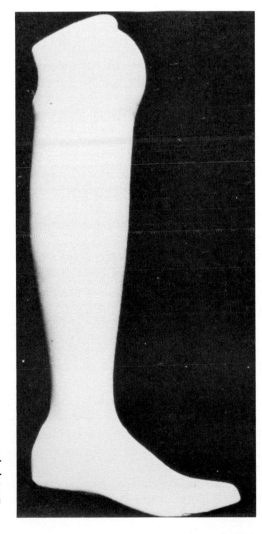

FIGURE 9-18. The PTB socket with supracondylar/suprapatellar (SC/SP) suspension. (From Stewart, RE: *Variants of the PTB (patellar-tendon-bearing) below-knee prosthesis.* **Bull Prosthet Res 10–13:129, 1970, with permission.)**

---

*In recent years in the United States and Canada, the term PTS has come to denote all PTB prostheses with high medial and lateral walls.

[3 in]) and those with knee instability due to ligamentous or muscular dysfunction. These patients would otherwise have received an auxiliary suspension such as a thigh corset.

ADVANTAGES

1. Less restrictive to circulation than the cuff.
2. Provides more medial-lateral stability at the knee than the cuff.
3. Easier to don than the removable wedge type.
4. Provides knee extension control (prevents genu recurvatum during stance phase without utilizing external components).
5. More cosmetic than the thigh corset.
6. Less maintenance and lower repair costs than suspension devices with straps, cuffs, corsets, or belts.
7. Larger areas of support; therefore, less unit pressure.

DISADVANTAGES

1. Patella enclosure may inhibit extreme knee flexion, thus inhibiting comfortable kneeling; the knee may pop out of the socket while kneeling.
2. The prosthesis may have a tendency to slip down when the knee is flexed 90 degrees and beyond, as the leg is lifted.
3. Difficult to get good suspension on an extremely obese limb.
4. Heavier than the PTB prosthesis, with a lower proximal trim line.
5. Cannot be used with a very long residual limb.

SUPRACONDYLAR (SC) WEDGE SUSPENSION

The concept of achieving suspension by placing a wedge above the medial femoral condyle between the stump and the socket (the Kondylenbettung Münster (KBM) Prosthese developed by Dr. Götz-Gerd Kühn) was brought to the United States from Münster, West Germany, by Carlton Fillauer in 1967. A wedge would not be necessary if the proximal walls of the prosthesis were flexible enough to allow donning by spreading them apart. It offers more medial-lateral stability than the ordinary PTB prosthesis by virtue of the higher medial and lateral brims.

ADVANTAGES

1. Less circulation restriction than the cuff.
2. Provides more medial-lateral stability at the knee than the cuff.
3. Less knee-flexion restriction and better suspension than with the cuff.
4. Functions better than cuff suspension for fitting shorter limbs.
5. The stump sock does not tend to wrinkle around the patella, as with the cuff suspension.
6. Suspension is as good in flexion as in extension.
7. More cosmetic than the cuff suspension.

DISADVANTAGES

1. Requires precision in positioning of the wedge and in construction of the wedge seat.

2. Some amputees require adjustment to the wedge.
3. May initially be difficult to don.
4. Difficult to use on short, obese limbs.

SUPRACONDYLAR WEDGE METHODS

Location

The wedge can be located between the insert and the socket, between the limb and the socket if an insert is not used, or it can be attached to the insert. Although a wedge can be located medially, laterally, or above the patella, the medial wedge is by far the most common. The medial wedge covers the medial aspect of the femoral condyle from just posterior to the patella to the posterior part of the femoral condyle (Fig. 9-19). The thicker part is placed just proximal to the medial femoral condyle (Fig. 9-20). The proximal brim of the medial wall has an indentation to accommodate the wedge and a lip that holds the wedge in position (Fig. 9-21).

Types

HARD OR SOFT. Hard removable wedges may be made of a material such as plastisol or a firm rubber. The medium size will fit most adults (Fig. 9-22). Polyurethane foam (used in the construction of heels for SACH feet) may be used to provide a soft, compressible wedge that is glued in place. Compression of the soft wedge allows passage of the femoral condyles.

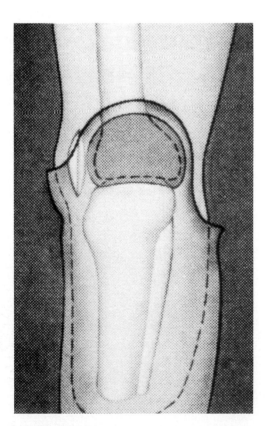

FIGURE 9-19. A medial view of a patellar-tendon-bearing prosthesis showing a medial supracondylar wedge in place. (From Fillauer, C: *Supracondylar wedge suspension of the P.T.B. prosthesis.* **Orthotics and Prosthetics 22:40, 1968, with permission.)**

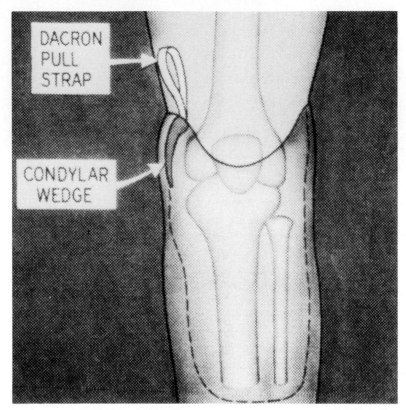

FIGURE 9-20. An anterior view showing the location of a medial supracondylar wedge. (From Fillauer, C: *Supracondylar wedge suspension of the P.T.B. prosthesis.* Orthotics and Prosthetics 22:40, 1968, with permission.)

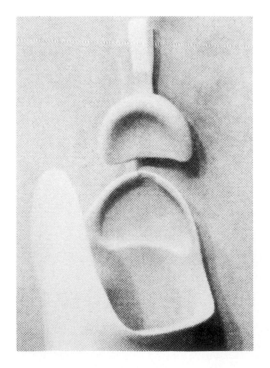

FIGURE 9-21. The proximal brim of the medial wall of the prosthesis is indented to retain the wedge in position. The wedge (above the prosthesis) is removed by using a loop of Dacron webbing. (From Fillauer, C: *Supracondylar wedge suspension of the P.T.B. prosthesis.* Orthotics and Prosthetics 22:41, 1968, with permission.)

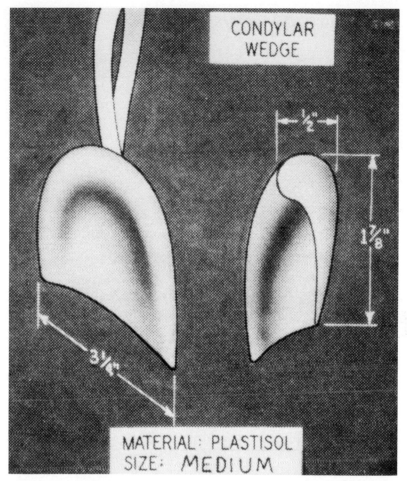

FIGURE 9-22. A supracondylar plastisol wedge used for suspension of the PTB prosthesis. *(Left)* A Dacron webbing loop facilitates removal from the socket. *(Right)* A cross-section view shows the comma shape, the thicker part being located proximal to the femoral condyle and the concave side of the wedge next to the convex condyle. (From Fillauer, C: *Supracondylar wedge suspension of the P.T.B. prosthesis.* Orthotics and Prosthetics 22:40, 1968, with permission.)

INFLATABLE WEDGE. Lincoln Baird invented another means of suspension, similar to the hard wedge designed by Fillauer, that involved an inflatable bulb that was placed superior to the medial femoral condyle (Fig. 9-23). This type of suspension was secure, comfortable, and reliable. It also offered built-in adjustability for day-to-day changes in edema, which was not offered by other suspension systems. The placement of the inflatable wedge was not as critical as that of the hard wedge because the inflatable wedge conformed to the shape of the condyle. The bulb was made of black neoprene and was inflated with a blood pressure bulb. The wedge-and-bulb system was filled with antifreeze for use in all climates. Because of problems with leakage, this type of wedge is no longer available.

DETACHABLE (REMOVABLE) MEDIAL BRIM. The detachable medial brim was designed for use with patients who have donning problems because of the extreme dis-

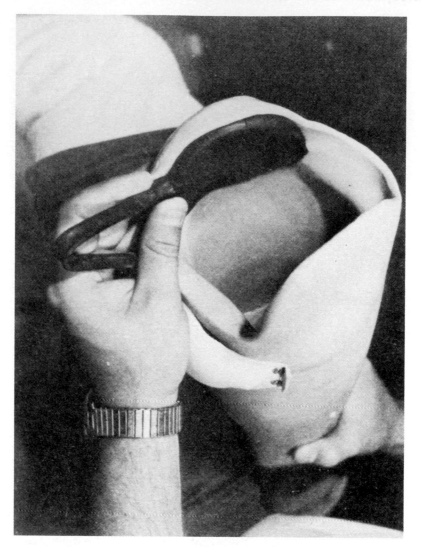

FIGURE 9-23. Baird's inflatable wedge supracondylar-type suspension, which is adjustable from 5 mm (0.2 in) to 25 mm (1 in). The medial lip of the socket, which holds the bulb in place, is reinforced. (From Staats, T: *Inflatable wedge suspension system.* Orthotics and Prosthetics 27:36, 1973, with permission.)

crepancy, usually 3.5 to 4 cm (1 3/8 to 1 1/2 in), between the mediolateral dimension at the supracondylar (A) and epicondylar (B) levels (Fig. 9-24). Extra-thick wedges are not always successful for managing this problem. The medial brim separates from the socket at the epicondylar level (the widest part of the knee, which is usually about midpatellar level). The hard socket is intact when the medial brim is in place. The hardware is placed in the center of the lamination of the socket. The medial brim is held on by a spring-ball assembly. The primary problem with the removable medial brim is pinching of the skin as the medial brim is reapplied. Also, amputees with limited hand function have difficulty removing the brim.

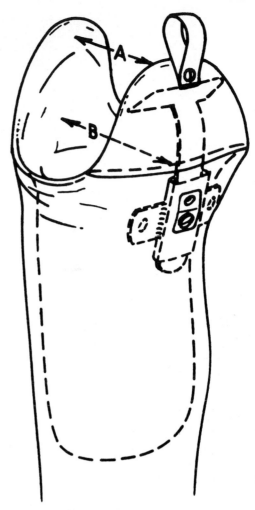

FIGURE 9-24. A patellar-tendon-bearing socket with a detachable medial brim. (From Fillauer, C: *A patellar-tendon-bearing socket with a detachable medial brim.* Orthotics and Prosthetics 25:27, 1971, with permission.)

MOLDED RUBBER SLEEVE SUSPENSION

The rubber sleeve is used as a suspension mechanism with any PTB prosthesis with or without the high medial and lateral walls (Fig. 9-25). The sleeve provides a friction grip to the prosthesis below the knee and the thigh above the knee. It helps to create an upward external force from the internal negative pressure created between the distal part of the limb and the bottom of the socket. The negative pressure creates a suction-type below-knee prosthesis. Patients have reported that the prosthesis feels lighter in weight, like a more intimate body part, and that piston action is minimal.

The sleeve is applied to the prosthesis in the area of the patella. It is rolled or pulled up to cover 5 to 10 cm (2 to 4 in) of the thigh above the stump sock. All air should be expelled from the sleeve and all creases and wrinkles removed. It has been recommended that the amputee keep several sleeves on hand and that they be cleaned with isopropyl alcohol and powdered with talcum. Potential problems are heat and perspiration, thus necessitating good hygiene.

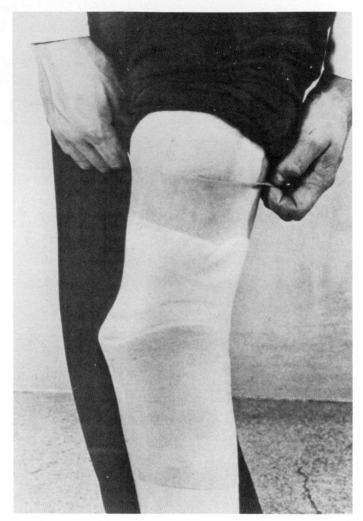

FIGURE 9-25. Molded rubber sleeve suspension of a PTB prosthesis. (From Giacinto, JP and McUmber, RA: *Fabrication of the silicone gel insert: Below-knee prosthesis and rubber sleeve suspension.* University of Michigan Medical Center, Ann Arbor, Michigan, 1976, p. 75, with permission.)

ADVANTAGE

1. Relatively simple to apply.

DISADVANTAGES

1. Sense of constriction.
2. Heat and perspiration buildup.
3. Relatively fragile.

SUPRAPATELLAR STRAP

Another method of suspending the PTB prosthesis is the suprapatellar strap. A piece of elastic webbing is attached to the brim of the medial and lateral walls. The strap passes just over the patella and helps to suspend the prosthesis. It is easy to don the prosthesis: the patient pulls the strap out with one hand and slips the residual limb into the socket.

BIBLIOGRAPHY

ALEXANDER, A: *Amputee's Guide: Below-the-Knee.* Medic Publishing Co, Issaquah, Washington, 1975.

ALLEN, RW AND VERHOFF, JR: *Supracondylar suspension patellar tendon bearing prosthesis: Its evaluation in unselected cases.* South Med J 63:59–61, 1970.

ANDERSEN, JG: *Below knee amputation.* Lepr Rev 47:51–55, 1976.

BAEHR, E AND SINEK, J: *A quick-change ankle disconnect for a below-knee amputation.* Orthot Pros 32:32–35, 1978.

BAKALIM, G: *Experiences with the PTB prosthesis.* Artificial Limbs 9:14–22, 1965.

BARCLAY, W: *Below-knee amputation-prosthesis.* In MURDOCH, G (ED): *Prosthetic and Orthotic Practice.* Edward Arnold & Co, London, 1970, pp 69–78.

BARNES, RW, SHANIK, GD, AND SLAYMAKER, EE: *An index of healing in below-knee amputations: leg blood pressure by Doppler ultrasound.* Surgery 79:13–18, 1976.

Below-Knee and Above-Knee Prostheses. A Report of a Workshop Sponsored by the Committee on Prosthetic Research and Development, Division of Medical Sciences, National Research Council, National Academy of Sciences, 1973.

BENNETT, L: *Transferring load to flesh. V. Experimental work.* Bull Prosthet Res 10-19:88–103, 1973.

BENNETT, L: *Transferring load to flesh.* Bull Prosthet Res 10–22:133–143, 1974.

BENNETT, L: *Transferring load to flesh. VII. Gel liner effects.* Bull Prosthet Res 10–21:23–53, 1974.

BENNETT, L: *Transferring load to flesh. VIII. Stasis and stress.* Bull Prosthet Res 10–23:202–210, 1975.

BERME, N, PURDEY, CR, AND SOLOMONIDIS, SE: *Measure of prosthetic alignment.* Artificial Limbs 2:73–75, 1978.

BICKEL, WH: *Amputations below the knee in occlusive arterial disease.* Surg Clin North Am 23:982–994, 1943.

BICKEL, WH AND GHORMLEY, RK: *Amputations below the knee in occlusive arterial disease.* Proc Mayo Clinic 18:361–367, 1943.

BLECK, EE, CANTY, TJ, AND DOOLITTLE, RC: *Below-the-knee, closed-end, soft socket.* J Bone Joint Surg 45A:967–976, 1963.

BLOCK, MA AND WHITEHOUSE, FW: *Below-knee amputation in patients with diabetes mellitus.* Arch Surg 87:682–689, 1963.

BOCHMANN, D AND THOMSON, HG: *The slip-socket prosthesis for juveniles: A new clinical application.* Inter-Clinic Info Bull 8:1–6, 1969.

BRADHAM, RR AND SMOAK, RD: *Amputations of the lower extremity: Used for arteriosclerosis obliterans.* Arch Surg 90:60–64, 1965.

BREAKEY, J: *Flexible below-knee socket with supracondylar suspension.* Orthot Pros 24:1–10, 1970.

BREAKEY, JW: *Criteria for use of supracondylar and supracondylar-suprapatellar suspension for below-knee prostheses.* Orthot Pros 27:14–18, 1973.

BREAKEY, JW: *Prefabricated below-knee sockets for the maturing stump.* Bull Prosthet Res 10–19:42–51, 1973.

BURGESS, EM: *The below-knee amputation.* Bull Prosthet Res 10–9:19–25, 1968.

BURGESS, EM: *The below-knee amputation.* Inter-Clinic Info Bull 8:1-22, 1969.

BURGESS, EM AND COLEMAN, E: *The cushion-socket below-knee prosthesis.* Clin Orthop 16:304–307, 1960.

BURGESS, EM AND ZETTL, JH: *Amputations below the knee.* Artificial Limbs 13:1–12, 1969.

BYERS, J, NITSCHKE, RO, AND GARDNER, HF: *Total-contact below-knee socket liners of "Cordo solution": Fabrication procedure.* Bull Prosthet Res 10–16:141–148, 1971.

CALDWELL, JL: *Inverted V-strap suspension for PTB prosthesis.* Artificial Limbs 9:23–26, 1965.

CANTY, TJ: *Amputations and recent developments in artificial limbs.* US Armed Forces Med J 3:1147–1152, 1952.

CHAVATZAS, D, BUDAK, D, AND JAMIESON, CW: *An assessment of value of long posterior flaps in below-knee amputations by skin blood pressure.* J Cardiovasc Surg 16:594–596, 1975.

CHILVERS, AS, ET AL: *Below and through knee amputations in ischaemic disease.* Br J Surg 58:824–826, 1971.

CHINO, N, ET AL: *Negative pressures during swing phase in below-knee prostheses with rubber sleeve suspension.* Arch Phys Med Rehabil 56:22–26, 1975.

CLAUGUS, CE, ET AL: *Amputations of the lower extremity for arteriosclerosis.* Arch Surg 76:992–996, 1958.

CLIPPINGER, FW AND TITUS, BR: *A "hard socket" patellar tendon bearing below-knee prosthesis.* Inter-Clinic Info Bull 4:16–18, 1965.

CONDON, RE AND JORDAN, PH, JR: *Below knee amputation for arterial insufficiency.* Surg Gynecol Obstet 130:641–648, 1970.

CRANLEY, JJ, ET AL: *Below-the-knee amputation for arteriosclerosis obliterans: With and without diabetes mellitus.* Arch Surg 98:77–80, 1969.

CUMMINGS, V: *Incorporation of a quadrilateral ischial weight-bearing thigh socket into a prosthesis for the below-knee amputee.* Arch Phys Med Rehabil 44:504–506, 1963.

DALE, WA AND CAPPS, W, JR: *Major leg and thigh amputations: Ten-year survey of results.* Surgery 46:333–342, 1959.

DEDERICH, R: *Stump correction by muscle-plastic procedure.* In *Prosthetics International, Proceedings of the Second International Prosthetics Course, Committee on Prostheses, Braces and Technical Aids, International Society for the Welfare of Cripples.* Copenhagen, 1960, pp 59–61.

DEDERICH, R: *Plastic treatment of the muscles and bone in amputation surgery: A method designed to produce physiological conditions in the stump.* J Bone Joint Surg 45B:60–66, 1963.

DEDERICH, R: *Technique of myoplastic amputations.* Ann R Coll Surg Engl 40:222–226, 1967.

DELAGI, EF AND LIPPMAN, HI (EDS): *Below-knee amputation.* NY State J Med 62:396–398, 1962.

DOLAN, CME: *The Army Medical Biomechanical Research Laboratory porous laminate patellar-tendon-bearing prosthesis.* Artificial Limbs 12:25–34, 1968.

ERAKLIS, A AND WHEELER, HB: *Below-knee amputations in patients with severe arterial insufficiency.* N Engl J Med 269:938–943, 1963.

ERIKSON, U AND LEMPERG, R: *Roentgenological study of movement of the amputation stump within the prosthesis socket in below-knee amputees fitted with a PTB prosthesis.* Acta Orthop Scand 40:520–529, 1969.

FAJAL, G: *Stump casting for the PTS below-knee prosthesis: Prothese tibiale supra condylienne.* Prosthet Int 3:22–24, 1968.

FILLAUER, C: *Supracondylar wedge suspension of the P.T.B. prosthesis.* Orthot Pros 22:39–44, 1968.

FILLAUER, C: *A patellar-tendon-bearing socket with a detachable medial brim.* Orthot Pros 25:26–34, 1971.

FLEER, B AND WILSON, AB, JR: *Construction of the patellar-tendon-bearing below-knee prosthesis.* Artificial Limbs 6:25–73, 1962.

FLEURANT, FW AND ALEXANDER, J: *Below knee amputation and rehabilitation of amputees.* Surg Gynecol Obstet 151:41–44, 1980.

FOORT, J: *The patellar-tendon-bearing prosthesis for below-knee amputees: A review of technique and criteria.* Artificial Limbs 9:4–13, 1965.

GALVAO, MSL: *An improved technique for below-knee amputation.* J Cardiovasc Surg 16:603–608, 1975.

GANGULI, S, BANERJEE, S, AND BOSE, KS: *A preliminary communication of fitting below-knee amputees with patellar-tendon-bearing prosthesis.* J Indian Med Assoc 59:145–152, 1972.

GANGULI, S, BOSE, KS, AND DATTA, SR: *Performance of BK amputees using PTB prostheses.* Acta Orthop Scand 46:123–134, 1975.

GANGULI, S AND DATTA, SR: *Studies in load carrying in BK amputees with a PTB prosthesis system.* J Med Eng Technol 1:151–154, 1977.

GARDNER, H: *A pneumatic system for below-knee stump casting.* Prosthet Int 3:12–14, 1968.

GAY, R AND HEARD, G: *Long posterior flap below-knee amputations for obliterative vascular disease of the lower limb.* Ir J Med Sci 141:25–30, 1972.

GIACINTO, JB: *The rubber sleeve suspension for below-knee prostheses.* Orthot Pros 30:17–19, 1976.

GIACINTO, JP AND MCUMBER, RA: *Fabrication of the silicone gel insert: Below-knee prosthesis and rubber sleeve suspension.* University of Michigan Medical Center, Ann Arbor, Michigan, 1976.

GILPIN, RE, DALE, GG, AND HARRIS, WR: *Canadian experiences with the patellar tendon bearing below-knee prosthesis.* J Bone Joint Surg 44B:795–799, 1962.

GOLDBERG, MJ AND GOLBRANSON, FL: *The fitting of a patellar tendon bearing prosthesis 47 years after the original below-knee amputation.* J Am Geriatr Soc 15:556–559, 1967.

HALL, CB: *Prosthetic socket shape as related to anatomy in lower extremity amputees.* Clin Orthop 37:32–46, 1964.

HAMONTREE, SE, TYO, HJ, AND SMITH, S: *Twenty months experience with the "PTS."* Orthot Pros 22:33–39, 1968.

HAMPTON, F: *Suspension casting for below-knee, above-knee and Syme's amputations.* Artificial Limbs 10:5–26, 1966.

HAMPTON, FL: *The suspension method for casting of below-knee stumps.* Prosthet Int 3:9–11, 1968.

HAMPTON, FL: *Prosthetic principles in the lower extremity amputee.* Orthop Clin North Am 3:339–347, 1972.

HARRIS, PD, SCHWARTZ, SI, AND DEWEESE, JA: *Midcalf amputation for peripheral vascular disease.* Arch Surg 82:381–383, 1961.

HAYES, RF: *A below-knee weight-bearing, pressure-formed socket technique.* Orthot Pros 29:37–40, 1975.

HICKS, L AND MCCLELLAND, RN: *Below-knee amputations for vascular insufficiency.* Am Surg 46:239–243, 1980.

HOAR, CS, JR AND TORRES, J: *Evaluation of below-the-knee amputation in the treatment of diabetic gangrene.* N Engl J Med 266:440–443, 1962.

HOOG, J: *An experimental below-the-knee prosthesis.* Phys Ther Rev 38:326–330, 1958.

HUGHES, J: *Below-knee amputation-biomechanics.* In MURDOCH, G (ED): *Prosthetic and Orthotic Practice.* Edward Arnold & Co, London, 1970, pp 61–67.

HUNTER-CRAIG, I, VITALI, M, AND ROBINSON, KP: *Long posterior-flap myoplastic below-knee amputation in vascular disease.* Br J Surg 57:62–65, 1970.

ISHERWOOD, PA: *Letter: Variation of stump volume after below-knee amputation.* Lancet 2:169, 1974.

JONES, RF: *Amputee rehabilitation: Basic principles in prosthetic assessment and fitting.* Med J Aust 2:290–293, 1977.

JONES, RF AND BURNISTON, GG: *A conservative approach to lower-limb amputations: Review of 240 amputees with a trial of the rigid dressing.* Med J Aust 2:711–718, 1970.

KATZ, K, ET AL: *End-bearing characteristics of patellar-tendon-bearing prostheses: A preliminary report.* Bull Prosthet Res 10–32:55–68, 1979.

KAY, HW: *Notes on the KBM prosthesis.* Inter-Clinic Info Bull 8:18–19, 1968.

KAY, HW AND NEWMAN, JD: *Report of a workshop on below-knee and above-knee prosthetics.* Orthot Pros 27:9–25, 1973.

KENDRICK, RR: *Below-knee amputation in arteriosclerotic gangrene.* Br J Surg 44:13–17, 1956.

KING, B, MCINTYRE, R, AND MYERS, K: *Below-knee amputation in peripheral arterial disease.* Aust NZ J Surg 45:301–304, 1975.

KOEPKE, GH, GIACINTO, JP, AND MCUMBER, RA: *Silicone gel below-knee amputation prostheses.* U Mich Med Cent J 36:188–189, 1970.

LAMBERT, CN: *Applicability of the patellar tendon bearing prosthesis to skeletally immature amputees.* Inter-Clinic Info Bull 3:7, 1964.

LIM, RC, JR, ET AL: *Below-knee amputations for ischemic gangrene.* Surg Gynecol Obstet 125:493–501, 1967.

LITTLE, JM, ET AL: *A trial of flapless below-knee amputation for arterial insufficiency.* Med J Aust 1:883–887, 1970.

LOON, HE: *Below-knee amputation surgery.* Artificial Limbs, 6:86–99, 1962.

LYQUIST, E: *Clinical study of the application of the PTB air-cushion socket.* Artificial Limbs 13:41–42, 1969.

LYQUIST, E: *Clinical study of the application of the PTB air-cushion socket.* Orthot Pros 23:159–160, 1969.

LYQUIST, E: *Recent variants of the PTB prosthesis (PTS, KBM, and air-cushion sockets).* In MURDOCH, G (ED): *Prosthetic and Orthotic Practice.* Edward Arnold & Co, London, 1970, pp 79–88.

MALONE, JM, ET AL: *Therapeutic and economic impact of a modern amputation program.* Bull Prosthet Res 10–32:7–17, 1979.

MARSCHALL, K AND NITSCHKE, R: *The P.T.S. prosthesis: Complete enclosure of the patella and femoral condyles in below knee fittings.* Orth Pros Appl J 20:123–126, 1966.

MARSCHALL, K AND NITSCHKE, R: *Principles of the patellar tendon supra-condylar prosthesis.* Orth Pros Appl J 21:33–38, 1967.

MCCOLLOUGH, NC, III: *The dysvascular amputee.* Orthop Clin North Am 3:303–321, 1972.

MCCONVILLE, BE, KENNEDY, EH, AND SCHOUTEN, M: *An evaluation of the patellar-tendon-bearing prosthesis.* Int Surg 47:377–381, 1967.

MOONEY, HV: *A treatment of the below-knee stump having intermittent breakdown.* Orth Pros Appl J 19:39–40, 1965.

MOONEY, V, ET AL: *The below-the-knee amputation for vascular disease.* J Bone Joint Surg 58A:365–368, 1976.

MOORE, WS, HALL, AD, AND LIM, RC, JR: *Below-knee amputation for ischemic gangrene: Comparative results of conventional operation and immediate postoperative fitting technic.* Am J Surg 124:127–134, 1972.

MOORE, WS, HALL, AD, AND WYLIE, EJ: *Below knee amputation for vascular insufficiency: Experience with immediate postoperative fittings of prosthesis.* Arch Surg 97:886–893, 1968.

MURDOCH, G: *Levels of amputation and limiting factors.* Ann R Coll Surg Engl 40:204–216, 1967.

MURDOCH, G: *Myoplastic techniques.* Bull Prosthet Res 10–9:4–13, 1968.

MURDOCH, G: *The "Dundee" socket for the below-knee amputation.* Prosthet Int 3:15–21, 1968.

MURDOCH, G: *The surgery of the below-knee amputation.* In MURDOCH, G (ED): *Prosthetic and Orthotic Practice.* Edward Arnold & Co, London, 1970, pp 45–60.

MURDOCH, G: *Amputation surgery in the lower extremity.* Prosthet Orthot Int 1:72–83, 1977.

MURPHY, EF: *The fitting of below-knee prostheses.* In KLOPSTEG, PE AND WILSON, PD (ED): *Human Limbs and their Substitutes.* Hafner Publishing, New York, 1954, pp 693–735.

MURPHY, EF AND WILSON, AB, JR: *Anatomical and physiological considerations in below-knee prosthetics.* Artificial Limbs 6:4–15, 1962.

MURRAY, DG *Below-knee amputation in the aged: Evaluation and prognosis.* Geriatrics 20:1033–1038, 1965.

PALOSCHI, GB AND LYNN, RB: *Major amputations for obliterative peripheral vascular disease, with particular reference to the role of below-knee amputation.* Can J Surg 10:168–171, 1967.

PARADYSTAL, T: *Amputation and prosthetic fitting in a patient with Guépar endoprosthesis.* Acta Orthop Scand 48:105–107, 1977.

PARRAS, G: *Interim B.K. patella tendon suspension prosthesis.* RALAS 15:2–4, 1974.

PEARSON, JR, ET AL: *Pressure variation in the below-knee patellar tendon bearing suction socket prosthesis.* J Biomech 7:487–496, 1974.

PEARSON, JR, ET AL: *Pressures in critical regions of the below-knee patellar-tendon-bearing prosthesis.* Bull Prosthet Res 10–19:52–76, 1973.

PEDERSEN, HE, LAMONT, RL, AND RAMSEY, RH: *Below-knee amputation for gangrene.* South Med J 57:820–825, 1964.

PERRY, T, JR: *Below-knee amputations.* Arch Surg 86:199–202, 1963.

PERSSON, BM: *Sagittal incision for below-knee amputation in ischaemic gangrene.* J Bone Joint Surg 56B:110–114, 1974.

PFALTZGRAFF, RE: *A simplified below-knee prosthesis.* Bull Prosthet Res 10–5:48–57, 1966.

PRIOROV, NN: *Amputation of the extremities and prosthesis in the U.S.S.R.* J Internat Coll Surgeons 8:13–19, 1945.

PRITHAM, CH: *Suspension of the below-knee prosthesis: An overview.* Orthot Pros 33:1–19, 1979.

QUIGLEY, MJ AND WILSON, AB, JR: *An evaluation of three casting techniques for patellar-tendon-bearing prostheses.* In *Selected Readings: A Review of Orthotics and Prosthetics.* American Orthotics and Prosthetics Association, Washington, DC, 1980, pp 178–191.

RADCLIFFE, CW: *The biomechanics of below-knee prostheses in normal, level, bipedal, walking.* Artificial Limbs 6:16–24, 1962.

RADCLIFFE, CW AND FOORT, J: *The Patellar-Tendon-Bearing Below-Knee Prosthesis.* Biomechanics Laboratory, University of California at San Francisco and Berkeley, 1961.

RECORD, EE: *Surgical amputation in the geriatric patient.* J Bone Joint Surg 45A:1742–1749, 1963.

REED, B, WILSON, AB, JR, AND PRITHAM, C: *Evaluation of an ultralight below-knee prosthesis.* Orthot Pros 33:45–53, 1979.

ROBB, HJ, JACOBSON, LF, AND JORDAN, P: *Midcalf amputation in the ischemic extremity: Use of lateral and medial flap.* Arch Surg 91:506–508, 1965.

ROBINSON, K: *Long-posterior-flap myoplastic below-knee amputation in ischaemic disease: Review of experience in 1967-71.* Lancet 1:193–195, 1972.

ROON, AJ, MOORE, WS, AND GOLDSTONE, J: *Below-knee amputation: A modern approach.* Am J Surg 134:153–157, 1977.

ROSENBERG, N: *Midleg amputation in patients with necrotic leg muscles.* Arch Surg 81:614–617, 1960.

ROSENFELDER, R: *The below-knee amputee with skin grafts.* J Am Phys Ther Assoc 50:1338–1346, 1970.

ROSENTHAL, AM: *The case for below-knee amputation.* J Einstein Med Cent 9:233–234, 1961.

RUBIN, G AND BYERS, JL: *A porous, flexible insert for the below-knee prosthesis.* In *Selected Readings: A Review of Orthotics and Prosthetics.* American Orthotics and Prosthetics Association, Washington, DC, 1980, pp 169–177.

RUBIN, G, NITSCHKE, RO, AND GARDNER, HF: *The supracondylar-suprapatellar PTB prosthesis.* Bull Prosthet Res 10–14: 102–106, 1970.

RUSKIN, AP, ROSNER, H, AND SAPERSTEIN, H: *Bent-knee prosthesis.* Geriatrics 25:109–114, 1970.

SAVANDER, GR AND KIM, KH: *Use of the soft liner in the preparatory plaster-of-Paris below-knee socket.* J Am Phys Ther Assoc 49:162–165, 1969.

SCHEINHAUS, A .AND RUBIN, G: *A modification of the porous below-knee soft socket insert.* Orthot Pros 32:3–5, 1978.

SEEBER, JJ, MAGILNER, A, AND REYES, T: *Radiologic technique to evaluate patellar-tendon-bearing prosthesis.* Arch Phys Med Rehabil 53:65–69, 1972.

SHEPLAN, L, LIBERMAN, B, AND SARMIENTO, A: *Patellar tendon bearing prostheses: Value of routine x-ray studies.* South Med J 62:1223–1226, 1969.

SHUMACKER, HB, JR AND MOORE, TC: *Leg and thigh amputations in obliterative arterial disease.* Arch Surg 63:458–465, 1951.

SILBERT, S: *Amputation below the knee for gangrene in the diabetic: Preliminary report.* Am J Dig Dis 11:394–401, 1944.

SILBERT, S: *Mid-leg amputations for gangrene in the diabetic.* Ann Surg 127:503–512, 1948.

SILBERT, S AND HAIMOVICI, H: *Results of midleg amputations for gangrene in diabetics.* JAMA 14:454–458, 1950.

SIMONS, BC, TRAUB, JE, AND ZETTL, JH: *University of Washington PTB suspension system.* Orth Pros Appl J 21:58–60, 1967.

SMITH, BC: *Amputation through lower third of leg for diabetic and arteriosclerotic gangrene.* Arch Surg 27:267–295, 1933.

SMITH, BC: *A twenty year follow-up in fifty below knee amputations for gangrene in diabetics.* Surg Gynecol Obstet 103:625–630, 1956.

SONCK, WA, COCKRELL, JL, AND KOEPKE, GH: *Effect of liner materials on interface pressures in below-knee prostheses.* Arch Phys Med Rehabil 51:666–669, 1970.

STAATS, T: *Inflatable wedge suspension system.* Orthot Pros 27:34–37, 1973.

STAROS, A AND GARDNER, HF: *Direct forming of below knee PTB sockets with a thermoplastic material.* Bull Prosthet Res 10–12:34–47, 1969.

STAROS, A AND GARDNER, HF: *Direct forming of below-knee PTB sockets with a thermoplastic material.* Artificial Limbs 14:57–64, 1970.

STAROS, A, ET AL: *Direct forming of below-knee patellar-tendon-bearing sockets with a thermoplastic material.* Orthot Pros 23:36–61, 1969.

STEWART, RE: *Variants of the PTB (patellar-tendon-bearing) below-knee prosthesis.* Bull Prosthet Res 10–13:120–134, 1970.

STROHM, BR AND OGG, L: *Patella tendon bearing–cuff suspension below-knee prosthesis: An evaluation procedure.* Phys Ther Rev 41:339–347, 1961.

SYMINGTON, DC, LOWE, PJ, AND MACKAY, S: *Semi-flexible sockets for amputation below the knee.* Arch Phys Med Rehabil 56:399–404, 1975.

Symposium on below-knee prosthetics. Orthot Pros 23:142–163, 1969.

TAFT, CB: *The patellar-tendon-supracondylar (PTS) prosthesis: Report of a preliminary study.* Inter-Clinic Info Bull 7:16–22, 1968.

TERMANSEN, NB: *Below-knee amputation for ischaemic gangrene: Prospective, randomized comparison of a transverse and a sagittal operative technique.* Acta Orthop Scand 48:311–316, 1977.

THOMPSON, RG: *The patellar tendon bearing total contact prosthesis for below-knee amputees.* Orth Pros Appl J 16:238–244, 1962.

THOMPSON, RG: *Amputation in the lower extremity.* J Bone Joint Surg 45A:1723–1734, 1963.

THOMPSON, RG: *"The decline and fall of the PTB": With apologies to Edward Gibbon (The Decline and Fall of the Roman Empire).* Orth Pros Appl J 19:21–22, 1965.

THOMPSON, RG: *PTB nomenclature.* Newsletter Amp Clinics 3:6–7, 1971.

THOMSON, HG AND BOCHMANN, D: *The skin-grafted below-knee stump: Can knee function be salvaged?* Can J Surg 13:37–40, 1970.

TOLSTEDT, GE AND BELL, JW: *Failure of below-knee amputation in peripheral arterial disease: Use of arteriography in determining site of election.* Arch Surg 83:934–936, 1961.

TRACY, GD: *Below-knee amputation for ischemic gangrene.* Pacif Med Surg 74:251–253, 1966.

VAGIAS, GJ AND HURWITZ, R: *Method of making patellar tendon-bearing pylon.* J Am Phys Ther Assoc 42:253–255, 1962.

VITALI, M: *Rehabilitation of the amputee.* Proc Roy Soc Med 59:1–3, 1966.

VONWERSSOWETZ, OF, PAINTER, CW, AND WRIGHT, DW: *Problems in fitting and alignment of the below the knee prosthesis.* Arch Phys Med Rehabil 36:345–348, 1953.

WARREN, R AND KIHN, RB: *A survey of lower extremity amputations for ischemia.* Surgery 63:107–120, 1968.

WILSON, AB, JR: *Recent advances in below-knee prosthetics.* Artificial Limbs 13:1–12, 1969.

WILSON, AB, JR: *A material for direct forming of prosthetic sockets.* Artificial Limbs 14:53–56, 1970.

WILSON, AB, JR: *Evaluation of synthetic balata for fabricating sockets for below-knee amputation stumps.* Artificial Limbs 14:58–67, 1970.

WILSON, AB, JR: *Evaluation of the patellar-tendon-bearing prothesis and its variations.* In MURDOCH, G (ED): *Prosthetic and Orthotic Practice.* Edward Arnold & Co, London, 1970, pp 105–114.

WILSON, AB, JR: *Limb prosthetics: 1970.* Artificial Limbs 14:1–52, 1970.

WILSON, AB, JR, PRITHAM, C, AND STILLS, M: *Manual for an Ultralight Below-Knee Prosthesis.* Rehabilitation Engineering Center, Moss Rehabilitation Hospital, Temple University, Philadelphia, 1977.

WILSON, AB, JR AND STILLS, M: *Ultra-light prostheses for below-knee amputees: A preliminary report.* Orthot Pros 30:43–47, 1976.

WILSON, LA AND LYQUIST, E: *Plaster bandage wrap cast: Procedure for the below-knee stump.* Prosthet Int 3:3–7, 1968.

WILSON, LA, LYQUIST, E, AND RADCLIFFE, CW: *Air-Cushion Socket for Patellar-Tendon-Bearing Below-Knee Prosthesis: Principles and Fabrication Procedures.* Biomechanics Laboratory, University of California at San Francisco and Berkeley, Technical Report 55, May, 1968.

WILSON, LA, LYQUIST, E, AND RADCLIFFE, CW: *Air-cusion socket for patellar-tendon-bearing below-knee prosthesis: Principles and fabrication procedures.* Bull Prosthet Res 10–10:5–34, 1968.

WITTECK, FA: *Some experience with patellar tendon-bearing below-knee prostheses.* Artificial Limbs 6:74–85, 1962.

WOLCOTT, LE AND KOEPKE, GH: *Experience with patellar tendon-bearing below-knee prosthesis with total contact socket.* Arch Phys Med Rehabil 43:474–476, 1962.

ZETTL, JH AND TRAUB, JE: *Premodified casting for the patellar-tendon-bearing prosthesis.* Artificial Limbs 15:1–14, 1971.

ZOTOVIC, B: *Experience with the air-cushion below-knee socket in Yugoslavia.* Orthot Pros 23:160–163, 1969.

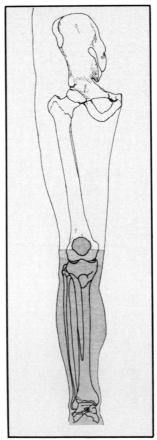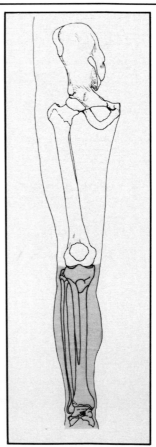

CHAPTER 10

KNEE DISARTICULATION (LEG [LEG], COMPLETE)

(THROUGH-THE-KNEE, THRU-KNEE, AT THE KNEE JOINT, EX-ARTICULATION)

TRANSCONDYLAR/SUPRACONDYLAR (LEG [LEG], COMPLETE)

(GRITTI-STOKES, KIRK, CALLANDER, AT THE KNEE)

POLYCENTRIC LINKAGE
MECHANISM
  CENTER OF ROTATION
  SWING CONTROL DEVICES
  OHC (ORTHOPAEDIC
  HOSPITAL IN COPENHAGEN,
  DENMARK) FOUR-BAR-

LINKAGE POLYCENTRIC
KNEE-DISARTICULATION
PROSTHESIS
FLUID-CONTROL KNEE
SYSTEM
  ADVANTAGES
  DISADVANTAGE

The earliest mention of amputation at the knee joint was made by the Father of Medicine, Hippocrates. Disarticulation seems to have been the form of amputation practiced at that time. Limb ablation was limited to cases of gangrene and was performed through dead tissue, carefully avoiding living tissue. After the technique of using ligatures to arrest hemorrhage was perfected, amputation was also performed in cases of accident and for diseases other than gangrene. The rules established by Hippocrates regarding amputation were rarely altered prior to the Middle Ages. Fabricius Hildanus, in 1581, allegedly performed an amputation at the knee joint following a leg fracture on a man from Dusseldorf.

In 1830, Velpeau, in his *Mémoire sur l'amputation de la jambe dans l'articulation du genou*, described an operative technique for amputation at the knee. He is credited with reintroducing the procedure to modern surgery. In France, amputation at the knee joint was opposed by Larrey and Dupuytren. Malgaigne, however, considered the procedure inconsiderately condemned and felt that it was preferable to amputation at the thigh.

The first disarticulation recorded in America was performed by Nathan Smith of New Haven in 1824. This publication actually preceded Velpeau's. Smith used an anterior flap, which included the patella and its tendon, and a posterior flap, which included the head of the gastrocnemius muscle, the tendons of the flexor muscles, and the popliteal vessels and nerves. Following the amputation, he described an immediate adhesive inflammation of the synovial membrane that resulted in ankylosis of the patella to the femur and thus offered a useful amputation limb.

M.L. Blaquière reported that he amputated the right leg at the femorotibial articulation in a 25-year-old Indian while in Mexico in 1833. Professor Pancoast of Philadelphia, in 1841, removed the leg of a woman, who was about 35 years old, at the knee joint. The procedure, described in *Treatise on Operative Surgery*, was performed in about 2 minutes.

Stephen Smith reported additional American cases in 1852, as did Thomas Markoe in 1856. Eight major advantages of knee disarticulation over above-knee amputation reported by Markoe still apply:

1. Disarticulation at the knee leaves a limb that is more useful for end-bearing and ambulation. Weight borne through the end of the bone after above-knee amputation may cause ulceration. The limb after disarticulation is capable of sustaining the body weight.
2. There is less shock with disarticulation because the amputation is farther from the trunk and is not through large muscle masses.
3. Dissection is less extensive although large flaps are exposed in a section at the knee joint; the femur is covered by a natural cartilaginous surface rather than by a denuded surface.
4. There is less risk of inflammation because in a section at the knee, no muscu-

lar interspaces are surgically exposed except for a small part of the proximal heads of the gastrocnemius.

5. Fewer ligatures are required.
6. Muscle action is easier because the muscles that move the limb are not divided.
7. No retraction of the cut muscles occurs after the wound is healed.
8. The bone is unwounded, without risk of dead bone, sequestra, and suppurative phlebitis.

Markoe supported the use of a long anterior flap and a short posterior flap. He noted that the most common mistake in performing the surgery had been in cutting the flaps too short and that amputation at the knee should under no circumstances be performed when amputation below the knee is equally safe.

During this time, disarticulations at the knee joint were favored in the hope of avoiding pyemia from osteomyelitis, which might occur if the bone were severed more proximally, leaving the bone marrow exposed. However, disarticulations required such long flaps for closure that the flaps were predisposed to gangrene. Also, there were pockets and recesses in the wound.

In 1866, James Syme of Edinburgh published a paper favoring amputation at the knee. He emphasized that it is safer than amputation at the thigh and that the skin over the bone becomes thicker, not thinner, enabling comfortable end weight-bearing. Syme's method of amputation at the knee was to excise some of the condyles; the limb would have the advantage of a large weight-bearing surface and would also offer a raw bone to which the soft parts could adhere. The supracondylar amputations introduced by Syme and, later, by Carden soon replaced disarticulations. Stephen Smith, however, found excision of some of the condyle unnecessary and objectionable.

Syme's early technique of the large posterior flap with muscle tissue from the calf fell into disuse. Carden's modification, utilizing a long anterior flap, replaced the Syme amputation at the knee. The patella was removed in both the Syme and Carden amputations.

John Brinton, in 1868, distinguished between amputation "at the knee joint" and amputation "at the knee." Amputation "at the knee joint" is a true disarticulation; at most, additional femoral articular cartilage or a small portion of the condyles is removed. Amputation "at the knee," known in England at that time as Carden's amputation, is a more extensive procedure, with section of the femur 2.5 to 6.5 cm (1 to 2½ in) above the joint articulation. This would include the Gritti-Stokes and Callander amputations of today.

Dr. William MacCormac, in 1870, supported Stephen Smith in his objection to amputation through the condyles. MacCormac felt that if the condyles were healthy, they should be retained. He pointed out that not only does the cartilage not interfere with healing, but if primary union for some reason does not occur, the cartilage-covered bone offers better safety than exposed cancellated tissue.

Amputation at the knee joint declined after anesthesia and asepsis came into use because the time saved was not as critical and the danger of opening bone marrow and muscle bellies was not as great as before. Through-knee disarticulation was abandoned mainly because the artificial-limb makers discouraged the site because a durable, efficient, cosmetic prosthesis did not exist. Thus, until World War II, the below-knee and above-knee amputations were the standard amputations primarily because the artificial limbs for these levels were non-critically accepted. In short, the surgeon was governed by the limitations of prostheses in choosing an amputation level. In the aged, however, who would probably never wear a prosthesis, the site of amputation was occasionally chosen for its simplicity, minimal danger of shock from hemorrhage, and ability to heal.

SURGICAL PROCEDURES

KNEE DISARTICULATION

Knee disarticulation is generally performed only when there is inadequate skin coverage for a below-knee amputation or when there is less than 4 cm (1 ½ in) of viable tibia remaining. Bone is not cut and muscle severance is minimal. Rehabilitation is enhanced by having a large horizontal end covered with soft tissue adapted to weight-bearing and a long lever under good muscular control. Also, a permanent prosthesis can be fitted early since the limb shrinks less than an above-knee limb; total end-bearing is usually tolerated 2 to 3 weeks after amputation. These characteristics make knee disarticulation particularly valuable to the elderly. It is specifically indicated for children because the distal femoral epiphysis is preserved during the growth period.

FLAPS

A variety of flaps have been described for knee disarticulation surgery: the circular cuff of Velpeau resulting in a vertical posterior scar, the double posterior flap and single anterior flap of Pancoast, Nathan Smith's equal anterior and posterior flaps, James Syme's larger posterior flap, and Carden's longer anterior flap. Techniques using medial and lateral flaps have also been described by Jørgen Evald Kjølbye and George Murdoch. In these procedures, the medial flap should be longer than the lateral flap for adequate coverage of the slightly larger and more prominent medial femoral condyle. Currently, long anterior and shorter posterior flaps placing the scar posteriorly are preferred by most surgeons.

OPERATION

ANTERIOR FLAP

The anterior flap is cut 7.6 to 10 cm (3 to 4 in) below the tibial plateau, which is about 2.5 cm (1 in) below the insertion of the patellar tendon, and parallel to the plateau more than halfway around the leg. A curved flap may impose tension over the femoral condyles, resulting in sloughing.

POSTERIOR FLAP

The posterior flap is cut 2.5 to 5 cm (1 to 2 in) below the posterior joint crease. Laterally, both the anterior and posterior flaps are cut proximal to the joint line.

PATELLAR TENDON

The patellar tendon is detached as long as possible at the tibial tubercle. It is later sutured to the cruciate ligaments for stability. The patella is retained in an effort to conserve the peripatellar arterial anastomosis and thus improve the chances of viability of the anterior flap. Also, if the patella is removed, the operation will be prolonged, there will be a decrease in the weight-bearing surface area, and the skin adapted for weight-bearing will be displaced.

The anterior capsule is divided. The cruciate ligaments are cut near the tibial attachment so they will be as long as possible. The gastrocnemius is divided near its origin. The hamstring tendons are divided at the level of the knee joint. The posterior capsule and popliteal vessels and nerve are divided. The vessels are ligated. The cartilage is not removed from the patella or the femoral condyles; therefore, the patella does not become fixed to the condyles. The patellar tendon is sutured to the cruciate ligaments or the posterior capsule, and the hamstring tendons are sutured to the cruciate ligaments, intercondylar notch, or remaining part of the capsule, offering active muscular control of the limb and thus the prosthesis. Remnants of the gastrocnemius muscle may be sutured into the intercondylar notch. The skin flap from the infrapatellar area is adapted for weight-bearing. It is important to have enough skin for loose closure to avoid skin breakdown with resulting infection and formation of a broad adherent scar. If there is insufficient skin for a loose closure, the posterior portion of the femoral condyles should be resected.

ADVANTAGES OVER ABOVE-KNEE AMPUTATIONS

1. Technically, it is a simple procedure. Since no bones are cut and muscles are severed at their insertions, hemostasis is easily obtained, shock occurs less frequently, and there is less edema, thus placing minimal stress on the patient.
2. The limb offers a broad, horizontal end-bearing surface. Most of the body weight can be transmitted through the end. The femoral condyles continue their customary function of weight-bearing, as do skin and soft tissue at the end of the limb.
3. Retaining the distal femoral epiphysis in children allows maximum longitudinal growth (80 to 90 percent of femoral growth).
4. The procedure can be performed rapidly (in about 30 minutes).
5. A prosthesis can be fitted early because there is little muscle atrophy. Early mobility is especially important for the elderly patient.
6. The bulbous distal limb may be used for suspension of the prosthesis. It provides excellent rotational stability between the residual limb and the socket.
7. Since the limb is longer, proprioceptive and kinesthetic feedback is better, which is especially important to elderly and blind patients.
8. The long anatomic lever arm and well-preserved musculature enable better balance and gait. The limb does not have the tendency to flex and abduct because of muscle imbalance, like the above-knee limb.
9. The patient can kneel without a prosthesis.
10. Medial-lateral stability can be maintained at minimal unit pressure because of the long limb.
11. The healing and rehabilitation success rates are high, while postoperative complications and mortality are low.
12. The final prosthesis will be lighter since it usually will not have to provide ischial weight-bearing or a pelvic band for suspension.
13. Phantom pain and residual limb pain are very rare.

DISADVANTAGES

1. The skin flaps are very long (unlike supracondylar or above-knee amputations), which may result in inadequate healing, especially if the vessels are diseased.
2. An oblique weight-bearing surface may remain after disarticulation because the femoral condyles are somewhat uneven. The skin may ulcerate over the longer condyle, which bears the greater weight.
3. The sutures securing the patellar tendon to the cruciate ligaments may not be strong enough for the powerful contraction of the quadriceps. Rigid ankylosis may be necessary.
4. Effusion in the reconstituted "knee joint" has been reported, but it is rare.
5. Fitting of a satisfactory prosthesis may be impossible if the hip motion is markedly limited or if a significant hip flexion contracture exists.
6. The broad femoral condyles impose limitations in socket design.
7. The space below the limb is inadequate for installation of an above-knee friction or fluid-control knee mechanism.

MODIFIED KNEE DISARTICULATION

A modified knee disarticulation is one in which the condyles are trimmed but the femoral length is retained. This was originally done in an attempt to make a less bulbous, more cosmetic limb. Condylar trimming is not performed on children whose distal femoral epiphyses have not closed. If a knee disarticulation is performed on young children, the length and width of condylar growth will be slowed, thus producing a conical limb without trimming the condyles.

PROCEDURE

Following a standard knee disarticulation, the patella is removed, retaining the patellar tendon and quadriceps expansion. Following a synovectomy, the medial, lateral, and posterior flares of the distal femur are removed (Fig. 10-1). The remaining articular cartilage is removed. The tendinous insertions of the anterior muscles are sutured over the distal end of the femur to the hamstrings or the anterior cruciate ligament.

ADVANTAGES OVER TRUE KNEE DISARTICULATION

1. Allows more prosthetic alignment adjustment, especially socket adduction.
2. Allows for a more cosmetic socket.
3. If the socket is set in flexion to accommodate a hip flexion contracture, flexion is less noticeable if the socket is not bulbous.

DISADVANTAGES

1. The limb may be unable to tolerate full body weight. Sometimes it cannot tolerate end-bearing. This necessitates proximal (ischial) weight-bearing, which in effect creates an overly long above-knee limb.
2. Added suspension is necessary because the bulbous characteristic of the limb is either gone or minimized.

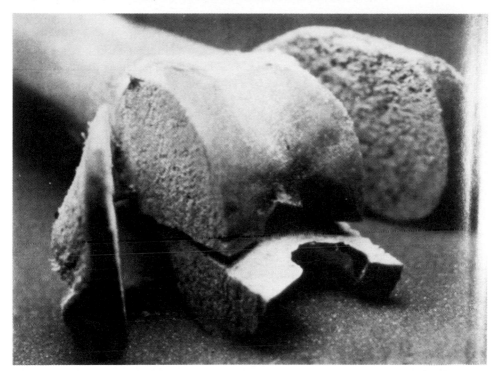

FIGURE 10-1. A demonstration of the lateral, medial, and posterior flare resections made in the surgical procedure. (From Utterback, TD and Rohren, DW: *Knee disarticulation as an amputation level.* J Trauma 13:116, 1973, with permission.)

TRANSCONDYLAR/SUPRACONDYLAR AMPUTATIONS

In 1845, James Syme reported two cases of amputation at the knee joint (transection through the condyles just above the articular surface) for tuberculosis of the knee joint. A long posterior flap from the calf was used to cover the end. In 1864, Carden reported a method of amputation at this level using an anterior flap after removal of the patella. In 1866, Syme commended Carden on the thicker flap, which was more serviceable and allowed weight-bearing as did the Syme amputation at the ankle. A variety of flaps have been described for transcondylar/supracondylar amputations, including lateral flaps, but some variation of the anterior-posterior flap has retained the greatest popularity.

Supracondylar amputation is indicated in cases of occlusive lesion in the vicinity of the bifurcation of the popliteal artery. If a below-knee amputation is performed under such circumstances, the limb usually ulcerates in a year or two.

GRITTI-STOKES AMPUTATION (STOKES' MODIFICATION OF GRITTI'S MODIFICATION OF CARDEN'S AMPUTATION)

Osteoplastic operation
Through femoral condyles
Patella fused to femur

In 1870, William Stokes published a modification of Gritti's method of amputation at the knee which he (Stokes) termed "supra-condyloid amputation of the thigh." Rocco Gritti of Milan, in 1857, had described his procedure of amputation through the knee using the patella in an osteoplastic flap to enable an end-bearing limb. Gritti's amputation was actually a modification of Carden's amputation at the knee. Stokes' method differs from the others in that the femur is sectioned higher (1.3 to 2 cm [1/2 to 3/4 in] above the anterosuperior edge of the condyloid cartilage). This level of femoral section does not, however, open the medullary canal. The cartilaginous surface of the patella is removed, which Stokes felt was necessary to get an osseous ankylosis between the femur and patella.

Stokes stated that the advantages of dividing the bone this high were as follows:

1. The face of the limb is covered with the portion of the flap that contains the patella.
2. The cut surface of the femur is perfectly and permanently covered by the patella.
3. The limb will not be inconveniently long for a prosthesis. The knee joint will have a more natural representation.

Stokes described the anterior flap as an oval flap from a point 2.5 cm (1 in) above either condyle, downward to the tibial tubercle, and upward to a point 2.5 cm (1 in) above the other condyle. A posterior flap that was at least one third the length of the anterior flap (rather than no flap) was felt to be necessary because the posterior tissues retract so much more than the anterior tissues.

Gritti's Amputation (1857)	Stokes' Modification (1870)
1. Femoral section is at the upper level of the epiphyseal line.	1. Femoral section is at least 1.3 cm (1/2 in) above the anterosuperior edge of the condyloid cartilage.
2. Cartilage from the back of the patella is removed.	2. Cartilage from the back of the patella is removed.
3. The flap is rectangular.	3. The flap is oval, not rectangular.
	4. The posterior flap is half the length of the anterior flap.

One advantage of the osseous ankylosis of the patella to the femur is that the extensor muscles have a firm point of fixation and are thus able to move the thigh more powerfully.

Knee disarticulation declined in use after it was first described because an acceptable prosthesis had not been designed and often the wound did not heal. This led to the support of a modification—the Gritti-Stokes amputation.

This amputation level is often selected over the above-knee procedure because it is less of an operative risk and the longer limb gives better sitting balance in cases of bilateral amputation and better prosthetic control in all instances.

OPERATION

The incision is U-shaped anteriorly. It begins at the adductor tubercle, passes downward anteriorly to cross the mid part of the tibial tubercle, and then goes upward laterally to a point corresponding to the adductor tubercle. The incision across the posterior aspect of the knee is convex distally (about 2.5 cm [1 in]).

With the knee joint acutely flexed, the collateral and cruciate ligaments are divided. The tibia is then dislocated forward as the posterior capsule and ligaments are divided. Using an anterior approach, the nerves and vessels in the popliteal fossa are divided and ligated. Posteriorly, the hamstring tendons are divided.

The distal femur is sectioned at the level of the adductor tubercle (the landmark most commonly used now). The articular surface of the patella is also sectioned (Fig. 10-2). A hole is bored through the lower end of the patella and the posterior lip of the patella through which sutures are passed, or the patellar tendon is sutured to the remnant of the posterior capsule to keep the patella in place over the cut end of the femur. The hamstring tendons are sutured to the popliteal, lateral, or anterior ligamentous structures to preserve their extensor function.

ADVANTAGES

1. Mortality is less than with mid-thigh amputations, probably because the operation can be performed rapidly, blood loss is minimal, and the muscle mass is uninjured.

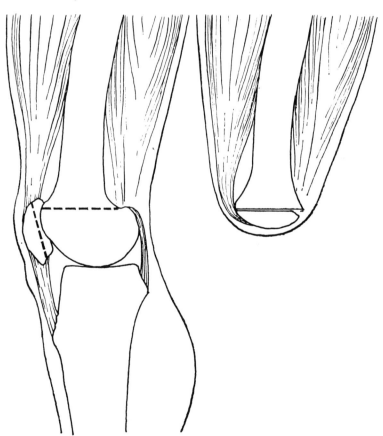

FIGURE 10-2. The Gritti-Stokes amputation. The dotted lines show the section of the femur and the patella. The remaining patella is fused to the distal femur. The resulting limb is conical. (From Newcombe, J: *Through-knee amputation.* Nursing Times 65:871, 1969, with permission.)

2. The superior genicular artery is preserved, so blood supply to the skin flaps is good.
3. Division is through skin, tendons, ligaments, and cancellous bone rather than through muscle; therefore, blood loss, shock, and hematoma formation are minimal compared with above-knee amputations. Circulation is better than if amputation is at the knee.
4. The major muscles that move the thigh are not divided and the limb is long, thus assuring good control of a prosthesis.
5. The limb is partially end weight-bearing because the patella and prepatellar skin are accustomed to weight-bearing.
6. Shrinkage is not a problem. A prosthesis can be fitted early.
7. The marrow cavity is not opened surgically.
8. The anterior flap is shorter than in knee disarticulation; therefore, there is less incidence of delayed healing.
9. Skin closure is easier than in through-knee amputations.
10. Healing is fast, by first intention usually, and reamputation is rare, thus making it an especially good procedure for elderly patients who are prone to respiratory, cardiac, or urinary complications if confined to bed.
11. Phantom limb sensation is minor.
12. The limb is not too bulbous and thus can be introduced into a rigid socket from above. Since the femur is sectioned within the flare of the condyles, the slightly bulbous distal limb can still be used for suspension.

DISADVANTAGES

1. The distal femoral epiphysis is not preserved; therefore, this procedure should not be chosen for children if disarticulation through the knee joint can be done.
2. The disarticulation limb is bulkier, giving better rotational control of a prosthesis than the long conical limb after Gritti-Stokes amputation.
3. The limb usually cannot tolerate total end weight-bearing because the patella gives a small surface area compared with the through-knee amputation. Most patients need ischial weight-bearing as well.
4. Complications associated with preserving the patella are as follows:
   - reduction of weight-transmitting surface
   - non-union to femur (the patella may be mobile if the articular cartilage is not completely removed)
   - avascular necrosis
   - pain; even if there is bony union between the femur and patella, the irregular shape of the patella can make end-bearing uncomfortable.
5. A posterior flap that is too short may result in suture line infection because of too much tension.
6. Joint sensation is lost.
7. The operation itself is more severe than knee disarticulation, with greater risk of interfering with the collateral circulation.
8. The end is not bulbous enough to aid suspension as well as the knee disarticulation amputation.
9. The length of the limb prevents the use of a standard knee unit within the dimensions of the normal leg.

KIRK AMPUTATION

| Tendoplastic operation |

In the supracondylar tendoplastic amputation of Kirk, the skin flaps are designed so that the anterior flap is longer than the posterior flap by a ratio of 4 to 1. The anterior flap is sectioned just below the upper margin of the patella and therefore does not include the patella. The suprapatellar bursa is carefully dissected out to avoid later accumulation of synovial fluid. The bone is sectioned 3.2 cm (1¼ in) above the articular surface on a plane that would be parallel to the floor if the patient was standing. Because of the normal valgus angle of the femur, if the bone is sectioned at a right angle to the long axis the lateral margin will be prominent and may be painful on weight-bearing. The quadriceps tendon is brought over the end of the bone and is sutured to the posterior fascia without tension.

CALLANDER AMPUTATION

| Tendoplastic operation |

In 1935, C. Latimer Callander described a new amputation at the distal thigh.

OPERATION

The skin incisions are slightly unequal anteriorly and posteriorly.

Anterior Flap

The incision begins at a point 5 cm (2 in) proximal to the most prominent part of the medial femoral condyle. The incision passes distally in the groove between the sartorius and vastus medialis muscles, over the medial epicondyle, and passes over the anterior surface of the tibia to the tibial tubercle. The thigh is then rolled medially, and the lateral incision is begun at a point 5 cm (2 in) proximal to the lateral femoral condyle. The incision passes distally in the groove between the tendon of the biceps femoris and the tensor fasciae latae muscle, over the lateral epicondyle, and over the anterior surface of the tibia to the tibial tubercle. This forms the outline of the anterior flap.

Posterior Flap

Incisions are made from each femoral epicondyle posteriorly, obliquely, and inferiorly to a point on the calf considerably distal to the level of the tibial tubercle on the anterior aspect of the leg or about midway the belly of the gastrocnemius muscle. The posterior amputation flap is thus a little longer than the anterior flap.

The sartorius, gracilis, semimembranosus, and semitendinosus muscles are divided at their tibial insertions. The adductor magnus tendon is severed at the adductor tubercle attachment. The popliteal artery and vein are ligated and divided. The tibial and common peroneal nerves are ligated and divided.

The lateral incision is deepened and the biceps femoris tendon is severed. The anterior incision is deepened and the quadriceps tendon is severed at the insertion into the tibial tubercle. The patella is dissected from the quadriceps tendon, taking care to preserve the tendon of the rectus femoris.

The femur is severed just proximal to the adductor tubercle. The cut end of the femur at this level is about the same size as the socket from which the patella has just been removed. The cut end of the femur is smoothed and rounded with a rasp. It is eventually fitted into the socket in the quadriceps tendon from which the patella was removed (Fig. 10-3).

The deep structures (tendons and aponeuroses) are not sutured to each other and are therefore not under tension and are not subject to consequent pressure necrosis.

The flaps, which appear exceedingly long, are brought loosely together and clipped. At that time, the flaps extend 2.5 cm (1 in) or more below the distal end of the femur and appear excessively redundant (Fig. 10-4).

Within the first 3 postoperative days, the hamstring muscles will contract enough to bring the suture line posteriorly to about the level of the limb end. As the posterior flap gradually retracts, the suture line is drawn proximal to the end of the bone. The femur becomes securely seated in the patellar fossa, creating an end-bearing limb through the rectus femoris tendon, prepatellar bursa, and tough overlying skin.

Length of the Amputation Flaps

Extensive retraction of the hamstring compared with the quadriceps muscles can be

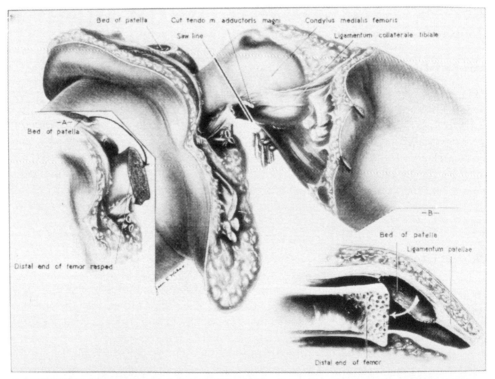

FIGURE 10-3. Medial view of the left thigh and knee during a Callander amputation. Note the long anterior and posterior flaps and the saw line for section of the femur. (A) The cut end of the femur will be covered with the patella fossa. (B) The anterior and posterior flaps are loosely approximated. As the posterior flap retracts, the patellar fossa lodges over the cut end of the femur. (From Callander, CL: A new amputation in the lower third of the thigh. JAMA 105:1750, 1935, with permission.)

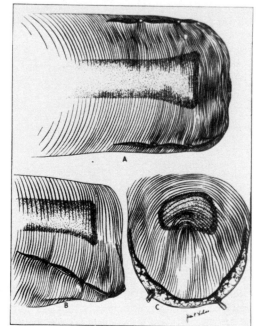

FIGURE 10-4. Transparent drawings show the remaining condylar flare and redundant tissue following a Callander amputation. *(A)* An anterior view. *(B)* A lateral view showing intermittent skin clips. *(C)* A distal vIew prior to the placement of skin clips. (From Callander, CL: *A new amputation in the lower third of the thigh.* JAMA 105:1751, 1935, with permission.)

expected. This occurs because the hamstring muscles originate from the pelvis except for the short head of the biceps femoris, which originates on the shaft of the femur. All of the quadriceps originates from the shaft of the femur except for the rectus femoris; thus, there is little tendency for the quadriceps to retract. The tensor fasciae latae muscle does not retract markedly because the muscle mass is so short. Thus, the anterior flap retracts very little and the posterior flap retracts to an extensive degree.

ADVANTAGES

1. The Callander procedure takes several precautions to ensure against infection:
   - The posterior flap is cut long enough to eliminate tension with the anterior flap at the suture line.
   - Muscles are sectioned at their tendinous insertions.
   - Incisions are made through natural intermuscular cleavage spaces to avoid section of muscle fibers.
   - No skin or subcutaneous tissue is dissected from the deep fascia.
2. Operative shock is avoided by controlling hemorrhage through early ligation of popliteal vessels and by severing muscles at their tendinous insertions rather than through muscle bellies.

DISADVANTAGES

1. If patella enucleation is not performed carefully, there may be damage to the genicular arteries, which will result in vascular impairment to the anterior flap.
2. Survival of the anterior flap is generally more tenuous than the posterior flap because the blood supply to the front of the limb is poorer than to the back.

DISADVANTAGES OF SUPRACONDYLAR COMPARED WITH KNEE DISARTICULATION AMPUTATION

1. Longer operative time.
2. Greater chance of bleeding.
3. Greater chance of infection.

PROSTHESES

SOCKETS

PLUG FIT SOCKET

The socket can be made of plastic laminate or molded of leather. A positive model is made from a cast of the limb, which is modified at the end to allow for an end-bearing pad. Polyester laminate is fabricated, or cowhide leather is cut to shape, soaked, and sewed onto the model. As it dries, the leather shrinks tightly to the model. The socket is lined with horsehide. Regardless of the material, a lengthwise anterior cutout that comes to a point about 7.6 cm (3 in) above the end (lower for knee disarticulations) is necessary to enable donning, because of the bulbous shape of the limb. The cutout is held together by a lace (Fig. 10-5), hooks and eyes, straps and buckles, or Velcro fasteners. The semirigid socket can be partially ischial-bearing and partially end-bearing to prevent ulceration of the distal skin. A resilient pad at the distal end helps to distribute weight evenly and absorbs high impact loads.

Suspension is usually achieved by the molded shape of the thigh-lacing corset above the femoral condyles; a waist belt or pelvic band may augment suspension. A knee control strap that attaches to the waist belt controls excessive heel-rise after toe-off and provides extension bias.

ADVANTAGES

1. The socket can be adjusted to minor changes in the size of the limb.
2. The socket is not completely rigid and feels more natural.
3. The socket itself conforms to the shape of the limb, which enhances the appearance.

DISADVANTAGES

1. The anterior part of the leather socket deforms easily under pressure, allowing too much flexibility of the socket as a whole.
2. The patient with weak, arthritic hands may not be able to lace the thigh corset tightly enough to ensure proper suspension or fit.
3. The plug fit often results in skin infections and ulcerations.
4. Tightness over the thigh from the use of laces can cause muscle atrophy.

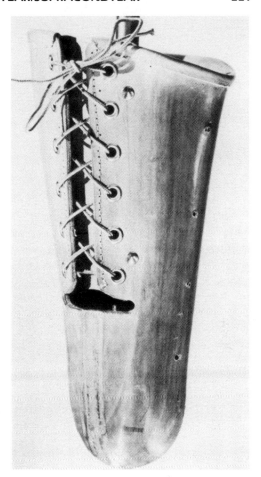

FIGURE 10-5. A leather socket with an anterior opening for a knee-disarticulation limb. (From Gardner, H: *Report: Basic steps in the fabrication of the through-knee socket.* Workshop on Knee-Disarticulation and Hip-Disarticulation Prostheses, March 1969, p. 7, with permission.)

MODIFIED QUADRILATERAL SOCKET

A modified quadrilateral inlet eliminates the plug fit and obtains some ischial weight-bearing. Suspension is obtained through supracondylar contouring rather than through the use of external straps and auxiliary suspension. The plastic socket may have an anterior removable panel secured with Velcro straps that allows insertion of the limb, or it may have an expandable, flexible, soft inner socket with a rigid outer shell, similar to the windowless Syme prosthesis.

ADVANTAGES

1. No external auxiliary suspension is necessary.
2. Pistoning is virtually eliminated.
3. Partial weight-bearing is carried through the ischial tuberosity, thereby reducing the forces through the femur and distal limb.

DISADVANTAGES

1. The socket opening and straps, if used, are uncosmetic.

2. The ischial tuberosity tends to fall off of the supporting shelf into the socket if the anterior opening is not supported by straps that do not deform under pressure.

KNEE UNITS

KNEE HINGES

A prosthesis with metal sidebars and heavy-duty uniaxial knee joints, similar to those used in braces, was used initially. The knee joints were located on either side of the femoral condyles so that knee flexion occurred at approximately the same level as the sound side. The joints had mechanical stops that could be placed to give some inherent stability in full knee extension. Locks were sometimes placed on the knee joint so that the patient had the option of walking with a locked knee or a free swinging action. A check-strap of leather or cord on the posterior aspect of the knee joint provided control for terminal-impact of the shank and protection for the mechanical extension stop by decelerating the shank in the latter part of the swing phase. If a true knee bolt was used, it had to be located well below the limb, resulting in a marked disparity in knee levels, which was especially apparent during sitting.

ADVANTAGES

1. The axis of motion occurs at approximately the same level as the sound side.
2. A mechanical lock can be used for stability in complete extension.

DISADVANTAGES

1. The side joints are bulky, uncosmetic, and lack the strength to withstand the torque placed on them by a vigorous or heavy walker.
2. Poor swing phase control.
3. The external knee control strap offers varying resistance as the elastic stretches and wears.
4. The posteriorly located, external knee check-strap makes the knee unstable if the check-strap is too tight and results in audible terminal-impact if it is too loose. The required fine adjustment varies as the material stretches or the adjustment screws loosen.

YOKE

The yoke system, which spans the posterior socket, was designed to make fluid knee controls available on the through-knee prosthesis. The fluid knee unit attaches to the bottom of the yoke. The arms of the yoke connect to the outside knee joint through brackets that allow the piston rod to pivot.

PROBLEMS

1. Mechanical failure of yoke or piston rod.
2. Noise.

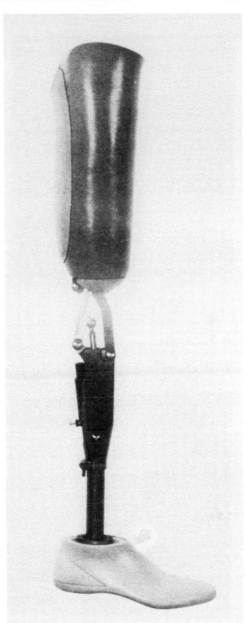

FIGURE 10-6. OHC four-bar-linkage polycentric knee unit in the extended position without a cosmetic cover. (From Lyquist, E: *The OHC knee-disarticulation prosthesis.* **Orthotics and Prosthetics 30:27, 1976, with permission.)**

POLYCENTRIC LINKAGE MECHANISM

The polycentric linkage mechanism was designed for the amputee with a knee disarticulation. It provides a knee mechanism that is located below the limb within the shank yet provides the center of rotation at the femoral condyles.

CENTER OF ROTATION

Since the unit is polycentric, the center of rotation between the shank and thigh changes as the knee flexes and extends. The center of knee rotation starts high, which improves the leverage for voluntary control of knee stability, and then descends rapidly with knee flexion to allow a greater range in knee flexion and a more normal appearance during sitting.

SWING CONTROL DEVICES

These can be added to the basic mechanism and are desirable. Either sliding friction or hydraulic swing control units may be used.

OHC (ORTHOPAEDIC HOSPITAL IN COPENHAGEN, DENMARK) FOUR-BAR-LINKAGE POLYCENTRIC KNEE-DISARTICULATION PROSTHESIS

This knee unit, developed by Erik Lyquist in Copenhagen, was the first of its kind (Fig. 10-6). The appearance of the OHC prosthesis is enhanced by several factors. The four bar linkage swings inward during knee flexion, leaving no protruding mechanical parts at any point of knee flexion. A semirigid plastic kneecap gives a natural appearance and

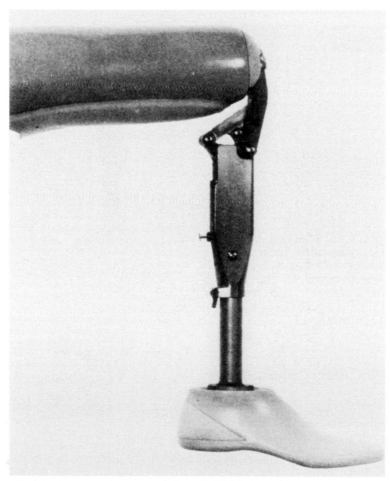

FIGURE 10-7. The OHC unit in flexion. (From Lyquist, E: *The OHC knee-disarticulation prosthesis.* Orthotics and Prosthetics 30:28, 1976, with permission.)

protects clothing. Cosmetic covers of either factory-molded or custom-shaped rubber cover the shank.

The OHC unit can also be used on above-knee prostheses. It is especially valuable to amputees with a short above knee residual limb because of the inherent stability. Knee flexion is limited to about 100 degrees (Fig. 10-7). The prosthesis is strong and lightweight owing to its aluminum construction.

FLUID-CONTROL KNEE SYSTEM

Knee disarticulation and supracondylar amputation levels were not very popular for many years due, at least in part, to the lack of swing phase control at the knee joints. Attempts were made at friction control, but these were not adequate because they were suitable for only one preset rate of cadence. The hydraulic units used for above-knee amputees could not be used for the knee-level amputations without causing a difference in knee height. A method to incorporate fluid-control knee mechanisms into the plastic or molded-leather socket for through-knee or supracondylar prostheses was thus

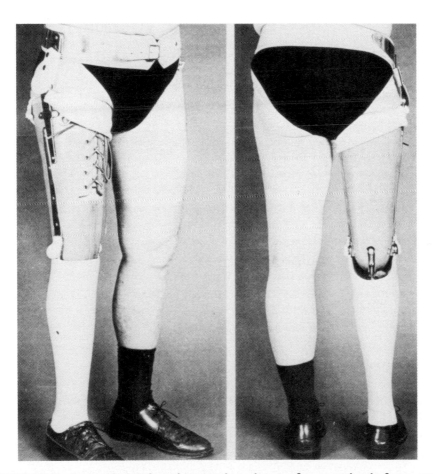

FIGURE 10-8. Anterolateral and posterior views of a prosthesis for a supracondylar amputation stump. A piston-type hydraulic or pneumatic knee mechanism may be used with a leather, anterior-lacing socket. (From Cortellino, J and Gardner, HF: *Hydraulic knee controls for knee-level amputations.* Bull Prosthet Res 10–11:62, 1969, with permission.)

developed. For example, the Dyna-plex hydraulic swing phase control was designed to be installed in the OHC four-bar frame. Additional material is designed into the posterior distal part of the socket (knee) area so the unit can be attached just posterior to the distal limb (Fig. 10-8). The outside knee joint is located at an imaginary axis through the knee of the prosthesis, and the piston rod of the fluid-control system functions about 3 cm (1⅕ in) posterior to the imaginary knee axis. The posterior wall must be at least 3.2 cm (1¼ in) thick for adequate strength.

ADVANTAGES

1. Enhances swing phase control.
2. May also offer extension bias (assistance to knee extension at the initiation of swing phase).
3. May offer a locking mechanism.

DISADVANTAGE

1. Adds weight to the prosthesis (about 1361 to 1814 g [3 to 4 lb]).

BIBLIOGRAPHY

BADDELEY, RM AND FULFORD, RM: A trial of conservative amputations for lesions of the feet in diabetes mellitus. Br J Surg 52:38–43, 1965.

BAR, A, SELIKTAR, R, AND SUSACK, Z: Pneumatic supracondylar suspension for knee-disarticulation prostheses. Orthot Pros 31:3–7, 1977.

BATCH, JW, SPITTLER, AW, AND MCFADDIN, JG: Advantages of the knee disarticulation over amputations through the thigh. J Bone Joint Surg 36A:921–929, 1954.

BAUMGARTNER, RF: Knee disarticulation versus above-knee amputation. Prosthet Orthot Int 3:15–19, 1979.

BAUMGARTNER, R: Failures in through-knee amputation. Prosthet Orthot Int 7:116–118, 1983.

BEACOCK, CJM, ET AL: A modified Gritti-Stokes amputation: Its place in the management of peripheral vascular disease. Ann R Coll Surg Engl 65:90–92, 1983.

BOTTA, P AND BAUMGARTNER, R: Socket design and manufacturing technique for through-knee stumps. Prosthet Orthot Int 7:100–103, 1983.

BRINTON, JH: On amputation at the knee-joint, and at the knee. Am J Med Sci 55:305–338, 1868.

BURGESS, EM: Disarticulation of the knee: A modified technique. Arch Surg 112:1250–1255, 1977.

CALLANDER, CL: A new amputation in the lower third of the thigh. JAMA 105:1746–1753, 1935.

CALLANDER, CL: Tendoplastic amputation through the femur at the knee: Further studies. JAMA 110:113–118, 1938.

CANTY, TJ: Amputations and recent developments in artificial limbs. US Armed Forces Med J 3:1147–1152, 1952.

CARDEN, HD: On amputation by single flap. Br Med J i:416–421, 1864.

CARNES, EH: Amputations, stumps and prostheses. War Med 1:656–663, 1941.

CHILVERS, AS, ET AL: Below- and through-knee amputations in ischaemic disease. Br J Surg 58:824–826, 1971.

CLEVELAND, M AND HAYWARD, OS: *Nathan Smith (1762–1829) on amputations.* J Bone Joint Surg 43A:1247–1254, 1961.

CORTELLINO, J AND GARDNER, HF: *Hydraulic knee controls for knee-level amputations.* Bull Prosthet Res 10–11:60–64, 1969.

CORTOLINO, J AND GARDNER, H: *Hydraulic knee controls of prostheses for thru-knee and supra-condylar amputation levels.* In *Report: Workshop on Knee-Disarticulation and Hip-Disarticulation Prostheses.* Subcommittee on Design and Development, Committee on Prosthetics Research and Development, Division of Engineering, National Research Council, National Academy of Sciences, National Academy of Engineering, San Francisco, 1969.

DALTON, DH, JR, McDOWELL, HA, AND LYONS, C: *Through-the-knee guillotine amputation.* Ann Surg 161:614–616, 1965.

EARLY, PF: *Rehabilitation of patients with through-knee amputation.* Br Med J 4:418–421, 1968.

ELOESSER, L: *Exarticulation at the knee joint.* Surg Clin North Am 6:407–411, 1926.

ELOESSER, L: *On sites and types of amputation and exarticulation together with some notes on technic.* Surg Clin North Am 13:9–18, 1933.

GARDNER, H: *Basic steps in the fabrication of the thru-knee socket.* In *Report: Workshop on Knee-Disarticulation and Hip-Disarticulation Prostheses.* Subcommittee on Design and Development, Committee on Prosthetics Research and Development, Division of Engineering, National Research Council, National Academy of Sciences, National Academy of Engineering, San Francisco, 1969.

GREEN, PWB, ET AL: *An assessment of above- and through-knee amputations.* Br J Surg 59:873–875, 1972.

GREENE, HG: *Amputation through the knee for the nonambulatory patient.* Surg Gynecol Obstet 140:771–773, 1975.

HAMPTON, FL: *Above-knee prostheses.* Orthop Clin North Am 3:359–372, 1972.

HARDING, HE: *Knee disarticulation and Syme's amputation.* Ann R Coll Surg Engl 40:235–237, 1967.

HARRIS, FE: *The through-knee amputation prosthesis.* In MURDOCH, G (ED): *Prosthetic and Orthotic Practice.* Edward Arnold & Co, London, 1970, pp 263–268.

HARRIS, RI: *Syme's amputation: Technical details essential for success.* J Bone Joint Surg 38B:614–632, 1956.

HARRIS, RI: *The history and development of Syme's amputation.* Artificial Limbs 6:4–43, 1961.

HOPKINS, JDP AND HARRIS, EE: *Knee disarticulation in arteriosclerotic limb.* Prosthet Int 2:4–7, 1965.

HOWARD, RRS, CHAMBERLAIN, J, AND MACPHERSON, AIS: *Through-knee amputation in peripheral vascular disease.* Lancet 2:240–242, 1969.

HUGHES, J: *Through-knee amputation biomechanics.* In MURDOCH, G (ED): *Prosthetic and Orthotic Practice.* Edward Arnold & Co, London, 1970, pp 259–261.

JACKSON, NJ AND HUNT, TE: *Supracondylar amputation of the lower limb.* Can J Surg 7:12–18, 1964.

JANSEN, K: *Management of the knee disarticulation.* In *Prosthetics International, Proceedings of the Second International Prosthetics Course, Committee on Prostheses, Braces and Technical Aids, International Society for the Welfare of Cripples.* Copenhagen, 1960, pp 103–104.

JONES, RN: *Letter.* Br Med J 2:1496, 1961.

KJØLBYE, J: *The surgery of the through-knee amputation.* In MURDOCH, G (ED): *Prosthetic and Orthotic Practice.* Edward Arnold & Co, London, 1970, pp 225–257.

KLASSON, DH: *Supracondylar amputation with functional stump.* J Int Coll Surg 38:547–550, 1962.

LISHMAN, IV: *The Gritti-Stokes amputation in peripheral vascular disease.* J R Coll Surg Edinb 10:212–220, 1965.

LUNT, R: *Through-knee amputation.* Br Med J 4:831, 1968.

LYQUIST, E: *The OHC knee-disarticulation prosthesis.* Orthot Pros 30:27–28, 1976.

LYQUIST, E: *Casting the through-knee stump.* Prosthet Orthot Int 7:104–106, 1983.

MACCORMAC, W: *On amputation through the knee-joint.* Dublin Quart J Med Sci 49:273–292, 1870.

MARKOE, TM: *Amputation at the knee joint.* NY State J Med 16:19–48, 1856.

MARTIN, P, RENWICK, S, AND THOMAS, EM: *Gritti-Stokes amputation in atherosclerosis: A review of 237 cases.* Br Med J 3:837–838, 1967.

MARTIN, P AND WICKHAM, JEA: *Gritti-Stokes amputation for atherosclerotic gangrene.* Lancet 2:16–17, 1962.

MAZET, R, JR AND HENNESSY, CA: *Knee disarticulation: A new technique and a new knee-joint mechanism.* J Bone Joint Surg 48A:126–139, 1966.

MCCOLLOUGH, NC, III: *The dysvascular amputee.* Orthop Clin North Am 3:303–321, 1972.

MIDDLETON, MD AND WEBSTER, CU: *Clinical review of the Gritti-Stokes amputation.* Br Med J 2:574–576, 1962.

MURDOCH, G: *Levels of amputation and limiting factors.* Ann R Coll Surg Engl 40:204–216, 1967.

MURDOCH, G: *Knee-disarticulation amputation.* Bull Prosthet Res 10–9:14–18, 1968.

MURDOCH, G: *Amputation surgery in the lower extremity.* Prosthet Orthot Int 1:72–83, 1977.

NAYMAN, J: *Gritti-Stokes amputation for obliterative arterial disease associated with gangrene.* Med J Aust 1:441–444, 1964.

NEUMAN, LA AND JONES, RA: *Supracondylar amputation in the aged.* Calif Med 95:88–91, 1961.

NEWCOMBE, J: *Through-knee amputation.* Nurs Times 65:871–874, 1969.

NEWCOMBE, JF AND MARCUSON, RW: *Through-knee amputation.* Br J Surg 59:260–266, 1972.

PRIOROV, NN: *Amputation of the extremities and prosthesis in the U.S.S.R.* J Internat Coll Surgeons 8:13–19, 1945.

RADCLIFFE, CW: *Polycentric linkages as prosthetic knee mechanisms for the through-knee amputee.* Presentation at the World Congress of ISPO, INTERBOR, and APO in Montreux, Switzerland, Oct 1974.

REEVES, MM AND QUATTLEBAUM, FW: *The lateral flap technique in supracondylar amputations.* Surg Gynecol Obstet 102:751–756, 1956.

Report: Workshop on Knee-Disarticulation and Hip-Disarticulation Prostheses. Subcommittee on Design and Development, Committee on Prosthetics Research and Development, Division of Engineering, National Research Council, National Academy of Sciences, National Academy of Engineering, San Francisco, 1969.

RICHARDS, JF, JR AND PIERCE, JN: *Knee disarticulation successfully fitted with a PTS socket.* Inter-Clinic Info Bull 16:7–10, 17, 1977.

ROGERS, SP: *Amputation at the knee joint.* J Bone Joint Surg 22:973–979, 1940.

ROGERS, SP: *Amputation through the knee joint: A physiologic amputation.* Miss Valley Med J 62:174–176, 1940.

ROGERS, SP: *Amputation at the knee joint.* J Bone Joint Surg 44A:1697–1698, 1962.

SEATON, DG, WILSON, LA, AND SHEPHERD, WG: *An approach to the prosthetic fitting of the long femoral stump.* Med J Aust 2:718–722, 1970.

SHACKLETON, ME: *The Gritti-Stokes amputation: A reappraisal.* NZ Med J 65:226–229, 1966.

SMITH, N: *On amputation at the knee-joint.* Am Med Rev, Philadelphia 2:370–371, 1825.

SMITH, S: *Amputation at the knee-joint (Operation by W. Parker).* NY State J Med 9:307–330, 1852.

SMITH, S: *Amputation at the knee-joint by modified lateral flaps.* Am J Med Sci 59:33–36, 1870.

STAATS, TB: *Technical Manual for the O.H.C. Polycentric Knee Disarticulation Prosthesis.* United States Manufacturing Company, 1981.

STOKES, W: *On supra-condyloid amputation of the thigh.* Med-chir Trans London 53:175–186, 1870.

SYME, J: *Amputation at the knee.* Lon and Edin Mon J Med Sci 5:337–341, 1845.

SYME, J: *On amputation at the knee.* Edin Med J 11:871–874, 1866.

TAYLOR, GW: *Amputation of the lower limb for ischaemic disease.* Proc R Soc Med 60:69–70, 1967.

THOMPSON, RG: *Amputation in the lower extremity.* J Bone Joint Surg 45A:1723–1734, 1963.

UTTERBACK, TD AND ROHREN, DW: *Knee disarticulation as an amputation level.* J Trauma 13:116–120, 1973.

VITALI, M: *Rehabilitation of the amputee.* Proc R Soc Med 59:1–3, 1966.

VITALI, M AND HARRIS, EE: *Prosthetic management of the elderly lower limb amputee.* Clin Orthop 37:61–81, 1964.

WEALE, FE: *The supracondylar amputation with patellectomy.* Br J Surg 56:589–593, 1969.

WILSON, AB, JR: *Limb prosthetics: 1970.* Artificial Limbs 14:1–52, 1970.

ZARRUGH, MY AND RADCLIFFE, CW: *Simulation of swing phase dynamics in above-knee prostheses.* J Biomech 9:283–292, 1976.

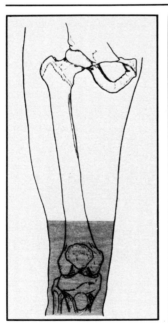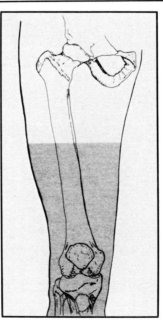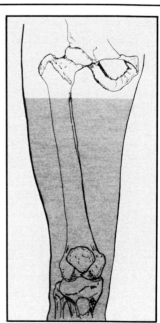

CHAPTER 11

ABOVE KNEE (AK)
(THIGH [Th], PARTIAL)

AMPUTATION LEVELS

**LONG AK (DISTAL ⅓) (THIGH [Th], PARTIAL [LOWER ⅓])
MID-THIGH (MIDDLE ⅓) (THIGH [Th], PARTIAL
   [MIDDLE ⅓])
SHORT AK (PROXIMAL ⅓) (THIGH [Th], PARTIAL
   [UPPER ⅓] [LESS THAN 5-CM (2-IN) LIMB])**

Historically, thigh amputations were the most common lower extremity amputations. In recent years, the ratio of mid-leg amputations to primary thigh amputations has increased. The major indications for primary above-knee amputation include: when gangrene has extended to the knee, or gas-forming infection has progressed toward the knee; recent thrombosis of the femoral or iliac artery without adequate collateral circulation for a mid-leg amputation; or when preservation of the knee is contraindicated because of disease. Modified above-knee amputations are performed for some malignant soft-tissue tumors that involve the adductor and hamstring muscles of the thigh. Although these muscles are completely removed, the procedure is less mutilating than an alternative hip disarticulation.

The only medical advantage of above-knee amputation over amputation below the knee is the greater chance of primary healing. An above-knee amputation should be considered if prosthetic rehabilitation is doubtful, if a prolonged convalescence presents a health threat, or if the healing capacity at the below-knee level is questionable.

OPERATION

The skin is marked at the proposed level of bone division. The skin flaps, which curve distally, are of equal anterior and posterior lengths whenever possible, but variations may be required. Incisions are made through the skin, subcutaneous tissue, and deep fascia along the skin flap lines. Thigh muscles and periosteum are divided cleanly to the bone at a length just beyond the most distal part of the skin flaps. If a myoplasty is performed, the thigh muscles are divided into four groups and are elevated from the femur back to the level of proposed bone section. The periosteum is raised from the bone back to the level of proposed bone section. The blood vessels are transected just proximal to the level of bone section. The nerves should be cut at a level that would ensure their being well covered by muscle and remote from the scar. If a neuroma becomes attached to the distal scar, it may displace during walking, causing pain. The femur is divided and the sharp peripheral edge of the cut femur is rounded with a rasp. If a periosteumosteoplasty is being performed, the medullary cavity is closed by suturing the periosteal flap over the end of the bone. Next, with the residual limb in a neutral position, the muscles are trimmed and sutured. The skin flaps are closed without undue tension.

ADVANTAGES OF ABOVE-KNEE AMPUTATION

1. The healing rate is greater than for the more distal amputations.

2. The residual limb is composed of a thick layer of soft tissue on all sides and is, therefore, somewhat easier to fit with a socket.
3. The average hospital stay is briefer for above-knee amputees than for below-knee amputees. This is probably because the healing rate is greater in above-knee amputees and fewer above-knee amputees are rehabilitated to walking with a prosthesis.
4. The average time taken to final rehabilitation with a prosthesis is shorter for an above-knee amputee than for a below-knee amputee. This is usually because the below-knee residual limb requires a more careful fit since there is less soft tissue present.

DISADVANTAGES OF ABOVE-KNEE AMPUTATION

1. Mortality is greater than for distal amputations. This may be due to the frailty of the patient subjected to above-knee amputation rather than to the shock of the operation per se.
2. Amputation through muscle bellies results in greater blood loss and a higher incidence of shock than amputation through tendinous insertions, as in a knee disarticulation.
3. Cut muscle bellies retract, atrophy, and lose their function. Myoplasty will prevent this problem; however, myoplasty is seldom performed.
4. Shaping of the residual limb to its final size takes longer than with other amputation sites.
5. Rehabilitation to walking with a prosthesis is less successful than with more distal amputations.
6. The limb is not end-bearing, as with a transcondylar or knee-disarticulation amputation.
7. In children, the distal femoral epiphysis is removed; thus, the final limb length may be very short at maturity. Another problem is that the bone may show overgrowth relative to the soft tissue. These problems do not exist following disarticulation.

MYOPLASTY AND MYODESIS

Myoplasty and myodesis are methods of reinserting divided muscles. In a myoplasty, the sectioned muscles are attached to opposing muscles; in a myodesis, the sectioned muscles are attached to the bone. If severed muscles are not sutured, they retract. The more distal the amputation, the greater the retraction. If the skin is adherent, puckering or wrinkling of the skin results as the muscles retract. In amputations through the thigh, muscle imbalance results. An abduction contracture is likely to develop if most of the adductor muscles have been severed. A flexion contracture may also develop since the hamstring muscles have been cut. Flexion and abduction contractures are more pronounced in the shorter limbs. Lack of functional muscle activity results in a disturbance of blood flow—venous stasis—especially in the terminal area. Local evidence on the skin includes small brown petechiae, black and blue discoloration, hyperkeratosis, or ulcerations. The skin is cooler than on the sound side and has less hair growth.

Myoplasty or myodesis helps to restore muscle balance, as well as circulation, by maintaining active muscle function. The hamstrings are thus able to assist in hip extension and thereby stabilize a prosthetic knee. Muscles are sutured slightly shorter than resting length for optimum efficiency. Thigh muscles, by being able to contract strongly, help reduce weight-bearing on the ischial seat. Myoplasty also produces a smoother, more rounded, cylindrical distal surface, which enhances fitting with a prosthesis. Because the surface area is larger, unit pressure is reduced and proprioception is enhanced. After myoplasty, phantom pain is usually decreased or nonexistent, and normal sensation often returns. Although there are many benefits from myoplasty, it is rarely performed by most surgeons.

DEDERICH METHOD

In 1963, Rolf Dederich of Bonn, West Germany, described a method of suturing the adductor muscles to the abductors and the iliotibial band over the end of the femur and anchoring them by passing some sutures through the periosteum in front of and behind the bone to prevent the muscles from slipping off of the end of the bone. This layer is covered at right angles by a second pair of muscles, the anterior and posterior thigh muscles, which are sutured to each other and to the underlying muscle layer. Redundancy or overlapping of the opposing muscles is avoided. This method is occasionally complicated by the muscle loops sliding off of the end of the bone or forming a painful bursa from movement of the muscle loop over the end of the bone. Excessive tension will cause the sutures to tear.

WEISS METHOD

The method described by Marion Weiss of Poland in 1966 differs in that the divided muscles are anchored level with the distal end of the bone by passing sutures through multiple drill holes in the bone. In the Weiss technique, the muscles do not slide off of the end of the bone and the limb is more tapered.

MURDOCH METHOD

George Murdoch's technique, developed in Dundee, Scotland, and described in 1968, is a combination of the Dederich and Weiss techniques. The muscles on the medial, lateral, and posterior sides of the thigh are attached to the bone by the Weiss technique (Fig. 11-1). The anterior thigh muscles are carried over the end of the bone and sutured to the hamstrings by the Dederich technique (Fig. 11-2).

PERIOSTEUMOSTEOPLASTY

In the normal limb, blood is forced into the medullary cavity during muscular contraction, which increases the intramedullary pressure. In 1959, H.E. Loon reported that if the cut end of the bone is left open after amputation, the intramedullary pressure will be zero and venous stasis will occur. Since a closed system is necessary for the hydrodynamic effect, closure of the cut end of the bone with periosteumosteoplasty is performed by some surgeons. In many cases, pain at the end of the limb is less following osteoplasty.

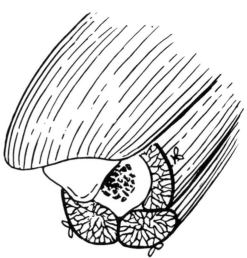

FIGURE 11-1. Murdoch technique: The adductor muscles and lateral and medial hamstrings are sutured to the bone. An anterior periosteal flap is used to cover the end of the bone to close off the medullary canal. The quadriceps is left long. (From Murdoch, G: *Myoplastic techniques.* Bull Prosthet Res 10-9:11, 1968, with permission.)

FRACTURE

Occasionally, above-knee amputees sustain fractures of the femoral neck, shaft, or intertrochanteric area. Successful results have been reported with open reduction and internal fixation with nails or compression plates. Care should be taken in the placement of the scar so that it does not interfere with the functional use of a prosthesis. If a femoral shaft fracture is treated closed and a malunion results, the malunion may be in a position so that adequate fitting cannot be obtained.

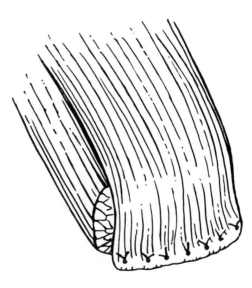

FIGURE 11-2. Murdoch technique: The quadriceps muscle is drawn over the end of the bone and sutured to the hamstrings. (From Murdoch, G: *Myoplastic techniques.* Bull Prosthet Res 10-9:11, 1968, with permission.)

MORTALITY

Within 30 days after an above-knee amputation, mortality is usually 15 to 30 percent. Most of these amputees are elderly and have generalized arteriosclerotic vascular disease. Many are hypertensive. The leading causes of death among recent amputees are myocardial infarction, strokes, pulmonary embolism, and sepsis. In contrast, the operative mortality for knee-disarticulation amputations is less than for above-knee amputations.

PROSTHESES

SOCKETS

PLUG-FIT

This socket predominated before the introduction of the quadrilateral socket in the 1950s. The plug-fit socket has a conical interior that is essentially the same shape as the exterior of the residual limb (Fig. 11-3). The socket is larger at the top and tapers to a small diameter distally. The circumference of the socket is usually the same as the circumference of the limb for which it was made. A socket that matches the limb circumference does not provide optimum pressure distribution because it does not make allowances for relative differences in tissue firmness. Greater pressure is applied to firm areas and less to soft areas with this type of socket. Because the end of the above-knee amputation limb is small and bony, it cannot tolerate the high unit pressure of full end weight-bearing. Breakdown of the soft tissues between the end of the bone and the socket would result. Weight-bearing in the plug-fit socket thus occurs around the entire socket on the remaining soft tissue of the residual thigh. Tissue, however, tends to be displaced upward, which causes fleshy rolls above the brim and muscular atrophy within the socket. Socket-limb pressure is not uniform because the residual limb is not uniformly firm throughout, especially when the muscles are active. Many amputees wear plug-fit sockets successfully. It is possible to keep the socket-limb pressures below the critical level because of the relatively large surface area of the above-knee amputation limb. This socket is suspended with a pelvic belt or shoulder suspenders.

QUADRILATERAL

Virtually all above-knee amputees are currently fitted with a quadrilateral socket, regardless of the type of suspension used, because it allows for better muscular control of the prosthetic leg and provides more comfort than a plug-fit socket. Although the distal end of the quadrilateral socket may either be open or may provide total contact, the latter has become very popular in recent years because it achieves better pressure distribution and more sensory feedback and promotes venous return.

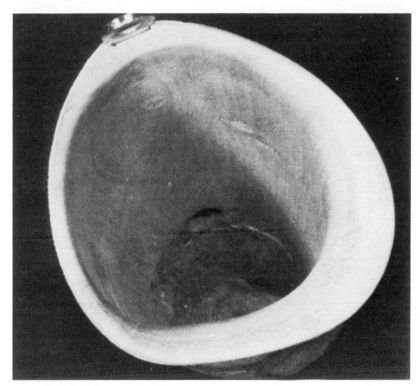

FIGURE 11-3. Plug-fit socket for above-knee prosthesis. (From *Orthopaedic Appliances Atlas, Vol 2, Artificial Limbs.* JW Edwards, Ann Arbor, Michigan, 1960, p 293, with permission.)

SOCKET SHAPE

The quadrilateral socket gets its name from the proximal shape, which is essentially quadrangular (Fig. 11-4). This shape is different from the cross-sectional shape of the limb. The socket is characterized by reliefs and bulges on the inner surface. Reliefs—or concavities—reduce pressure on relatively firm tissue, such as tendons, muscles, and bony prominences. The socket allows space for muscle contraction and thus reduces disuse atrophy and subsequent loss of function. The socket's bulges—or convexities—press on soft areas of the limb to provide load-sharing. Variations in shape depend on the muscular development of the individual residual limb (Fig. 11-5).

POSTERIOR WALL

The inner surface of the posterior wall of the socket is a flat surface that slants anteriorly as it goes distally so the limb is set in initial flexion. Below the brim, the socket is contoured for the hamstring muscles. The posterior wall provides the surface against which the limb pushes to keep the trunk erect and to maintain knee extension. The outer surface of the posterior wall is flat to prevent rolling so that the wearer may sit in a stable manner. The exterior is padded to protect the socket surface, absorb the sound of impact on a chair, and protect the wearer's clothing from friction against a chair.

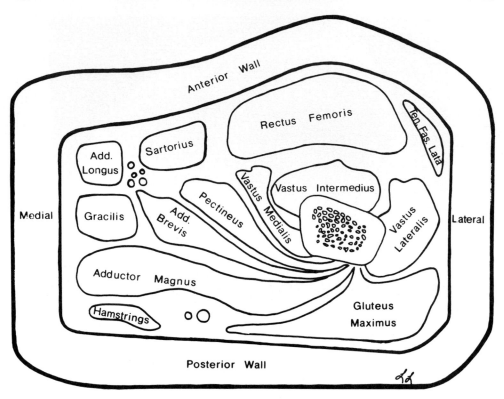

FIGURE 11-4. Cross section through an above-knee quadrilateral socket at the level of the ischial tuberosity.

POSTERIOR BRIM

The brim of the posterior wall is horizontal, parallel to the floor. The ischial seat, a thickening of the medial part of the posterior brim under the ischial tuberosity, provides the major weight-bearing area. Medially, the proximal wall slants upward and posteriorly so as not to produce excessive pressure on the hamstring tendons. The lateral part of the brim, the gluteal shelf, contacts the gluteus maximus for additional weight-bearing and has a slanted relief to permit gluteal bulging during walking. If the muscle is firm, the proximal posterior wall may flare as much as 10 degrees, or as little as 7 degrees if it is soft. In very muscular limbs, the ischial seat may be reduced in size because more weight is borne on the well-developed muscles of the thigh.

MEDIAL WALL

The medial wall is vertical and parallel to the sagittal plane. The wall prevents medial movement of the residual limb within the socket, especially during mid-stance. The wall forces the thigh laterally against the lateral wall, which allows the abductors to maintain a level pelvis. A relief channel with a generous proximal flare is provided in the anteromedial corner of the socket for the adductor longus tendon. The anterior-posterior (AP) measurement is the horizontal length of the medial wall at the ischial level, which should be approximately 1.3 cm (½ in) minus the actual distance from the

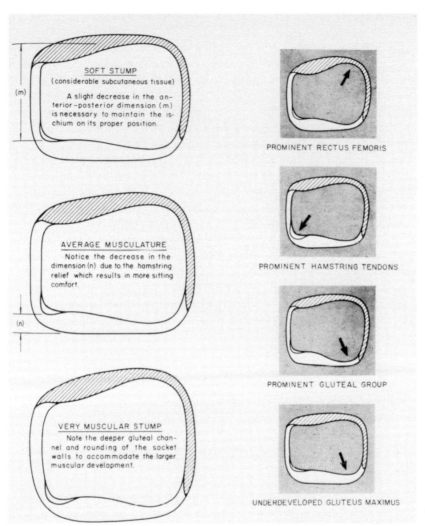

FIGURE 11-5. The influence of muscular development on the shape of the quadrilateral socket at the ischial level. (From Radcliffe, CW: *Functional considerations in the fitting of above-knee prostheses.* Artificial Limbs 2:47, 1955, with permission.)

ischial tuberosity to the adductor longus tendon. This will maintain the ischium on the ischial seat. The medial wall should be high enough to contain the soft tissues of the medial thigh, obviating an adductor roll.

MEDIAL BRIM

The brim of the medial wall is horizontal and at the same height as the posterior brim. If there is marked tissue redundancy, the medial brim may be slightly lower than the posterior brim but no more than 0.3 to 0.6 cm (1/8 to 1/4 in). The socket should not press on the pubic ramus.

ANTERIOR WALL

The weight line passes anterior to the ischial tuberosity and thus tends to rotate the pelvis forward, causing the tuberosity to slide off of the ischial seat. A high anterior wall provides counterpressure to check this movement. A convexity on the anterior wall, Scarpa's bulge, is located over Scarpa's (the femoral) triangle. Scarpa's bulge exerts posteriorly directed forces on the limb to maintain the ischial tuberosity on its seat. Scarpa's triangle, which is bordered by the inguinal ligament proximally, the adductor longus tendon medially, and the sartorius muscle laterally, can sustain appropriately applied pressure for a prolonged period of time. The amount of pressure exerted depends upon the distance between the anterior and posterior walls and the contour of the bulge, which should occupy the medial two thirds of the anterior wall, with the apex of the bulge in the same sagittal plane at the same height as the ischial seat. The AP dimension is critical for proper fit. The anterior wall is about 6.5 cm (2 1/2 in) higher than the posterior wall. If the anterior wall is too low, a roll of flesh will bulge over the top of the brim. For very short residual limbs, the anterior wall may be even higher. A high wall provides a relatively large surface for the distribution of forces. Too high an anterior wall, however, limits hip flexion and presses on the anterior superior iliac spine during sitting. The prosthesis may even be pushed off if suction suspension is being used. The anterior brim is flared from the inside out so that it will not cause inguinal pressure when the amputee sits. A channel for the rectus femoris muscle is provided in the anterolateral aspect of the socket.

LATERAL WALL

The lateral wall is as high as the anterior wall. For the very short residual limb, the lateral wall is extended proximally above the greater trochanter to increase stability and control. On the inside of the socket, the wall inclines medially as it goes distally, that is, the limb is set in about 10 degrees adduction, to enhance function of the hip abductors. This simulates the adduction angle of the sound femur. Reliefs are often provided over the distal lateral end of the femur and the greater trochanter. The lateral wall is contoured to distribute pressure evenly over the lateral side of the residual limb as the limb is drawn forcefully against the wall by contraction of the gluteus medius and minimus muscles during the stance phase of gait. Mediolateral pelvic stability is maintained by pressure of the femur against the lateral wall of the socket. Unit counterpressure against the lateral aspect of the residual limb is less with a long limb than with a short limb. Lateral trunk bending toward the prosthetic side during stance phase will lessen the force against the limb. The upper portion of the lateral wall curves slightly inward to enclose the greater trochanter. This prevents lateral displacement of the limb, which would allow the pubic ramus to slip into the socket, resulting in discomfort.

Inadequate support on the lateral side will permit the pelvis to drop on the normal side, resulting in an uncomfortable crotch pressure as the pubic ramus contacts the medial brim. The amputee usually compensates by leaning over the prosthesis and walking with a list, or by walking with a wide base gait, which results in side-to-side swaying.

INITIAL FLEXION ANGLE

The socket is set in initial flexion to enable the amputee to more effectively use the hip extensors and thus to keep the trunk erect and assist voluntary control of the prosthetic knee. If flexion is inadequate, the amputee will experience increased lumbar lordosis as the prosthesis is extended. Initial socket flexion also aids in the use of the ischial and gluteal areas for weight-bearing and maintains the tuberosity on the ischial seat.

In normal locomotion, one leg is located 15 degrees posterior to a vertical line from the hip axis when a normal stride is taken with the other leg. This 15 degrees is obtained by a composite of 3 degrees of anterior pelvic tilt, 5 degrees of extension at the hip, and 7 degrees of knee flexion (Fig. 11-6).

In the above-knee amputee, the prosthetic knee is maintained in complete extension from heel-strike to toe-off; thus, the normal 7 degrees of knee flexion is lost. Only 8 degrees of displacement of the leg behind the vertical line from the hip occurs if 3 degrees of anterior pelvic rotation is maintained (Fig. 11-7).

Since the amputee cannot flex the prosthetic knee to obtain the 15 degrees of extension, posterior to vertical, stride length on the sound side is shortened. The remaining 7 degrees must come from some source other than the knee if normal gait is to be simulated. Above-knee amputees are able to anteriorly rotate the pelvis up to 10 degrees over a long period of time without any apparent strain to the lumbar spine. If anterior pelvic rotation is increased from 3 degrees to 10 degrees to compensate, then the hip-ankle angle will be able to come to 15 degrees posterior to the vertical line.

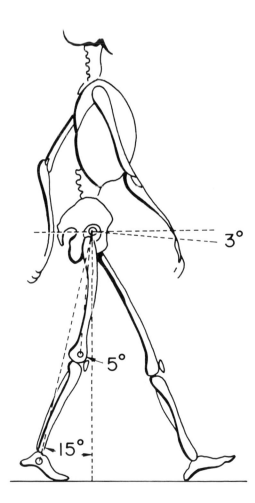

FIGURE 11-6. The right ankle is 15 degrees posterior to a vertical line from the hip axis during a normal stride. The pelvis anteriorly rotates 3 degrees and the thigh extends 5 degrees. The remaining 7 degrees are due to knee flexion. (From Hampton, FL: *Prosthetic principles in the lower extremity amputee.* Orthop Clin North Am 3:343, 1972, with permission.)

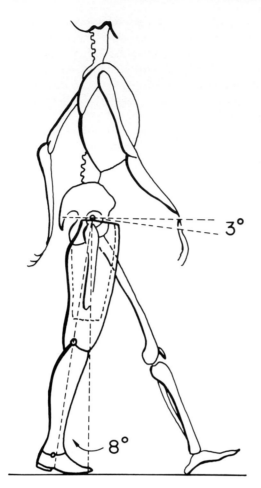

FIGURE 11-7. The above-knee amputee is attempting to walk with the normal 3 degrees of anterior pelvic rotation and 5 degrees of hip extension. The prosthetic knee remains in complete knee extension. The ankle is only 8 degrees posterior to the vertical because the 7 degrees of knee flexion is lost. Stride length with the sound leg is shortened. (From Hampton, FL: *Prosthetic principles in the lower extremity amputee.* Orthop Clin North Am 3:344, 1972, with permission.)

If the amputee does not have 5 degrees of extension at the hip because of a flexion contracture, or if the prosthesis is not designed to compensate for this problem, then the lumbar spine will go into an excessive lordosis as a normal-length stride is taken on the sound side. To avoid excessive arching of the back, the amputee has to shorten the stride length on the sound side. If the lumbar spine has been fused and an excessive lordosis cannot occur, then the amputee will be forced to walk with a short stride on the sound side if hip extension is less than 5 degrees on the amputated side.

The socket is set in about 5 degrees of initial flexion for those who have normal hip extension. This position puts a slight stretch on the gluteus maximus, which enables it to contract more efficiently, thus improving hip extension force. The formula used to calculate the amount of initial flexion that should be built into the socket is as follows:

Initial Socket Flexion = Fixed Flexion Contracture at the hip minus 10 degrees (pelvic tilt) plus 15 degrees (desired hip-to-ankle line posterior to vertical).

$$\text{ISF} = \text{FFC} - 10 \text{ degrees} + 15 \text{ degrees}$$

If the amputee has a hip flexion contracture, then initial flexion in the socket can compensate for the contracture. For example, for a 5-degree flexion contracture, 10

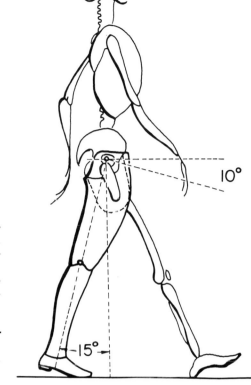

FIGURE 11-8. Compensatory anterior pelvic tilt to 10 degrees allows the prosthetic ankle to move 15 degrees posterior to the vertical line. With a short limb, a 30-degree flexion contracture can be accommodated for by 35 degrees of initial socket flexion. (From Hampton, FL: *Prosthetic principles in the lower extremity amputee.* Orthop Clin North Am 3:344, 1972, with permission.)

degrees of initial flexion should be built into the socket. With very short residual limbs, it is possible to build in as much as 35 degrees of initial flexion, which would accommodate a 30-degree hip flexion contracture (Fig. 11-8). If the residual limb is long, initial flexion may be limited to no more than 5 degrees without an unsightly bulge in the anterior part of the socket and a compromise of knee stability.

ADDUCTION ANGLE

When the amputee bears weight on the prosthesis, the femur is pulled laterally by the hip abductors. The amputated femur moves within a mass of tissue before it is stabilized against the lateral wall. If the socket is not set in adduction, the excursion of the gluteus medius is exhausted before the muscle can act to prevent the pelvis from dropping excessively on the sound side. If the socket is set in adduction, the amputated femur can move laterally only slightly when the gluteus medius contracts.

Adduction of the limb also places the hip abductors on stretch, which enhances their function. The adductors are relaxed when the socket is set in adduction and thus can be flattened against the medial wall, helping to avoid an adductor roll.

The adduction angle of the lateral wall should accommodate the adduction angle of the femur and should place the prosthetic heel about 5 cm (2 in) from the heel of the sound foot. The amount of adduction possible and the amount needed increase the more proximal the amputation. However, the above-knee amputee with a short limb length usually cannot tolerate the high unit pressure, so the abductors have to be limited by setting the socket in more abduction rather than adduction. To compensate, the amputee has to lean over the prosthesis somewhat to shift the weight line closer to the support line, resulting in excessive side sway. Abduction contractures are common, especially with the shorter limbs, and are very difficult to correct. Severe abduction deformity can make proper alignment impossible without excessive pressure on the limb. Abduction contractures are often accompanied by flexion and outward rotation of the femur, particularly if the limb is short.

MEDIOLATERAL STABILITY

Mediolateral stability is obtained by a medial position of the foot to the socket, an adducted position of the residual limb, and firm support to the residual limb by the lateral wall of the socket to allow efficient use of the hip abductors.

SUSPENSION

The quadrilateral socket may be suspended by suction alone, suction with auxiliary suspension (Silesian bandage or pelvic belt), or suspension without suction (Silesian bandage, pelvic belt, shoulder suspenders, or a combination of these). The quadrilateral socket offers more versatility in choices of suspension than does the plug-fit socket.

DISTAL SOCKET DESIGNS

Distal Chamber or Open-Ended

In this design, the distal end of the residual limb does not contact the socket (Fig. 11-9). The space—or air chamber—in the lower end of the socket may be closed or opened. If the air chamber is closed with a valve, then suction suspension can be obtained. Some amputees have problems with the open-ended suction-type socket. Skin appears to be less tolerant of suction than of positive pressure. The suction space is unphysiologic, creating what has been called a "pneumothorax" in the prosthetic system. If the distal chamber is open, other suspension methods must be used. The bottom of the socket is usually about 5 cm (2 in) below the residual limb.

    Edema may develop in the distal limb because of proximal constriction impairing venous return. Stretching of the skin over the distal end of the bone along with the distal edema can result in dermatologic disorders, such as verrucous hyperplasia, and eventual ulceration. The greater the amount of soft tissue at the end of the limb, the greater the potential amount of swelling. For this reason, it has been recommended by some prosthetists that the end of the limb be covered with skin and fascia only when the open-ended socket is to be used.

Total Contact

In the total-contact socket, all of the limb, including the distal end, contacts the socket. Although the distal limb provides some support, it is not enough to be called end weight-bearing. It does, however, reduce proximal pressure significantly. A special one-way valve for expulsion of air is positioned near the bottom of the socket, usually in the distal anteromedial corner.

    The total-contact socket promotes venous return and helps to prevent edema by acting as an external pump. During stance phase, the pressure between the limb and the socket increases and venous return is aided. During swing phase, the pressure is

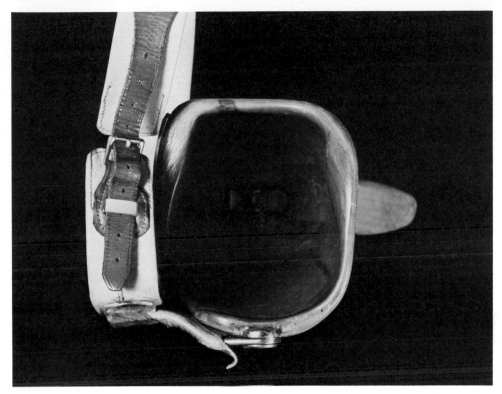

FIGURE 11-9. Above-knee prosthesis with open-ended quadrilateral socket.

negative and blood flows back into the limb. Even when the amputee is sitting, the lack of space at the end of the limb prevents edema. The total-contact socket gives a more uniform distribution of pressure and thus improves comfort and minimizes the possibility of tissue damage. The intimate fit of the socket to the contours of the residual limb enhances suspension, no matter which method is used. The total contact allows optimum use of suction suspension. It enables better control of the prosthesis through better sensory feedback and less relative motion between the residual limb and the socket. The intimate fit limits residual limb motion and thus the tendency to stretch the skin over the distal end of the bone. Excessive perspiration is sometimes a problem with total contact.

The distal socket can be either hard (plastic or wooden socket without an end pad) or soft. The hard end is more hygienic and does not alter in contour after years of use. A soft pad, usually of foam or sponge rubber, is used if the distal end of the residual limb is particularly sensitive. The pad allows femoral displacement without painful impingement and enables total contact during swing phase as well as stance phase.

SUSPENSION DEVICES

SILESIAN BANDAGE OR BELT

The Silesian bandage attaches, via a swivel connection, to the lateral wall of the prosthesis just proximal and posterior to the greater trochanter. The webbing belt passes across the pelvis posteriorly, goes between the iliac crest and the trochanter, and attaches to the anterior midline of the prosthesis at the height of the ischial tuberosity (Fig. 11-10). The anterior attachment may be bifurcated or may have a single attachment. The double attachment is the original Silesian bandage and the single attachment is a modification. In the original version, a D-ring is attached to the anterior end of the belt. A yolk passes through the D-ring and is attached at two points on the anterior socket. The bandage should not bind or cause excessive restriction when the amputee walks or sits. It is more comfortable and weighs less than the pelvic belt.

In addition to suspension, the Silesian bandage may be used to stabilize the above-knee prosthesis against rotation and abduction. Although the bandage prevents lateral displacement of the socket, it does not increase mediolateral stability during stance phase. Because of the high attachment on the lateral wall and low attachment on the anterior wall, stabilization without restriction of movement is possible.

The Silesian bandage is most often used as auxiliary suspension with the suction socket, particularly in warm climates where a build-up of perspiration can result in a loss of suction. In such cases, the amputee benefits psychologically from the feeling of security gained by having a belt around the pelvis. After a transition period, the amputee may gain enough confidence to use suction suspension only.

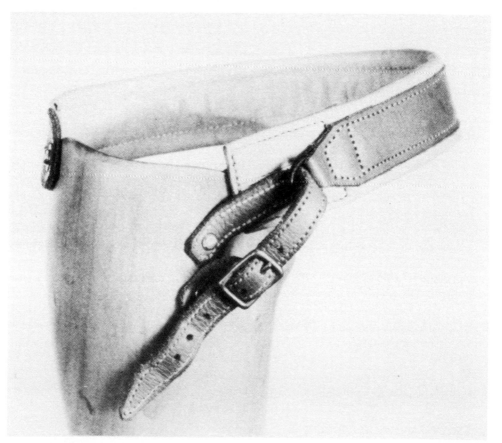

FIGURE 11-10. Silesian bandage for suspension of above-knee prosthesis. (From *Orthopaedic Appliances Atlas, Vol 2, Artificial Limbs.* JW Edwards, Ann Arbor, Michigan, 1960, p 209, with permission.)

PELVIC BELT

The pelvic belt is made of either leather and metal (usually aluminum) or polypropylene. It is connected to the prosthesis by a metal or polypropylene hip joint that is fastened to the superior lateral aspect of the socket. The axis of the hip joint is located about 2.5 cm (1 in) above and 1.3 cm (½ in) ahead of the greater trochanter, which corresponds to the axis of the normal hip joint (Fig. 11-11). The joint center should clear the lateral brim. The hip joint may be as much as 4 cm (1½ in) above the trochanter if the skeletal structure is large, or as little as 1.3 cm (½ in) if the skeletal structure is small. The hip joint should move in a plane parallel to the line of progression. A few degrees (2 to 3) of inward rotation may be tolerated. The pelvic belt encircles the pelvis between the iliac crest and the greater trochanter. The upper arm of the joint should be curved inwardly to fit snugly between the iliac crest and the trochanter. The belt should conform to the contour of the pelvis, distributing pressure evenly.

The belt not only suspends the prosthesis, but also helps to control rotation and augments mediolateral stability. Even a poorly aligned prosthesis may be worn with some degree of success with pelvic-belt suspension. The hip joint tends to restrict motions of the hip and, if improperly set, can cause discomfort when the amputee sits. It is sometimes difficult to fit the amputee with sitting comfort without sacrificing stability. Hip joints can tear or stain clothing. Noise, wear, and occasional breakage create

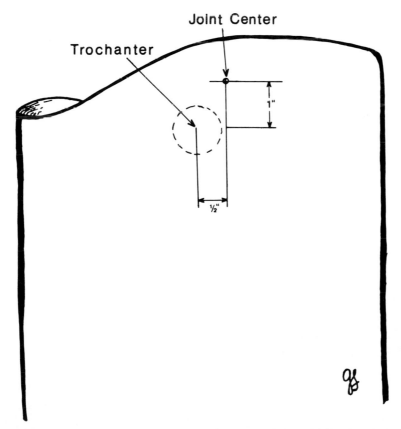

FIGURE 11-11. The axis of the hip joint of the pelvic band is located above and ahead of the greater trochanter of the femur.

maintenance problems. Pistoning usually exceeds that with suction sockets. Perspiration tends to be absorbed by the leather, which becomes unsanitary and can cause skin problems. The appearance is bulkier than with suction suspension, and the prosthesis weighs 0.5 to 1.4 kg (1 to 3 lb) more. Since rotation is prevented by the belt, rotational forces sometimes result in belt breakage. Faulty prosthetic alignment is more easily tolerated than with suction suspension only. The amputee's gait is usually poorer than when a suction socket is worn.

SUCTION

The first suction socket was patented by Dubois Parmelee of New York in 1863 (Fig. 11-12). In Germany, its use was rather widespread by the 1930s. In the United States,

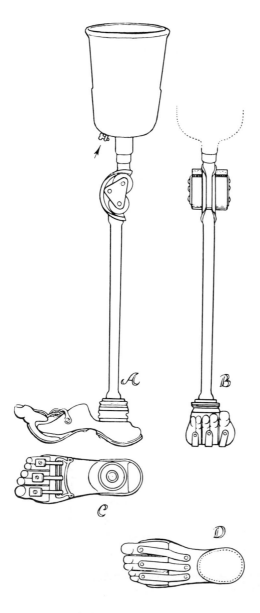

FIGURE 11-12. The D.D. Parmelee prosthesis with suction socket. (From *Historical development of artificial limbs.* In *Orthopaedic Appliances Atlas, Vol 2, Artificial Limbs.* JW Edwards, Ann Arbor, Michigan, 1960, p 11, with permission.)

however, it was not prevalent until the late 1940s. Suction suspension may be used with either the total-contact or the closed distal air chamber socket. The valve at the distal-medial (or lateral) aspect of the socket allows air to be expelled from the socket upon weight-bearing. Adjustments can be made to change the air leakage rate. If the leakage rate is too great, there may be excessive pistoning or loss of suspension. Edema may result if the leakage rate is too small.

During the swing phase of gait, negative pressure within the socket augmented by muscle tension holds the socket on the residual limb. The unsupported prosthesis will slowly slip if the amputee completely relaxes the muscles of the residual limb. A negative pressure of 105.5 g per sq cm (1 $\frac{1}{2}$ lb per sq in) is sufficient to suspend the prosthesis. Greater suction increases the feeling of security but can cause edema. Positive pressure develops during stance phase, which helps to control edema and gives the amputee a sense of "walking on air." Too much positive pressure tends to push the residual limb out of the socket.

No sock is worn with the suction socket, but a donning sock is used to help pull the residual limb down into the socket. The sock is removed by pulling it through the valve hole. Since suction suspension requires that residual limb muscles control the prosthesis to a greater extent than is the case with other modes of suspension, proper alignment is critical. Minimal alignment stability is needed because muscular control of the prosthesis is greater. Also, more sophisticated knee mechanisms can be used because of the finer neuromuscular control. Limb muscles usually become hypertrophic when the amputee uses a suction socket, rather than becoming atrophic as with other types of suspension. To avoid edema of the limb, enlarging the socket to accommodate hypertrophied muscles may eventually be necessary. Better suction is obtained by having proper socket contours than by having a tight fit. A close, accurate fit is essential because the socket must be airtight. If much difficulty is encountered in removing the donning sock, then the fit is too tight.

If the amputee has a very short residual limb, obtaining suspension with suction will be difficult, although limbs as short as 7.6 cm (3 in) from the perineum have been fitted successfully. It is usually necessary to use auxiliary suspension, such as a pelvic belt or Silesian bandage, with suction in marginal cases. A cylindrical limb with only slight tapering maintains better suction than a conical limb. A large flabby mass of soft tissue beyond the end of the bone is very undesirable and may require surgical revision before a suction socket can be used successfully.

If the amputee is timid or initially reluctant to use suction suspension alone, then a Silesian bandage may be prescribed for auxiliary suspension. Auxiliary suspension is usually discarded after adaptation. If the amputee fails to adapt to the suction suspension with a Silesian bandage, then conversion to pelvic-belt suspension is common.

A suction socket is contraindicated if there are marked volumetric fluctuations in the residual limb. The amputee should maintain a stable body weight. Since the musculature of the residual limb hypertrophies during training, a slight weight reduction can be tolerated during this time. If excessive subcutaneous fat is present, the limb will shrink considerably after the amputee wears the socket for a while, thus necessitating a liner or a new socket.

Many failures in the use of the suction socket have been attributed to psychological or emotional difficulties. Amputees who are impatient, unreasonable, easily discouraged, or uncooperative will likely be poor candidates for a suction socket. The amputee and clinical personnel must be willing to devote the time necessary for adequate fitting and training.

The suction socket is sometimes difficult to don correctly. Suction may "choke" the end of the residual limb, causing skin irritation. The socket may be uncomfortable in the sitting position. If some suction is lost, the socket may make an objectionable noise when weight is put on the prosthesis. Perspiration is a problem with all suction sockets, especially in warm climates.

The suction socket is more cosmetic and comfortable than other forms of suspension because the bulk and weight of external belts and straps are eliminated and the amputee walks in a more natural manner. The amputee has more freedom of motion, particularly the lack of restraint to rotation, and less interference with clothing. The amputee is required to use the remaining musculature of the limb more than with other suspension devices. Many amputees claim that the suction socket prosthesis feels more a part of them than non–suction socket prostheses and offers better control and proprioception. Piston action between the socket and limb is reduced. The alternating pressure variation improves limb circulation. No medical difficulties have been attributed to the long-term effect of reduced pressure on the limb. If the suction socket is unsuccessful, it can easily be converted to pelvic belt suspension. Most failures are due to the lack of experience or expertise on the part of the prosthetist or to improper training of the amputee.

SHOULDER SUSPENDERS

Shoulder suspenders are used only rarely, primarily in cases where the amputee has worn a prosthesis for many years and refuses a more modern suspension system. Occasionally, suspenders are a last resort when other means of suspension cannot be used or are inadequate. Shoulder-harness suspension was generally replaced by pelvic-belt suspension in the 1940s.

BIBLIOGRAPHY

APPOLDT, FA, BENNETT, L, AND CONTINI, R: *The results of slip measurements in above-knee suction sockets.* Bull Prosthet Res 10–10:106–112, 1968.

APPOLDT, FA, BENNETT, L, AND CONTINI, R: *Tangential pressure measurements in above-knee suction sockets.* Bull Prosthet Res 10–13:70–86, 1970.

BADDELEY, RM AND FULFORD, JC: *A trial of conservative amputations for lesions of the feet in diabetes mellitus.* Br J Surg 52:38–43, 1965.

Below-Knee and Above-Knee Prostheses. A Report of a Workshop Sponsored by the Committee on Prosthetics Research and Development, Division of Medical Sciences, National Research Council, National Academy of Sciences, 1973.

BERME, N, PURDEY, CR, AND SOLOMONIDIS, SE: *Measure of prosthetic alignment.* Artificial Limbs 2:73–75, 1978.

BIEDERMANN, WG: *Management of short above-knee amputees.* Orthot Pros 30:21–29, 1976.

BIEDERMANN, WG: *Management of short above-knee amputees.* In *Selected Readings: A Review of Orthotics and Prosthetics.* The American Orthotic and Prosthetic Association, Washington, DC, 1980, pp 206–215.

BRADHAM, RR AND SMOAK, RD: *Amputations of the lower extremity: Used for arteriosclerosis obliterans.* Arch Surg 90:60–64, 1965.

BURGESS, EM: *The stabilization of muscles in lower extremity amputations.* J Bone Joint Surg 50A:1486–1487, 1968.

CANTY, TJ: *Amputations and recent developments in artificial limbs.* US Armed Forces Med J 3:1147–1152, 1952.

CANTY, TJ: *Construction, Fitting and Alignment for the U.S. Navy Soft Closed End Plastic Above-Knee Socket.* Navy Prosthetic Research Laboratory Amputation Center, U.S. Naval Hospital, Oakland, California, 1955.

CARP, L: *Midthigh amputations for arteriosclerotic and diabetic gangrene: Analysis of one hundred thirteen consecutive amputations in one hundred eight patients, 1939-1952.* Arch Surg 66:115–125, 1953.

CHODERA, JD: *Czechoslovakian above-knee socket design.* In MURDOCH, G (ED): *Prosthetic and Orthotic Practice.* Edward Arnold & Co, London, 1970, pp 219–224.

CHODERA, JD: *Relation between the anatomical properties and output of the thigh stump.* In MURDOCH, G (ED): *Prosthetic and Orthotic Practice.* Edward Arnold & Co, London, 1970, pp 181–189.

CLAUGUS, CE, ET AL: *Amputations of the lower extremity for arteriosclerosis.* Arch Surg 76:992–996, 1958.

COLT, JD AND LEE, PY: *Mortality rate of the above-the-knee amputation for arteriosclerotic gangrene: A critical evaluation.* Angiology 23:205–210, 1972.

COOL, JC: *Linear valves for small flows.* Med Biol Eng 8:165–169, 1970.

DALE, WA AND CAPPS, W, JR: *Major leg and thigh amputations: Ten-year survey of results.* Surgery 46:333–342, 1959.

DEDERICH, R: *Stump correction by muscle-plastic procedure.* In *Prosthetics International, Proceedings of the Second International Prosthetics Course, Committee on Prostheses, Braces and Technical Aids, International Society for the Welfare of Cripples.* Copenhagen, 1960, pp 59–61.

DEDERICH, R: *Plastic treatment of the muscles and bone in amputation surgery: A method designed to produce physiological conditions in the stump.* J Bone Joint Surg 45B:60–66, 1963.

DEDERICH, R: *Technique of myoplastic amputations.* Ann R Coll Surg 40:222–227, 1967.

DILLARD, JE: *A.K. air-cushion sockets.* Orthot Pros 24:32–34, 1970.

ERBACK, JR: *Hydraulic prostheses for above-knee amputees.* J Am Phys Ther Assoc 43:105–110, 1963.

ERIKSON, U AND JAMES, U: *Roentgenological study of certain stump-socket relationships in above-knee amputees with special regard to tissue proportions, socket fit and attachment stability.* Ups J Med Sci 78:203–214, 1973.

FICKE, AJ AND OWENS, WF: *Femoral shaft fractures and the above-knee amputee: Use of the compression plate. A report of three cases.* Clin Orthop 87:200–203, 1972.

FOORT, J: *Adjustable-brim fitting of the total-contact above-knee socket.* Biomechanics Laboratory, University of California at San Francisco and Berkeley, 1963.

FREED, MM AND CHARETTEE, EE: *Rehabilitation after amputation of the lower extremity for malignancy.* Arch Phys Med Rehabil 45:564–570, 1964.

FULFORD, GE: *The surgery of the above-knee amputation.* In MURDOCH, G (ED): *Prosthetic and Orthotic Practice.* Edward Arnold & Co, London, 1970, pp 171–179.

GANGULI, S, ET AL: *Ergonomics evaluation of above-knee amputee-prosthesis combinations.* Ergonomics 17:199–210, 1974.

GARDNER, HF AND CLIPPINGER, FW, JR: *A method for location of prosthetic and orthotic knee joints.* Artificial Limbs 13:31–35, 1969.

GREEN, PWB, ET AL: *An assessment of above- and through-knee amputations.* Br J Surg 59:873–875, 1972.

HADDAN, CC AND THOMAS, A: *Status of the above-knee suction socket in the United States.* Artificial Limbs 1:29–39, 1954.

HALL, CB: *Prosthetic socket shape as related to anatomy in the lower extremity amputee.* Clin Orthop Rel Res 37:32–46, 1964.

HALL, R AND SHUCKSMITH, HS: *The above-knee amputation for ischemia.* Br J Surg 58:656–659, 1971.

HAMPTON, F: *Suspension casting for below-knee, above-knee, and Syme's amputations.* Artificial Limbs 10:5–26, 1966.

HAMPTON, FL: *Above knee prostheses.* Orthop Clin North Am 3:359–372, 1972.

HAMPTON, FL: *Prosthetic principles in the lower extremity amputee.* Orthop Clin North Am 3:339–347, 1972.

HANGER, HB: *Above-Knee Socket Shape and Clinical Considerations: A Guide for Physicians.* Committee on Prosthetic-Orthotic Education, National Research Council, Washington, DC, 1964.

HANSEN-LETH, C AND REIMANN, I: *Amputations with and without myoplasty on rabbits with special reference to the vascularization.* Acta Orthop Scand 431:68–77, 1972.

HINTERBUCHNER, C, SAKUMA, J, AND LEVY, D: *Hydraulic swing and stance phase control for above-knee amputees.* Arch Phys Med Rehabil 56:179–182, 1975.

HOLSTEDT, GE AND BELL, JW: *Sepsis and survival after above-knee amputation for peripheral vascular disease.* Am J Surg 103:372–375, 1962.

HUSTON, CC, ET AL: *Morbid implications of above-knee amputations: Report on a series and review of the literature.* Arch Surg 115:165–167, 1980.

HYDRA-CADENCE: *Guidebook.* U.S. Manufacturing Co., Glendale, CA.

JONES, RF AND BURNISTON, GG: *A conservative approach to lower-limb amputations: Review of 240 amputees with a trial of the rigid dressing.* Med J Aust 2:711–718, 1970.

KAY, HW AND NEWMAN, JD: *Report of a workshop on below-knee and above-knee prosthetics.* Orthot Pros 27:9–25, 1973.

KEGEL, B AND BYERS, JL: *Amputee's Manual: Mauch S-N-S knee.* Medic Publishing, Bellevue, WA, 1977.

KLEIN, R: *Knee instability my foot!* Med J Aust 2:856–859, 1971.

LEWIS, EA: *Fluid-controlled knee mechanisms: Clinical considerations.* Bull Prosthet Res 10 3:24–56, 1965.

LI, W: *Ankle-knee synchronous in a new endoskeletal above-knee prosthetic mechanism: A preliminary report.* Arch Phys Med Rehabil 57:479–481, 1976.

LYQUIST, E: *The above-knee prosthesis.* In MURDOCH, G (ED): *Prosthetic and Orthotic Practice.* Edward Arnold & Co, London, 1970, pp 199–211.

MAUCH, HA: *Stance control for above-knee artificial legs: Design considerations in the S.N.S. knee.* Bull Prosthet Res 10–10:61–72, 1968.

MAUCH, HA: *The development of artificial limbs for lower limbs.* Bull Prosthet Res 10–22:158–166, 1974.

McCOLLOUGH, NC, III: *The dysvascular amputee.* Orthop Clin North Am 3:303–321, 1972.

MURDOCH, G: *Levels of amputation and limiting factors.* Ann R Coll Surg Engl 40:204–216, 1967.

MURDOCH, G: *Myoplastic techniques.* Bull Prosthet Res 10–9:4–13, 1968.

MURDOCH, G: *Amputation surgery in the lower extremity.* Prosthet Orthot Int 1:72–83, 1977.

MURDOCH, G: *Above-knee amputation: An "ideal" situation.* Prosthet Orthot Int 3:13–14, 1979.

Orthopaedic Appliances Atlas, Vol 2, Artificial Limbs. JW Edwards, Ann Arbor, Michigan, 1960.

POETS, R: *The fitting of the above-knee stump.* In *Selected Readings: A Review of Orthotics and Prosthetics.* American Orthotics and Prosthetics Association, Washington, DC, 1980, pp 218–223.

RADCLIFFE, CW: *Alignment of the above-knee artificial leg.* In KLOPSTEG, PE AND WILSON, PD: *Human Limbs and Their Substitutes.* Hafner Publishing, New York, 1954, pp 676–692.

RADCLIFFE, CW: *Functional considerations in the fitting of above-knee prostheses.* Artificial Limbs 2:35–60, 1955.

RADCLIFFE, CW: *Functional considerations in the fitting of above-knee prostheses.* In *Selected Articles from Artificial Limbs.* Robert E. Krieger, Huntington, New York, 1970, pp 5–30.

RADCLIFFE, CW: *Biomechanics of above-knee prostheses.* In MURDOCH, G (ED): *Prosthetic and Orthotic Practice.* Edward Arnold & Co, London, 1970, pp 191–198.

RADCLIFFE, CW: *Prosthetic-knee mechanisms for above-knee amputees.* In MURDOCH, G (ED): *Prosthetic and Orthotic Practice.* Edward Arnold & Co, London, 1970, pp 225–249.

RADCLIFFE, CW: *Above-knee prosthetics.* Prosthet Orthot Int 1:146–160, 1977.

RADCLIFFE, CW, JOHNSON, NC, AND FOORT, J: *Some experience with prosthetic problems of above-knee amputees.* Artificial Limbs, 4:41–75, 1957.

RADCLIFFE, CW AND LAMOREAUX, LW: *The UC-BL Four-Bar Polycentric Knee for the Above-Knee Amputee.* Biomechanics Laboratory, Department of Mechanical Engineering, University of California at Berkeley, 1974.

RECORD, EE: *Surgical amputation in the geriatric patient.* J Bone Joint Surg 45A:1742–1749, 1963.

RUBIN, G: *Some problems of the above-knee amputee.* Bull Hosp Joint Dis 31:53–68, 1970.

SHUMACKER, HB, JR AND MOORE, TC: *Leg and thigh amputations in obliterative arterial disease.* Arch Surg 63:458–465, 1951.

STENER, B: *Amputation through the lower thigh with removal of the adductor and hamstring muscles: An alternative to hip joint disarticulation in certain cases of malignant soft-tissue tumor.* Clin Orthop 80:133–138, 1971.

THIELE, B, JAMES, U, AND STOLBERG, E: *Neurophysiological studies on muscle function in the stump of above-knee amputees.* Scand J Rehabil Med 5:67–70, 1973.

THOMPSON, JK, UDE, RH, AND BERMAN, BL: *Rehabilitation of a patient with a left above-knee amputation, a flaccid stump, and a flaccid left upper extremity.* Phys Ther 51:782–784, 1971.

THOMPSON, RG: *Amputation in the lower extremity.* J Bone Joint Surg 45A:1723–1734, 1963.

THORNDIKE, A: *Suction socket prosthesis for above-knee amputees.* Am J Surg 78:603–613, 1949.

THORNDIKE, A AND EBERHARD, HD: *Suction socket prosthesis for above-knee amputations.* Am J Surg 80:727–731, 1950.

THORNDIKE, A: *End results in suction socket prosthesis for above-knee amputees.* Am J Surg 89:919–923, 1955.

TIMM, OK: *Total-Contact Above-Knee Sockets.* Department of Medicine and Surgery, Prosthetic and Sensory Aids Service, Veterans Administration, Washington, DC, 1963.

TITNER, H: *Fitting and fabrication of a prosthesis for a severe flexion contracture: Case study.* Bull Prosthet Res 10–19:84–87, 1973.

TOLSTEDT, GE AND BELL, JW: *Sepsis and survival after above-knee amputation for peripheral vascular disease.* Am J Surg 103:372–375, 1962.

TOSBERG, WA: *Relationship of socket shape to anatomy and biomechanics.* In *Prosthetics International, Proceedings of the Second International Prosthetics Course, Committee on Prostheses, Braces and Technical Aids, International Society for the Welfare of Cripples.* Copenhagen, 1960, pp 109–110.

TOSBERG, WA: *Prosthetic management of the proximal A-K amputations.* In *Prosthetics International, Proceedings of the Second International Prosthetics Course, Committee on Prostheses, Braces and Technical Aids, International Society for the Welfare of Cripples.* Copenhagen, 1960, pp 111–112.

VITALI, M: *Rehabilitation of the amputee.* Proc R Soc Med 59:1–3, 1966.

WARREN, R AND KIHN, RB: *A survey of lower extremity amputation for ischemia.* Surgery 63:107–120, 1968.

WILSON, AB, JR: *Recent advances in above-knee prosthetics.* Artificial Limbs 12:1–27, 1968.

WILSON, AB, JR: *Limb prosthetics: 1970.* Artificial Limbs 14:1–52, 1970.

WOLTERS, BJ: *Follow-up survey study of a group of elderly above-knee amputees.* Arch Phys Med Rehabil 42:68–72, 1961.

WONG, GE: *A device for applying above-knee total-contact sockets.* Artificial Limbs 16:65–67, 1972.

ZETTL, JH: *The PRS above-knee casting fixture.* Artificial Limbs 14:75–76, 1970.

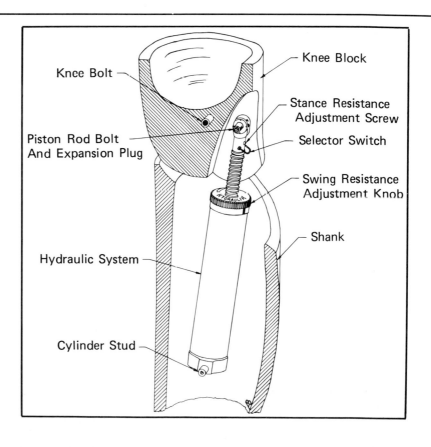

Knee Bolt

Knee Block

Piston Rod Bolt
And Expansion Plug

Stance Resistance
Adjustment Screw

Selector Switch

Swing Resistance
Adjustment Knob

Hydraulic System

Shank

Cylinder Stud

CHAPTER **12**

KNEE MECHANISMS

CLASSIFICATIONS

SWING PHASE CONTROL MECHANISMS

DEFINITIONS
CONSTANT RESISTANCE
VARIABLE RESISTANCE
CADENCE RESPONSIVE RESISTANCE
SLIDING (MECHANICAL) FRICTION
FLUID MECHANISMS
HYDRAULIC TYPES
PNEUMATIC TYPES
FLUID VERSUS SLIDING (MECHANICAL) FRICTION SYSTEMS

STANCE PHASE CONTROL MECHANISMS

MANUAL LOCKS
ALIGNMENT
FRICTION BRAKES
POLYCENTRIC LINKAGES
FLUID RESISTANCE DEVICES

KNEE EXTENSION CONTROLS (CORDS, TENDONLIKE PASSIVE STRAPS, "ARTIFICIAL TENDONS," BACK CHECK)

EXTENSION AIDS

INTERNAL TYPE
ADVANTAGES
DISADVANTAGES
EXTERNAL TYPE
ADVANTAGES
DISADVANTAGES

CLASSIFICATION OF COMMERCIALLY AVAILABLE UNITS

UNRESTRICTED, NONADJUSTABLE KNEE

EXAMPLE UNITS

SWING PHASE CONTROL ONLY

CONSTANT, SLIDING (MECHANICAL) FRICTION
EXAMPLE UNITS
VARIABLE FRICTION
EXAMPLE UNIT
NORTHWESTERN DISC FRICTION UNIT
VARIABLE, CADENCE RESPONSIVE RESISTANCE
EXAMPLE UNITS
DUPACO "HERMES" HYDRAULIC UNIT
HYDRA-CADENCE
ADJUSTMENTS

257

SWING AND STANCE PHASE CONTROL	STANCE CONTROL
CONSTANT, SLIDING (MECHANICAL) FRICTION SWING CONTROL WITH FRICTION UNDER WEIGHT-BEARING STANCE CONTROL	EXAMPLE UNIT HENSCHKE-MAUCH "HYDRAULIK" SWING-N-STANCE (S-N-S) CONTROL SYSTEM
EXAMPLE UNITS	SWING CONTROL

VARIABLE, FRICTION SWING CONTROL WITH FRICTION UNDER WEIGHT-BEARING OR POSTERIOR KNEE DISPLACEMENT STANCE CONTROL	STANCE CONTROL
	   MANUAL LOCK
	   YIELDING, ADJUSTABLE RESISTANCE
	ADJUSTMENTS
	   SWING RESISTANCE

EXAMPLE UNITS	SETTING EXTENSION RESISTANCE SETTING FLEXION RESISTANCE
VARIABLE, CADENCE RESPONSIVE SWING CONTROL WITH FLUID	STANCE RESISTANCE SELECTOR SWITCH

The knee mechanism should serve two main objectives: the restoration of as near normal function and appearance of gait as possible. Durability and conservation of energy are desired features.

CLASSIFICATIONS

Knee mechanisms are designed to give either no mechanical knee control, swing phase control only, stance phase control only, or both swing and stance phase control.

SWING PHASE CONTROL MECHANISMS

DEFINITIONS

1. *Constant resistance:* The amount of resistance does not vary during the swing phase regardless of the angle of knee flexion or the speed of the cadence. The amount of resistance can be preset at one of many levels.
2. *Variable resistance:* A preset level of resistance that varies as a function of the knee angle.
3. *Cadence responsive resistance:* A preset level of resistance that varies as a function of the velocity of knee movement.

SLIDING (MECHANICAL) FRICTION

Sliding friction—the force that resists the movement of one body that is in contact with another—is constant regardless of velocity. Friction, usually applied by a clamp around the knee bolt, resists motion of the shank. The friction resists flexion as much as it resists extension. Since the friction is the same regardless of the speed of gait, the amputee will be able to walk at only one cadence with optimum security and ease. Faster cadences will result in excessive heel-rise; the gait will be irregular in rhythm (vaulting on the sound side) as the amputee waits for the foot to lower; and terminal-impact at complete knee extension will be jarring and uncomfortable. An extension aid will limit heel-rise, but it will magnify terminal-impact. If the amputee walks too slowly, the friction will be relatively too great, resulting in inadequate heel-rise during early swing phase. There is also a danger that the knee may not reach full extension at heel-strike. Nevertheless, most knee units are of the sliding friction type because of their relative simplicity and lower cost.

FLUID MECHANISMS

Fluid systems are cadence responsive and function smoothly without exhibiting the "stickiness" seen in maladjusted sliding friction systems. They consist of a fluid-filled cylinder joined to the knee bolt by a piston.

HYDRAULIC TYPES

Most fluid systems are hydraulic. Because the liquid—oil—is incompressible, the resistance to piston motion results from fluid flow through one or more orifices. The resistance to fluid flow depends on the viscosity and density of the fluid, the size and smoothness of the channel, and the speed of movement. Viscosity is the degree to which a fluid resists flow under an applied force. The higher the viscosity, the greater the resistance to flow. As the temperature decreases, the viscosity increases, and thus the resistance to flow is greater. Nevertheless, once the piston is set in motion, sufficient heat is generated internally to restore the viscosity to its normal level.

Density is the mass per unit volume of a substance. The mass of the fluid itself affects the flow rate through a channel.

Fluid flow is either laminar or turbulent. When the particles move in a streamlike fashion parallel to each other, it is called laminar flow. Laminar flow resistance is directly proportional to speed. Turbulent flow is a random whirlpool movement of particles. Turbulent flow resistance is proportional to the speed squared and is thus suitable for knee units for rapid cadence responsiveness.

PNEUMATIC TYPES

Pneumatic units use air, which is compressible, as the "fluid." Resistance is offered by air compression plus air flow through orifices. Pneumatic units are simpler than hydraulic units, with no possibility of a leak that could soil clothing. They are also lighter in weight and cost less. However, because air is less dense and less viscous than oil, pneumatic units provide less cadence control than do hydraulic units.

FLUID VERSUS SLIDING (MECHANICAL) FRICTION SYSTEMS

Fluid	*Sliding (Mechanical)*
1. Smooth, consistent flow.	1. Excessive heel-rise and terminal impact if amputee walks at a faster cadence than preset level of resistance.
2. Cadence responsive.	2. Changes in walking speed not compensated for by unit.

3. Resistance does not change as a result of long-term use (does not need frequent adjustments).
4. Indicated for amputees who change walking speed over a wide range, usually the younger and highly active amputee.
5. Should be serviced by manufacturer only except for pneumatic and some newer hydraulic units.
6. More expensive.
7. Risk of oil leaks (hydraulic units only).

8. Noise if unit malfunctions.

9. Sealed unit.
10. Capable of operating at higher resistance settings than most sliding friction units.
11. Units with hydraulic stance control are usually aligned with the knee at or anterior to the trochanter-ankle (TA) line (stability is inherent in the unit). Units with hydraulic swing control only are aligned with the knee bolt somewhat posterior to the TA line, however, not as far back as with mechanical friction systems.

3. Loosens as amputee walks (needs frequent adjustments).

4. Indicated for amputees who walk at a single cadence, usually geriatric amputees or others who are not very active.
5. Usually serviced by prosthetist.

6. Less expensive.
7. No risk of leaks; however, grease on bushing can stain clothing.
8. Noise of terminal-impact may be present even without malfunctions unless damper is installed.
9. Debris clogs mechanism.
10. Maximum potential resistance setting is lower than most fluid units.
11. Usually aligned with the knee posterior to the TA line to ensure stability.

STANCE PHASE CONTROL MECHANISMS

MANUAL LOCKS

Once it is engaged, a manual lock prevents knee motion until the lock is manually disengaged. Locking is accomplished by a rod that passes through a slot at the knee. Some locks are spring loaded to engage automatically when the knee is extended. Manual locks offer absolute security against knee flexion at all times whenever the lock is engaged. However, the swing phase is unnatural. Such a unit must be unlocked when the amputee sits.

ALIGNMENT

Alignment is the conventional means of providing knee stability during the stance phase. The knee axis is placed posteriorly so that the load line is in front of the knee axis during the critical time in gait (from heel-strike to mid-stance). The greater the alignment stability, however, the more difficulty encountered in initiating hip and knee flexion at the end of the stance phase. Therefore, alignment stability is set individually.

Some knee units are mechanically stable independent of alignment stability with either a friction or hydraulic braking device.

FRICTION BRAKES

In these devices, an increase in friction between two surfaces during early stance phase causes resistance to knee flexion. The increased friction may be accomplished by the contact of two surfaces with high coefficients of friction (wedging or rubbing of surfaces) or by the tightening of a friction band about a brake drum. The application of body weight during the stance phase is necessary to bring the surfaces together or tighten the belt about the drum. Many friction-brake devices function even if the knee is flexed as much as 25 degrees. If the amputee is reluctant to bear substantial weight through the prosthesis, then the unit will not function safely, as designed. During level walking, the prosthetic knee will not bend until weight has been transferred to the sound leg. In contrast, the normal knee starts to bend before weight is shifted to the other leg. Since the units are designed to lock the knee upon weight application, they hinder the amputee who attempts to walk downhill, descend stairs step over step, or perform any other maneuver that requires knee flexion under load.

POLYCENTRIC LINKAGES

A polycentric unit provides rotation around more than one axis by means of four or more bar linkages. The unit displaces the center of rotation posteriorly, thus increasing the extension moment on the knee during most of the stance phase. The linkage also shifts the axis proximally, requiring less hip extension to maintain knee extension during stance phase. The displacement of the center of knee rotation, and thus the knee stability obtained by the use of these linkages, depends on the angular position of the knee rather than on the amount of weight borne through the unit, as with the frictional devices. Since the center of rotation changes as the knee flexes, they are called polycentric devices. The polycentric knee is inherently stable when loaded. Rotation of the knee axis results in a relative shortening of the shank during swing phase, which prevents toe stubbing.

Swing control is poor in polycentric knees unless the unit incorporates a hydraulic or pneumatic cylinder.

FLUID RESISTANCE DEVICES

In the one commercially available hydraulic stance control unit, the orifices through which oil flows during swing phase are almost closed at heel-strike. A small amount of fluid "leaks" past a valve, giving a high, yet yielding, resistance to knee flexion. The leakage rate can be adjusted to control the amount of yield under various loads. The valve opens when a hyperextension moment is placed on the knee during mid-stance. This enables the transition into swing phase.

KNEE EXTENSION CONTROLS (CORDS, TENDONLIKE PASSIVE STRAPS, "ARTIFICIAL TENDONS," BACK CHECK)

These cords or straps are designed to imitate the action of the hamstring muscles and to control or limit knee extension.

EXTENSION AIDS

Extension aids are devices that facilitate knee extension and resist knee flexion. They have been available since the mid-1800s. In a passive way, they simulate the action of the quadriceps muscle.

These aids tend to conserve energy by limiting knee flexion, and thus heel-rise, during early swing phase and by assisting knee extension during late swing phase. If not properly adjusted, the aid causes terminal-impact as the knee reaches full extension.

INTERNAL TYPE

This aid is an integral component of the knee mechanism. A common aid is a "kicker stick," "hickory stick," or extension lever that is located in the shank and is pivoted at a point just behind and below the knee bolt. The spring or elastic webbing loaded stick offers knee extension bias during swing phase. After about 60 degrees of knee flexion, the internal aid holds the knee flexed, keeping the foot safely back during sitting.

ADVANTAGES

1. Knee kept flexed when amputee kneels and sits.
2. Good appearance; it is contained within the prosthesis rather than being placed externally, as is the "kick strap."
3. Low maintenance.

DISADVANTAGES

1. Tends to be noisy if maladjusted.
2. Difficult to adjust.

EXTERNAL TYPE

These are externally applied devices of two basic types: (1) an elastic strap that passes through the anterior wall of the socket to a roller at the knee that acts as a kick strap, similar to the stick control; and (2) an adjustable elastic webbing strap that attaches to the socket anteriorly and passes anterior to the knee and is attached distally to the anterior shank. The external type generally provides higher extension forces than does the internal type.

External aids may not relax when the knee is flexed acutely, creating a hazard to others and an awkward appearance. When suction socket suspension is used, the upper end of the strap is attached high on the anterior portion of the socket. The strap acts as the vastus muscles by crossing only one joint—the knee joint. In this case, flexion of the knee creates high tension on the strap. This problem can be minimized by using an inverted Y strap. As the knee is flexed, the branches of the Y slip around the knee. This reduces the extension bias when the knee is flexed substantially, yet provides significant extension bias at or near complete knee extension.

If suspension is obtained with a pelvic band, then the proximal end of the strap is connected to the pelvic band. When the amputee sits, the strap is slackened at the hip as it is stretched at the knee. In this case, the strap acts more like the rectus femoris muscle, which crosses both the hip and knee joint and is therefore not as tight when the knee is flexed. After maximum knee flexion (heel-rise) during swing phase, the elastic extension strap offers an anterior force on the shank to return the knee to extension. The acceleration of the knee toward extension allows the amputee to walk at a faster cadence than if extension were obtained only by pendulum action of the shank. If the knee extension aid is too tight, the amputee may circumduct the prosthesis or vault on the sound leg during swing phase on the prosthetic side.

ADVANTAGES

1. Simple design.
2. Easy to adjust.

DISADVANTAGES

1. Requires frequent adjustment.
2. Poor cosmetic appearance.
3. May not relax when the knee is flexed acutely, especially if suspension is by suction and the upper end of the strap is attached to the anterior part of the socket.

CLASSIFICATION OF COMMERCIALLY AVAILABLE UNITS

UNRESTRICTED, NONADJUSTABLE KNEE

Friction in these knee mechanisms is minimal, being only that inherent in the bolt and bushing assembly. Accessories may include an extension aid or a manual knee lock. These are referred to as one-cadence knee mechanisms because they swing at the speed determined by their mass movement of inertia. Unless the lock is engaged, terminal-impact and excessive heel-rise are seen if the gait exceeds the natural frequency of the limb. To have a safe gait, the amputee must take very short steps at a low cadence so that the shank and foot have time to return to the fully extended position. These are suitable for patients who walk very little. They are lighter in weight and less expensive than most other knee units.

EXAMPLE UNITS

Otto Bock 3P4 with manual lock
Kolman Endo Free Knee
Hosmer System I

SWING PHASE CONTROL ONLY

Knee motion is controlled during the swing phase by either sliding or fluid resistance systems. Since heel-rise is restrained and shank motion is retarded, longer steps at higher cadences are possible. In all cases, resistance is adjustable. The units rotate about a single axis or a polycentric linkage.

CONSTANT, SLIDING (MECHANICAL) FRICTION

In these knee units, the amount of resistance to swing of the knee at a particular setting is constant. The amount of resistance can be adjusted by tightening or loosening the friction adjustment screw; once set, it does not change resistance according to the speed of walking, nor does it change resistance owing to the knee angle. The amount of friction depends on the coefficients of friction of the two surfaces that come together and the force of the clamp. Because these units constantly wear, the resistance level has to be adjusted frequently. They are, however, low in initial cost and relatively simple to adjust and maintain. Stability during stance is obtained by aligning the knee joint posterior to the weight (TA) line and by an active posteriorly directed force of the residual limb against the posterior wall of the socket.

EXAMPLE UNITS

> Ohio Willow Wood #10, 11, 22, 81
> Wagner 319, 98B, 320
> Standard Wood Knee
> Bock 3P-1, 3K-9, 3R-16, 3R-17, 3R-18, 3P-19, 3R-19 Modular Polycentric, 3R-20
>   Modular Polycentric, 3P-21, 3R-22, 3P-25, 3P-48, 3P-49, 3P-50
> Bock Endoskeletal Single Axis Knee
> Kolman Single Axis Endoskeletal Knee
> I.P.O.S. Knees
> Hosmer Mechanical Knee, AK 4-Bar Polycentric, KD 4-Bar Polycentric
> US Mfg. Co 2L-103, 2L-104, 2L-105, 5M-300-7, 5M-300-8

VARIABLE FRICTION

These knee units permit adjustment of the amount of resistance to knee motion. The amount of resistance varies according to the angular position of the knee (variable resistance). The variation is accomplished by concentrically mounted friction disks or by eccentric bearing surfaces that come into play successively. Resistance increases as maximum heel-rise is approached and just prior to complete knee extension (to minimize terminal-impact), which produces a more natural gait. Resistance does not vary with the walking cadence. This type of knee may require more maintenance and may be noisier than the constant friction units.

EXAMPLE UNIT

Northwestern Disc Friction Unit

NORTHWESTERN DISC FRICTION UNIT

The Northwestern disc friction unit, developed at Northwestern University Prosthetic Research Center, consists of multiple-disk friction brakes. The different angular sizes of the disks provide a stepped alteration of resistance as the knee flexes and extends during swing phase.

VARIABLE, CADENCE RESPONSIVE RESISTANCE

These are the most sophisticated swing phase control units. All of them are pneumatic or hydraulic piston/cylinder arrangements. The amount of resistance is adjustable. At a particular setting, the resistance varies with the knee angular velocity.

Unlike sliding friction knee units, fluid knee mechanisms adapt to different speeds of walking. Their inherent cadence responsiveness produces a smoother, quieter, better gait. Fluid resistance units can operate at higher resistance settings than most mechanical friction units and thus may be indicated for vigorous patients with long residual limbs. As with all knee units, however, the amputee requires a custom-made socket and suspension, which remains the most important determinant of the walking pattern. Resistance to fluid flow (fluid friction, viscosity) varies with the square of the velocity. This results in little resistance to swing at low velocities and great resistance at high velocities. For example, if the velocity is doubled, the resistance is increased four times. An extension bias spring is preloaded in the direction of extension as an integral part of hydraulic systems.

Pneumatic systems provide a somewhat lower resistance than the hydraulic systems. An air spring, formed by compressing air in the cylinder, controls extension.

EXAMPLE UNITS

> Hosmer Pneumatic, Hosmer System II
> Dupaco "Hermes" Hydraulic
> Hydra-Cadence Hydraulic
> Kingsley-Mortensen Hydra Nu-Matic (HNM) 2101, HF 25 Hydra-Flex, HL 2102
> Hydra Nu-Matic with Lock

DUPACO "HERMES" HYDRAULIC UNIT

The Dupaco "Hermes" hydraulic swing phase control unit consists of a single axis knee bolt and a hydraulic cylinder mechanism. Separate adjustments control resistance to knee flexion and extension. Excessive heel-rise is controlled by the resistance to knee flexion during swing phase. Terminal-impact is avoided by resistance to knee extension during late swing phase. Resistance increases at the end of range and as the speed of walking increases. This device is the only one that uses an oil with silicone, which changes very little with normal temperature variation, thus making temperature compensation unnecessary. Units that do not use silicone may be stiff on cold mornings because the oil has thickened slightly; however, after a few movements of the piston in the cylinder, the oil reverts to its usual viscosity. Flexion and extension resistance can be adjusted independently by two screws at the top of the cylinder, one for extension adjustment and one for flexion adjustment. Clockwise rotation of the screw increases resistance.

HYDRA-CADENCE

The original Hydra-Cadence knee/foot assembly system was designed by Jack Stewart, an engineer employed by the Vickers Corporation, and was hence called the Stewart-Vickers hydraulic leg. In 1959, the name was changed to the Hydra-Cadence leg (Fig. 12-1). The current device, which consists of a single-axis knee with hydraulic resistance, a hydraulically controlled ankle, and a cosmetic foam cover, can be used with any above-knee or hip-disarticulation socket and any type of suspension. When the knee reaches 20 degrees of flexion at the beginning of swing phase, a rod from the knee unit descends to dorsiflex the ankle. At heel-strike, the single-axis ankle exhibits low hydraulic resistance to plantarflexion. Therefore, the foot makes full contact with the ground quite rapidly, as if it had a very soft heel bumper. This feature increases the knee's stability, but some amputees are aware of foot slap. The effect of rapid plantarflexion, which minimizes the tendency of the knee to buckle, is especially apparent when going downhill. An internal spring automatically extends the shank whenever the foot is lifted from the floor, unless the knee is flexed more than 20 degrees. This feature adds safety when taking small steps.

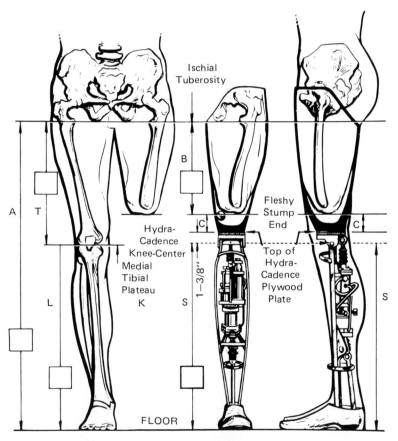

FIGURE 12-1. The Hydra-Cadence unit offers hydraulic resistance in swing phase at the knee, automatic ankle dorsiflexion at and beyond 20 degrees of knee flexion, and hydraulic resistance to plantarflexion. (From *Hydra-Cadence Guidebook*. Hydra-Cadence, Glendale, California, 1961, p 8, with permission.)

Ankle dorsiflexion during swing phase is designed to prevent toe-stubbing during the swing phase of gait and thus prevent the need to vault (plantarflex excessively on the sound side to clear the prosthesis). This feature is not found in any other unit. No properly adjusted prosthetic foot of correct length should drag during swing phase, assuming proper prosthetic length and adequate suspension. As opposed to other ankle units, the Hydra-Cadence's relatively large dorsiflexion range allows the seated amputee to bring the prosthetic foot farther back under a chair and yet keep the heel on the floor.

Adjustments

The position of the ankle is adjustable. Adjustments can be made for differences in heel heights. Although the heel of a high-heeled boot can be accommodated, the stiff upper portion of the boot will interfere with dorsiflexion. The adjustment knob is located within the shank and therefore is not convenient for temporary adjustments to go up or down inclines. Clockwise rotation of the knob plantarflexes the foot.

The Hydra-Cadence unit provides resistance by fluid flow through a single orifice. The greatest resistance occurs at an intermediate range in both flexion and extension rather than at the extremes of range when knee motion is to be stopped. Resistances to flexion and extension cannot be adjusted independently.

Swing phase resistance can be changed through adjustment of a valve that can be reached through a small hole in the back of the cosmetic cover. Valve adjustment affects both flexion and extension resistance simultaneously. Clockwise rotation increases resistance.

SWING AND STANCE PHASE CONTROL

CONSTANT, SLIDING (MECHANICAL) FRICTION SWING CONTROL WITH FRICTION UNDER WEIGHT-BEARING STANCE CONTROL

Constant, sliding friction is provided for swing phase control about a single-axis knee. Stance phase control is obtained by friction under weight-bearing. Body weight applied during the stance phase causes the two friction surfaces to come together as the knee block descends, thus resisting any further knee flexion or extension even if the knee is flexed up to 25 degrees. However, the knee will buckle if it is flexed beyond about 25 degrees before sufficient weight is borne on the prosthesis to engage the braking mechanism. The knee block is able to descend under weight-bearing by compressing a spring. The range of compression is adjustable. Stability during stance phase is also achieved by alignment of the knee posterior to the TA line. Stability is inherent in the mechanism and does not depend so much on the amputee's strength or coordination. This type of knee prevents knee flexion during weight-bearing, which prohibits descending stairs using the jackknife technique and makes going down inclines a problem. These knees are used for people who need stability.

EXAMPLE UNITS

Kolman Safety Knee (Fig. 12-2)
Kolman Endo Safety Knee
Bock Endo Safety Knee

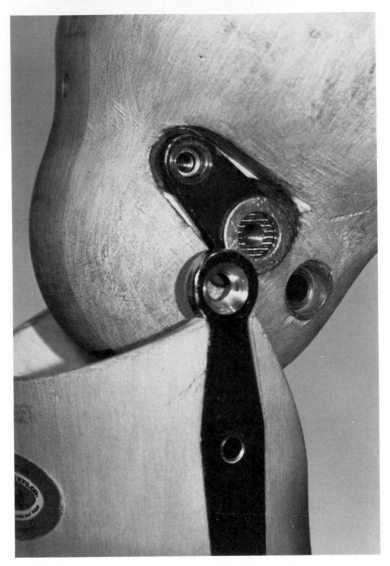

FIGURE 12-2. The Kolman Safety Knee unit offers sliding friction swing control, and stance control by friction under weight-bearing. (From *Selection and Application of Knee Mechanisms: Program Guide.* Veterans Administration, Washington, DC, 1976, p 57, with permission.)

Bock 3P23 (Fig. 12-3), 3P-24, 3L-11, 3R-15
Wagner 200 Safety Knee, 205
Teufel Secura
USMC 5M-300-6 Modular Safety Knee

VARIABLE, FRICTION SWING CONTROL WITH FRICTION UNDER WEIGHT-BEARING OR POSTERIOR KNEE DISPLACEMENT STANCE CONTROL

Variable friction is provided during swing phase. Stance phase control is obtained by an

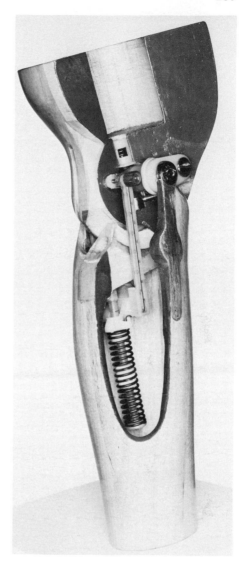

FIGURE 12-3. The Bock 3P23 knee unit offers sliding friction swing control, and stance control by friction under weight-bearing. (From *Selection and Application of Knee Mechanisms: Program Guide.* Veterans Administration, Washington, DC, 1976, p 54, with permission.)

increase of friction between the surfaces during weight-bearing or a posterior displacement of the center of knee rotation to produce an extension rather than flexion moment on the knee during weight-bearing. These knee mechanisms are polycentric devices consisting of four (or more) bar linkages.

EXAMPLE UNITS

Kolman Endoskeletal Polycentric
Lang Polycentric

VARIABLE, CADENCE RESPONSIVE SWING CONTROL WITH FLUID STANCE CONTROL

Variable, adjustable, cadence responsive resistance is provided during swing phase. Fluid resistance is also used during stance phase.

EXAMPLE UNIT

Henschke-Mauch S-N-S (Fig. 12-4)

HENSCHKE-MAUCH "HYDRAULIK" SWING-N-STANCE (S-N-S) CONTROL SYSTEM

The Henschke-Mauch S-N-S system, which was commercially introduced in 1968, can be used with any type of socket, suspension, or foot. The unit, designed by Dr. Ulrich Henschke and Hans Mauch, can function in any one of three different ways: with swing and stance control operational, with only swing control operational, or with the knee manually locked.

Swing Control

The swing control is designed to provide a natural appearing gait at various cadences. There is hydraulic swing resistance to both flexion and extension. To simulate the action of the knee flexors, fluid flow is progressively restricted toward the end of swing phase. The amount of resistance lowers somewhat as the temperature increases; thus, less energy is utilized during hot weather. A built-in temperature compensation mecha-

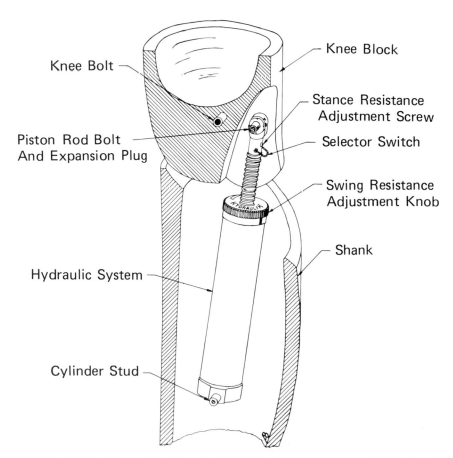

FIGURE 12-4. The Henschke-Mauch S-N-S knee unit can provide hydraulic resistance in swing and stance phases.

nism keeps the yielding speed rather constant despite viscosity changes in the hydraulic fluid. A built-in extension bias assists extension when the knee is slightly flexed.

Stance Control

The Henschke-Mauch hydraulic unit provides two types of stance control.

MANUAL LOCK. A manually operated lever locks the knee against flexion. This may be desirable when the amputee stands or sits for long periods. Unlike other manual locks, the amputee can engage the lock with the knee flexed. This enables the amputee to obtain a stable flexed attitude of the knee, which may be useful when driving a car. The accelerator pedal can be depressed with the prosthetic foot without risk of inadvertent knee flexion.

YIELDING, ADJUSTABLE RESISTANCE. This high phasic resistance to knee flexion while the limb is weight-bearing is utilized when walking on level surfaces or when descending stairs or inclines. A hyperextension moment of at least one tenth of a second on the knee releases the yielding resistance. This force occurs naturally just after mid-stance as the amputee rolls onto the ball of the foot. By automatically disengaging the high resistance to flexion, the knee can flex to initiate swing phase. As knee flexion nears maximum during swing phase, the high level of resistance is reinstated. Thus, if toward the end of swing phase the toe is stubbed and the amputee starts to fall, the high resistance to flexion retards flexion so much that the knee bends very slowly, allowing the wearer to recover.

Adjustments

The rate of yield of the hydraulic fluid can be adjusted for the individual amputee to produce optimum control of swing and stance.

SWING RESISTANCE. Swing resistance is adjusted with the stance control turned off. Resistance to forward swing or knee extension and backward swing or knee flexion can be adjusted independently. Low settings for both flexion and extension usually suit the new amputee. Even at the lowest settings, swing resistance is comparable to a sliding friction unit adjusted to moderately high friction. Resistance is gradually increased as the amputee learns to control the prosthesis. If a heavier shoe is worn, more resistance may be required. Adjustments are made by turning the serrated cap.

Setting Extension Resistance. The relationship of the cylinder to the black line under the serrated knob indicates the amount of extension resistance. When the marker is positioned to the extreme left (by turning the serrated ring), extension resistance is maximum (Fig. 12-5A). Extension resistance is minimum when the marker is at the extreme right (Fig. 12-5B, C) and moderate when the marker is in the center (Fig. 12-5D).

Setting Flexion Resistance. Resistance to flexion is indicated by the relationship of the letters in HYDRAULIK on the top of the serrated knob to the black line (marker). If the letter "H" is over the marker, then resistance to flexion is minimum (see Fig. 12-5A, C). If the serrated knob is turned clockwise until the letter "K" is over the marker, then the unit is set for maximum flexion resistance (see Fig. 12-5D).

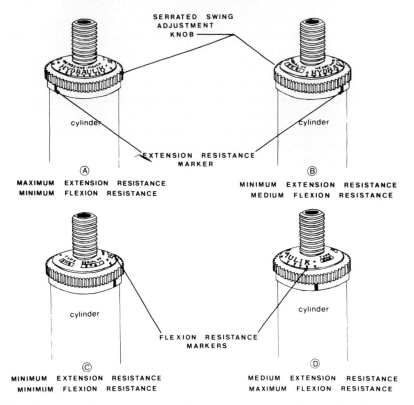

FIGURE 12-5. Flexion and extension resistance settings for the Henschke-Mauch S-N-S knee unit.

STANCE RESISTANCE. The amount of stance resistance determines how quickly the knee bends when weight is borne on it. This adjustment is made by turning a screw (using an Allen wrench) clockwise for maximum stability and counterclockwise for faster bending. Maximum stability is usually appropriate in early gait training.

SELECTOR SWITCH. With the prosthesis in the upright position, the selector switch (stirrup-shaped lever) is used to select the mode of operation desired.

> *To activate:*
> 1. *Swing and stance control:* The selector switch is placed in the *down position.* This is used for most activities.
> 2. *Swing phase control only:* The selector switch is lifted to the *up position* while a hyperextension moment of one tenth of a second or longer is placed on the knee. The amputee does this by placing the prosthetic leg behind the sound leg while bearing weight on the ball of the prosthetic foot. For activities such as bicycling, it is desirable to eliminate the stance control.
> 3. *Positive knee lock:* The selector switch is placed in the *up position* while the prosthetic knee does not have a hyperextension moment on it. The amputee may be standing with the prosthesis ahead of the sound leg, with a straight or bent knee, or may be sitting with the knee flexed when the selector switch is raised. The knee is then fully extended to engage the lock and will remain positively locked until the lever is lowered.

Special skill is required for proper installation and maintenance of fluid-controlled units. Also, the amputees need special training to realize the maximum benefit from the units. The cost of the fluid-controlled units exceeds that of sliding friction ones. Consequently, they should be prescribed only for amputees who need sophisticated swing control at various speeds, and in the case of the S-N-S unit, sophisticated stance control as well. There is no terminal-impact at the end of swing phase, as with frictional knees; therefore, those few amputees who have learned to rely on this sensory cue may have difficulty switching to the fluid-controlled mechanism.

BIBLIOGRAPHY

Clinical Application Study of the Dupaco "Hermes" Hydraulic Control Unit. Technical Report (TR-4). Research and Development Division, Prosthetic and Sensory Aids Service, Veterans Administration, New York, 1965.

Clinical Application Study of the Henschke-Mauch "HYDRAULIK" Swing Control System: Technical Report (TR-3). Research and Development Division, Prosthetic and Sensory Aids Services, Veterans Administration, New York, 1964.

Clinical Application Study of the Hydra-Cadence Above-Knee Prosthesis: A Technical Report (TR-2). Research and Development Division, Prosthetic and Sensory Aids Service, Department of Medicine and Surgery, Veterans Administration, New York, 1963.

ERBACK, JR: *Hydraulic prostheses for above-knee amputees.* JAPIA 43:105–110, 1963.

GARDNER, HF AND CLIPPINGER, FW, JR: *A method for location of prosthetic and orthotic knee joints.* Artificial Limbs 13:31–35, 1969.

HAMPTON, FL: *Above knee prostheses.* Orthop Clin North Am 3:359–372, 1972.

HINTERBUCHNER, C, SAKUMA, J, AND LERY, D: *Hydraulic swing and stance control for above-knee amputees.* Arch Phys Med Rehabil 56:179–182, 1975.

Hydra-Cadence Guide Book. Hydra-Cadence Inc, Glendale, Calif, Sept 1961.

Hydra-Cadence Manual. Hydra Cadence Inc, Glendale, Calif.

KEGEL, B AND BYERS, JL: *Amputee's Manual: Mauch S-N-S knee.* Medic Publishing, Bellevue, Wash, 1977.

LEWIS, EA: *Elements of Training with the Mauch S.N.S. System for Above-knee Amputees.* Research and Development Division, Prosthetic and Sensory Aids Service, Veterans Administration, New York.

LEWIS, EA: *Fluid-controlled knee mechanisms: Clinical considerations.* Bull Prosthet Res 10–3:24–56, 1965.

LEWIS, EA: *Clinical evaluation of a pneumatic knee system: The University of California-biomechanics laboratory swing-control unit.* Bull Prosthet Res 10–15:85–94, 1971.

LEWIS, EA AND BERNSTOCK, WM: *Clinical Application study of the Henschke-Mauch HYDRAULIK Model "A" swing and stance control system.* Bull Prosthet Res 10–10:35–60, 1968.

LI, WK: *Ankle-knee synchronous in a new endoskeletal above-knee prosthetic mechanism: A preliminary report.* Arch Phys Med Rehabil 57:479–481, 1976.

Manual for the Henschke-Mauch "Hydraulik" Swing-N-Stance Control System (Type S-N-S) (Standard Length) for Above-knee Prostheses. Mauch Laboratories, Dayton, Ohio, 1974.

Manual for the Henschke-Mauch "Hydraulik" Swing-N-Stance Control System (Type S-N-S) for Above-Knee Prostheses. Mauch Laboratories, Dayton, Ohio, 1976.

MAUCH, HA: *Stance control for above-knee artificial legs: Design considerations in the S-N-S knee.* Bull Prosthet Res 10–10:61–72, 1968.

MAUCH, HA: *The development of artificial limbs for lower limbs.* Bull Prosthet Res 10–22:158–166, 1974.

McKENZIE, DS: *Knee controls for artificial legs.* In KENEDI, RM (ED): *Biomechanics and Related Bio-Engineering.* Pergamon Press, Oxford, 1965, pp 433–441.

McLAURIN, CA: *Polycentric knees.* Inter-Clinic Info Bull 8:9–11, 1969.

MURPHY, EF: *The swing phase of walking with above-knee prostheses.* Bull Prosthet Res 10–1:5–39, 1964.

RADCLIFFE, CW: *Prosthetic-knee mechanisms for above-knee amputees.* In MURDOCH, G (ED): *Prosthetic and Orthotic Practice.* Edward Arnold & Co, London, 1970, pp 225–249.

RADCLIFFE, CW: *Above-knee prosthetics.* Prosthet Orthot Int 1:146–160, 1977.

RADCLIFFE, CW AND LAMOREUX, L: *UC-BL pneumatic swing-control unit for above-knee prostheses: Design, adjustment, and installation.* Bull Prosthet Res 10–10:73–89, 1968.

RADCLIFFE, CW AND LAMOREUX, LW: *The UC-BL Four-Bar Polycentric Knee for the Above-Knee Amputee.* Biomechanics Laboratory, Department of Mechanical Engineering, University of California at Berkeley, 1974.

RADCLIFFE, CW AND RALSTON, HJ: *Performance Characteristics of Fluid-Controlled Prosthetic Knee Mechanisms.* Biomechanics Laboratory, University of California at San Francisco and Berkeley, No. 49, 1963.

Selection and Application of Knee Mechanisms: Program Guide. Veterans Administration, Washington, DC, 1976.

Selection and Application of Knee Mechanisms: Program Guide. Veterans Administration, Washington, DC, 1980.

STAROS, A: *The principles of swing-phase control: The advantages of fluid mechanisms.* Prostheses Braces Techn Aids, 13:11–19, 1964.

STAROS, A AND MURPHY, EF: *Properties of fluid flow applied to above-knee prosthesis.* Bull Prosthet Res 10–1:40–65, 1964.

STAROS, A AND PEIZER, E: *Northwestern University intermittent mechanical friction system (disk-type).* Artificial Limbs 9:45–52, 1965.

THOMPSON, RG AND COMPERE, CL: *Clinical appraisal of the Otto Bock knee mechanism.* Orth Pros Appl J 12:29–32, 1958.

WALLACH, J AND SAIBEL, E: *Control mechanism performance criteria for an above-knee leg prosthesis.* J Biomech 3:87–97, 1970.

WILSON, AB, JR: *Recent advances in above-knee prosthetics.* Artificial Limbs 12:1–27, 1968.

WILSON, AB, JR: *Limb prosthetics: 1970.* Artificial Limbs 14:1–52, 1970.

ZARRUGH, MY AND RADCLIFFE, CW: *Simulation of swing phase dynamics in above-knee prostheses.* J Biomech 9:283–292, 1976.

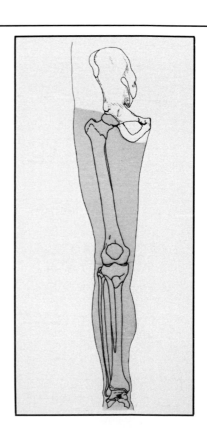

CHAPTER 13

HIP DISARTICULATION (THIGH [Th], COMPLETE)

(FEMORAL EXARTICULATION, THROUGH-THE-HIP)

William Kerr is reported to have performed the first surgical disarticulation at the hip in 1774 on an 11-year-old girl who had a tumor of the thigh. An account of a hip disarticulation that was successfully performed by Walter Brachear of Kentucky in 1806 for a comminuted compound fracture of the femur in a 17-year-old boy was reported by later authors. Brachear is said to have performed a mid-thigh amputation, ligated the major vessels, and then disarticulated the femur through a lateral exposure without anesthesia or antiseptics.

Sir Astley Cooper performed a hip disarticulation at Guy's Hospital, London, in 1824 on a 40-year-old man who had received an above-knee amputation some years before. Removal of the limb took 20 minutes, with an additional 15 minutes for ligation of major vessels and dressing application. The patient is reported to have fainted during the operation, but he survived the procedure.

Early hip disarticulations were usually performed for disease, but from the time of the French Revolution and the Napoleonic Wars until the end of the American Civil War, most of the cases reported were the result of battle wounds rather than disease. Dominique-Jean Larrey, the famous French surgeon and personal physician to Napoleon, performed seven disarticulations. Some of Larrey's indications for hip disarticulation in military surgery were as follows:

1. a limb that is torn off or severely lacerated close to the joint, making amputation in the continuity impossible
2. a rupture of the femoral artery or sciatic nerve secondary to a fracture in the area of the trochanters
3. massive gangrene extending near the hip joint from extensive soft-tissue wounds.

These indications were still valid at the time of the American Civil War.

During World War II, most of the 56 reported military hip disarticulation amputations were the result of extensive trauma (complete or nearly complete severance and major arterial injury). Amputations due solely to major arterial injury are less frequent now because of improved techniques in vascular repair and grafting. The incidence of gas gangrene has been reduced by prompt and thorough débridement and the use of antibiotics. It has been estimated that 0.5 percent of the surgical amputations performed in the American Civil War and 0.4 percent of those performed in World War II were hip disarticulations.

Indications for hip disarticulation in the non-military setting were stated by Velpeau in 1839: any incurable degeneration of the femur (comminuted fracture, necrosis, caries, osteosarcoma) above its shaft, and gangrene or any other disease that has progressed high on the thigh as long as the bones of the pelvis are not involved. Current indications are usually malignant tumors of the femur or thigh, extensive vascular disease with gangrene, severe decubitus ulcers with associated osteomyelitis of the femur in the paraplegic, and failed surgical procedures about the hip, usually with irreversible nerve lesions, nonunions, infection, and joint deformities. Not all malignant growths of the upper thigh require such drastic treatment. In some cases, the growth can be removed with wide excision.

SURGICAL PROCEDURES

LARREY PROCEDURE

Larrey, who was undoubtedly one of the most skilled surgeons of his time, is said to have completed the entire procedure in 14 to 15 seconds after ligating the femoral vessels. Without the benefit of anesthesia or the knowledge of asepsis, the amputation had to be performed as fast as possible. For speed, he used only four knife strokes:

1. A knife was inserted between the base of the femoral neck and the tendinous attachments of the lesser trochanter until it emerged posteriorly. The medial flap was cut by making an oblique downward stroke.
2. The medial flap was raised to expose the capsule, which was cut.
3. The thigh was abducted to expose the interarticular ligament, which was cut.
4. The lateral flap was then cut with a downward and outward stroke.

The remaining arteries were ligated, the muscles were not sutured, and the skin was approximated with a few sutures.

Although the speed of Larrey's method lessened shock, the muscles were sectioned through their richly vascular bellies, which contributed to hemorrhage and shock.

OLLIER OF LYONS (1859) PROCEDURE

> Subperiosteal hip disarticulation

The subperiosteal hip disarticulation was originally devised by Ollier and was later performed by James Shutter of London in 1881. A circular amputation was made at the junction of the middle and upper thirds of the thigh. The vessels were ligated. Through a longitudinal incision on the lateral thigh, the remaining portion of the femur was dissected out of the periosteum, which was peeled from the bone up to the intertrochanteric line. The periosteum was left in the flaps. The residual periosteum allowed muscle attachment; eventually, cartilaginous material (resembling a tough fibrous stalk) regenerated in the periosteum. The residual limb could be moved powerfully enough to move a prosthesis. This procedure fell into disuse at about the turn of the century because of undesirable, uncontrolled bone growths under the periosteal cuff. It was also technically difficult to strip the periosteum from healthy bone, and retaining the periosteum was not desirable for disarticulation performed for malignancies.

BOYD PROCEDURE

> Posterior (gluteal) flap
> Anterior suture line

In 1947, Harold Boyd at the Campbell Clinic, Memphis, described a method of anatomic hip disarticulation that utilized principles advocated by Callander and Kirk:

> *Callander* suggested reducing the incidence of shock by detaching the muscles at their origin or insertion rather than cutting through the muscle itself.

> *Kirk* described removing all muscles from the limb by detaching them at their origin, except for one muscle flap.

The Boyd technique involves dissecting along fascial planes and dividing the muscles at their pelvic origins or femoral insertions to minimize shock. Closure without tension is permitted because all muscles have been removed, except for the large gluteal flap that cushions the distal torso.

The incision begins at the anterior superior iliac spine and curves distally and medially (almost parallel with the inguinal ligament) to a point 5 cm (2 in) below the adductor muscle origins. The femoral vessels and nerve are ligated. The incision is continued posteriorly around the thigh 5 cm (2 in) distal to the ischial tuberosity and laterally 8 cm (3¹/₇ in) distal to the greater trochanter then curves proximally to meet the original incision line below the anterior superior iliac spine (Fig. 13-1).

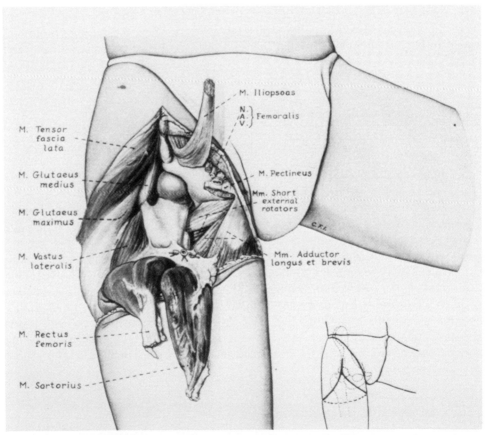

FIGURE 13-1. The stage of anatomic disarticulation following ligation of the femoral vessels and nerve, and detachment of the sartorius, rectus femoris, pectineus, and iliopsoas muscles. Inset shows the line of the incision. (From Boyd, HB: *Anatomic disarticulation of the hip.* Surg Gynecol Obstet 84:346, 1947, with permission.)

The sartorius and rectus femoris muscles are detached at their origins. The pectineus muscle is cut 0.6 cm (¼ in) from the pubis. The iliopsoas muscle is detached distally, followed by a proximal detachment of the adductors and gracilis muscle. Branches of the obturator artery are ligated. The obturator externus muscle is severed at its femoral insertion, as are the gluteus medius and minimus muscles. Next, the fascia lata is divided with the lowest fibers of the gluteus maximus. After ligation of the sciatic nerve, the short rotators are detached distally and the hamstring muscles are severed from the ischial tuberosity. Incision of the capsule and division of the ligamentum teres complete the disarticulation (Fig. 13-2).

The gluteal flap is brought anteriorly and the gluteal muscles are sutured to the pectineus muscle and point of origin of the adductors. Skin closure follows. A posterior flap with an anterior scar has several merits:

1. The scar is well removed from lateral or terminal pressure areas, making it the incision of choice for the use of the Canadian hip-disarticulation prosthesis.
2. The scar is placed so that fecal contamination of the wound is unlikely.

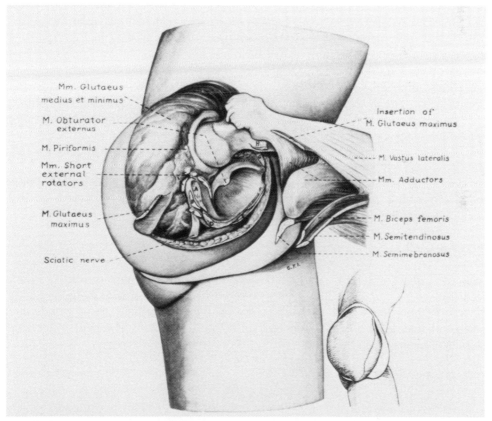

FIGURE 13-2. The stage of anatomic disarticulation following separation of the gluteus muscles from their insertions, division of the sciatic nerve, detachment of the short rotators, and severance of the hamstring muscles from the ischial tuberosity. Inset shows the residual tissue after wound closure. (From Boyd, HB: *Anatomic disarticulation of the hip.* Surg Gynecol Obstet 84:347, 1947, with permission.)

GEORGIADE, PICKRELL, AND MAGUIRE PROCEDURE (1956)

> Anterior (thigh) flap
> Posterior suture line

This procedure was devised for patients with multiple pressure sores over the greater trochanters, ischial tuberosities, and sacrum (e.g., paraplegics). These patients usually have a history of numerous hospitalizations for recurrent decubitus ulcers with repeated efforts at both conservative and surgical treatments (primary closure, split-thickness graft, and full-thickness flap coverage*) that have failed. They are usually from the lower socioeconomic stratum, poorly motivated toward rehabilitation, and are predominately bedridden. The ischial, trochanteric, and sacral areas are extensively scarred or ulcerated and draining. Anemia and osteomyelitis are often present, as are partially fused joints. Nutrition is generally poor.

In this procedure, the anterior thigh, a source of well-vascularized tissue, is used for flap coverage of the damaged trochanteric and ischial areas (Fig. 13-3A). For cases that also involve the sacrum, incision 12²/₃ cm (5 in) below the tibial tubercle with preservation of the skin and all underlying subcutaneous tissue, muscle tissue, and blood supply on the anterior leg has been reported. After removal of the femur (Fig. 13-3B), attention is directed to removing the ulcers and scarred areas over the sacral, ischial, and trochanteric areas. Excision is wide and includes all sinus tracts. Portions of the ischial tuberosity and sacrum may be removed. The soft-tissue flap (tissue that previously composed the anterior thigh and upper portion of the lower leg) is rotated posteriorly, trimmed to fit the defect, and sutured (Fig. 13-3C). The tissue that was previously on the anterior leg below the knee would now be covering the sacrum. Postoperatively, the patient is maintained in the prone position. The proximal femur (above the trochanter) may be retained for better sitting stability and pressure distribution. If this is done, the skin flap must extend well below the knee to acquire enough skin for closure without tension over the sacral area.

Wounds usually close more successfully in patients with flaccid paralysis than those with spastic paralysis. Spasticity may place tension on the flaps and sutures, resulting in wound dehiscence.

ADVANTAGES

Sources of infection (arthritis of the hip, osteomyelitis of the femur) can be removed. Skin defects that cannot be successfully treated by more conservative methods can be closed. Without the weight of the legs, the paraplegic is usually more mobile and attains a higher level of independence than before the surgery. The patient's general spasticity, especially in the abdominal muscles and bladder, decreases.

DISADVANTAGES

The main objection is that amputation of both lower extremities is extremely unaes-

---

*Note: Skin grafts over the bony prominences are often preceded by resection of the bone. Resection of the ischial tuberosities frequently leads to diverticula of the urethra. This is thought to occur because the cavity in which the urethra is normally located is gone and the perineum assumes a flatter shape. Arthritis of the hip can appear following trochanteric or ischial tuberosity resection if the hip joint is inadvertently opened.

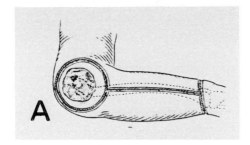

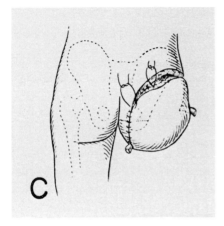

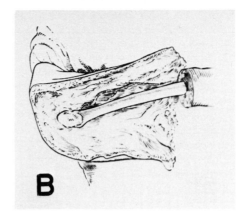

FIGURE 13-3. *(A)* The large trochanteric ulcer is circumscribed by a large incision. A mid-lateral thigh incision leaves the anterior tissue for a flap. *(B)* The total femur is removed. *(C)* The flap is sutured posteriorly. (From Georgiade, N, Pickrell, K, and Maguire, C: *Total thigh flaps for extensive decubitus ulcers.* Plast Reconstr Surg 17:221–222, 1956, with permission.)

thetic. Deformed limbs and chronic sores, however, are often more disfiguring than the surgical result. Another problem is that the patient loses sitting stability.

If patients have been debilitated for a long time, as is the case with many patients who undergo hip disarticulation surgery, they often exhibit extreme vasomotor instability and lowered blood volume. Measures should be taken to minimize blood loss and avoid hypovolemic shock (Table 13-1).

VARIATIONS

1. Angerer's procedure: This is a two-stage operation in which the femoral vessels are ligated 1 or 2 days before the disarticulation. It has been used for patients who are in poor condition. This method was designed to reduce blood loss and thus avoid shock.
2. Injection of the sciatic nerve with procaine followed by section of the nerve at the start of the operation rather than toward the end, after the nerve has been subjected to excessive tension, has been recommended as a precaution to avoid shock.
3. Radical groin (deep iliac) dissection is performed when the inguinal nodes are involved, most often for melanoma.
4. An anterior racquet incision (Fig. 13-4) is used for hip joint disarticulation, rather than the incision from the anterior superior iliac spine described by Boyd.

TABLE 13-1. METHODS USED TO AVOID SHOCK

1. Gentle handling of the tissues by the surgeon during surgery
2. Layer-by-layer dissection
3. Section of muscles at their femoral insertions or pelvic origins (relatively avascular areas) rather than through the vascular muscle bellies
4. Injection of the sciatic nerve with procaine and early section of the nerve
5. A two-stage operation in which the femoral vessels are ligated a day or two before the disarticulation
6. Speedy surgery
7. Elevation of the leg after ligation of the artery to allow drainage of the leg before ligation of the vein
8. Constant administration of whole blood during the operation, with transfusions in excess of measured blood loss
9. Use of an elastic wrap around the limb to conserve circulating blood volume (applied several hours before the operation) except in cases of melanoma, where tumor cells might be disseminated into the blood stream
10. Meticulous attention to hemostasis during surgery

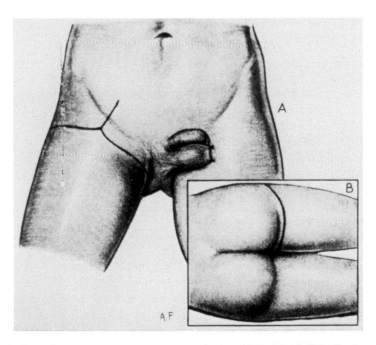

FIGURE 13-4. *(A)* **An anterior racquet incision for hip joint disarticulation, which begins just above the mid-portion of the inguinal ligament. The lateral incision goes just above the greater trochanter. The medial incision is somewhat higher, being located several centimeters below the genitocrural fold.** *(B)* **The medial and lateral incisions join posteriorly just below the infragluteal fold in an almost transverse line. (From Pack, GT and Ehrlich, HE:** *Exarticulation of the lower extremities for malignant tumors: Hip joint disarticulation (with and without deep iliac dissection) and sacro-iliac disarticulation (hemipelvectomy).* **Ann Surg 123:974, 1946, with permission.)**

5. In 1949, H.J. Seddon and J.T. Scales described an above-knee amputation with the remaining femur being enucleated and replaced by an internal prosthesis (Fig. 13-5) for long-standing chondromatous dysplasia of the femur. Today, it is possible to replace the upper part of the femur and hip, as well as the lower femur and knee, by endoprostheses and preserve the extremity distal to the femur.

POSTOPERATIVE COMPLICATIONS OF HIP DISARTICULATIONS

Postoperative complications may include massive hemorrhage, hematoma formation, or sequestration of small pieces of bone. Wound infection is rare. If it does occur, it is usually following removal of an ulcerated and infected tumor that required radical groin dissection. The surgical wound is also in close proximity to the anus, which may introduce a variety of organisms. Phantom limb and phantom pain may be present. Anemia is rare following hip disarticulation, although it is quite frequent following hemipelvectomy.

MORTALITY

In cases of cancer, if hip disarticulation is performed as a palliative measure in the late stage after other measures (wide excision, radiation, chemotherapy) have failed, then the mortality is generally higher than if it is performed early (symptoms of less than 6 months) as a cure. Hemipelvectomy is usually only indicated for malignancy proximal to the hip joint; when compared to hip disarticulation for malignant growths of the upper thigh, it presents no great difference as far as the surgery or postoperative disability are concerned and does offer a better chance for cure. Therefore, some surgeons consider hemipelvectomy to be the procedure of choice for soft-tissue or osteogenic malignancies of the upper thigh, as well as the pelvis.

The prognosis following hip disarticulation depends on the type, location, and extent of the tumor, the presence of metastases, and previous treatment measures (radiation, chemotherapy, local excisions, and conservative amputations). A better survival rate can be expected if the procedure is performed for early or moderately advanced, surgically untreated, malignant tumors of the thigh rather than for well-advanced cases that have been subjected to one or more local excisions and conservative amputations. Usually, both the physician and the patient procrastinate in making the decision for such a drastic, deforming amputation. While this reluctance is understandable, it does reduce the chance of long-term survival.

VERY SHORT THIGH AMPUTATION OR HIP DISARTICULATION

In cases of malignancy, usually the soft tissue and bone are radically removed. In cases of trauma or disease other than cancer, the surgeon may have a choice between a very short thigh amputation or a hip disarticulation.

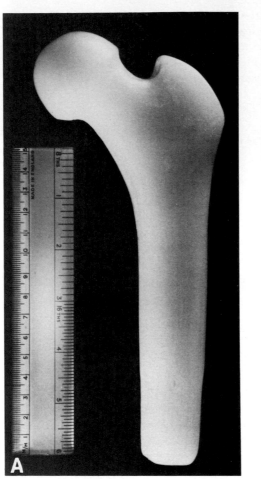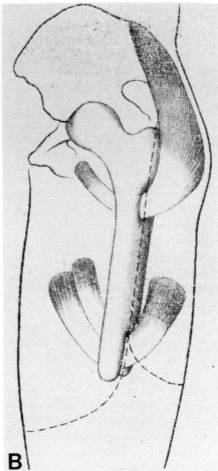

FIGURE 13-5. A mid-thigh amputation with prosthetic replacement of the remnant of femur by an internal prosthesis that was designed by Dr. J.T. Scales. *(A)* The polythene prosthesis. *(B)* The prosthesis in position. (From Seddon, HJ and Scales, JT: *A polythene substitute for the upper two thirds of the femur.* Lancet 2:795, 1949, with permission.)

In 1930, Verrall stated that if the distance below the greater trochanter is less than $12^2/_3$ cm (5 in), a hip-disarticulation prosthesis is used. In 1949, Slocum noted that when the amputation approaches the level of the lesser trochanter, the hip-joint function is inadequate and a hip-disarticulation prosthesis should be fitted. As artificial limbs and surgical procedures improve, higher thigh amputations can be fitted with modified above-knee prostheses. The success of using an above-knee prosthesis for high thigh amputations depends on the volume of remaining soft tissue as well as the length of remaining bone. An extreme example is a 15-cm (6-in) soft-tissue residual limb, in which the femur had been completely removed, that was successfully fitted with an above-knee suction socket prosthesis. It is therefore not accurate to give an absolute measurement for the shortest thigh segment that can successfully move an above-knee prosthesis, because success is also dependent upon the volume of the soft tissues. In general, the residual limb should be 8.5 to 13.6 cm ($3^1/_3$ to $5^1/_3$ in) in length from the perineum to permit movement of the prosthesis and to allow for about 2 to 3 cm (⁴/₅ to 1¹/₅ in) of pistoning. Success has been reported, however, with a suction socket above-knee prosthesis fitted on a limb 4 to 5 cm (1¹/₂ to 2 in) on the medial side.

Efforts have been made to surgically lengthen a femur that was too short to permit the use of an above-knee prosthesis. This has been done successfully by a homoplastic graft from the fibular diaphysis.

PROSTHESES

HISTORIC LIMBS

SAUCER TYPE

This prosthesis was basically an above-knee prosthesis with a saucer-shaped socket on top of the thigh section (Fig. 13-6).

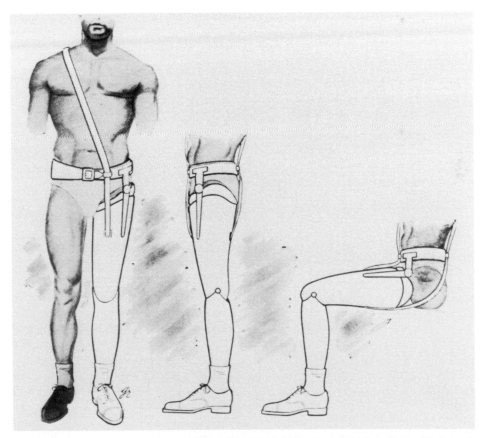

FIGURE 13-6. The saucer-type hip-disarticulation prosthesis. (From McLaurin, CA: *The evolution of the Canadian-type hip-disarticulation prosthesis.* Artificial Limbs 4:23, 1957, with permission.)

SUSPENSION

A pelvic band with a single-axis hip joint was used by some patients.

HIP JOINT

The single-axis hip joint was placed well forward of the anatomic hip to provide some stability. Locks, usually at the hip and knee, would engage automatically in full extension and required manual release for sitting.

TILTING-TABLE PROSTHESIS

This prosthesis was heavier than the saucer type but gave additional support (Fig. 13-7).

SOCKET

A leather socket was designed to fit the torso.

SUSPENSION

The socket was attached by a belt around the pelvis and sometimes a strap over the shoulder. This method of suspension was insecure and often allowed the socket to twist.

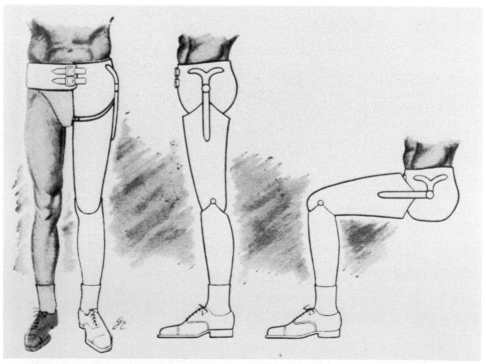

FIGURE 13-7. The tilting-table hip-disarticulation prosthesis. (From McLaurin, CA: *The evolution of the Canadian-type hip-disarticulation prosthesis.* Artificial Limbs 4:23, 1957, with permission.)

HIP JOINT

The single-axis hip joint, which joined the socket to the thigh section, was located lateral to the acetabulum. The hip joint was not strong enough to withstand the angular forces; therefore, the socket was designed to make contact with the medial edge of the thigh section in order to distribute weight-bearing. This made sitting lopsided. The hip and knee joints were locked during walking. Without locks, there was little control of the prosthesis.

PROBLEMS

The limb had to be advanced either by pelvic rotation or relative motion between the stump and the socket. The gait was unphysiologic and fatiguing. Excessive prosthetic weight and pistoning necessitated a shoulder strap. The pelvic band suspension was insecure and often allowed the socket to twist. The location of the hip joint (between the socket and the thigh piece) made sitting lopsided.

CANADIAN-TYPE HIP-DISARTICULATION PROSTHESIS

This prosthesis, which was introduced in the early 1950s by Colin McLaurin at the Prosthetic Service Centre at Sunnybrook Hospital in Toronto and was modified slightly through the years, is used almost universally.

SOCKET

The socket is sometimes called a bucket because of its shape. Functionally, it provides suspension, weight-bearing, and containment. An intimate fit is necessary for pelvic control of the prosthesis, comfortable support of the body weight, and adequate suspension. The amputee actually sits in the socket, as was done in the prototypes. Weight-bearing usually occurs on the ischial seat, although all of the ipsilateral pelvis contacts the socket. The weight-bearing area of the socket is constructed of rigid plastic laminate. The socket indents over the ipsilateral iliac crest. This indentation and a band-like extension of the socket (made flexible to permit easy donning) around the opposite iliac crest act to suspend the socket and prevent rotation (Fig. 13-8). If the socket is not sufficiently stabilized over the iliac crests, then excessive pistoning will occur. Reliefs are provided over the anterior and posterior iliac spines, the spinous processes of the vertebrae, and any other sensitive areas, such as surgical scars (Fig. 13-9).

The medial aspect of the socket is cut away to provide clearance for the normal leg and the genitalia. There should be no undue pressure on the pubic ramus. If pressure is intolerable with full weight on the socket, then the ischial seat and other weight-bearing areas should be enlarged for clearance of the ramus. Pressure over the soft tissue of the abdominal area is necessary for proper function (the leg is advanced by a posterior pelvic tilt). Better contact is made in the abdominal area if the cast is wrapped with the patient supine.

Variations of socket design include a *full socket* with an anterior opening, lateral opening, or anterior-lateral opening, and a *diagonal socket* with a lateral opening. The full socket includes both iliac crests for suspension and provides the best anterior-posterior stability in walking. It is preferred for the heavy person with soft residual

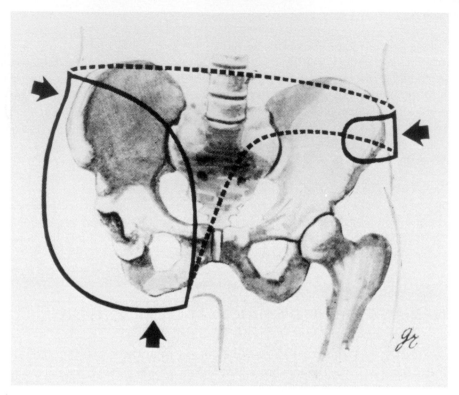

FIGURE 13-8. Anterior view of the Canadian-type hip-disarticulation prosthesis socket showing points of firm contact at the ipsilateral ischial tuberosity and iliac crest and the contralateral iliac crest. (From McLaurin, CA: *The evolution of the Canadian-type hip-disarticulation prosthesis.* Artificial Limbs 4:27, 1957, with permission.)

tissue. The diagonal socket works well only for the person with normal or lean build and firm residual tissue.

The diagonal socket exposes the pelvis down to the level of the anterior superior iliac spine on the amputated side. A flexible strap that extends over the crest of the ilium achieves suspension. The diagonal socket is cooler and easier to make, and it provides excellent suspension adjustment. It is less restrictive and more comfortable for sitting.

The anterodistal area of the surface of the socket is enlarged for attachment of the hip joint.

HIP JOINT

The hip joint is a broad hinge. A long bolt is used rather than the smaller single-axis joint used in older prostheses. Alignment stability is provided by the joint being located below and anterior to the axis of the normal hip. Ordinarily, no lock is needed. The axis of the hip-joint bearing is perpendicular to the line of progression and parallel to the floor. A posterior bumper (hip bumper or extension stop) controls the amount of hip extension. When the socket is pressed against the bumper, the vertebral spine should be in its natural position. The full-width hip joint resists lateral movement because of its strong connection between the prosthetic thigh and the socket.

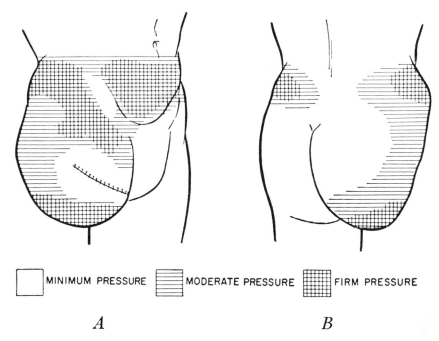

MINIMUM PRESSURE   MODERATE PRESSURE   FIRM PRESSURE

A   *B*

FIGURE 13-9. Distribution of weight when wearing the Canadian-type hip-disarticulation prosthesis. Areas of pressure provide support and stabilization. *(A)* Relief is provided over the surgical incision and the anterior superior iliac spine. *(B)* Relief is provided over the sacral area and posterior superior iliac spine. (From Radcliffe, CW: *The biomechanics of the Canadian-type hip-disarticulation prosthesis.* Artificial Limbs 4:37, 1957, with permission.)

THIGH

The prosthetic thigh should be parallel to the normal thigh and as close to the midline as possible.

KNEE UNIT

Since the amputee cannot stabilize the knee by extending the hip, stability is provided by posterior alignment of the knee rather than by a lock. The load transmitted between the socket and the ankle passes in front of the knee joint. Friction or hydraulic knee units enhance swing characteristics.

HIP FLEXION CONTROL STRAP (ELASTIC CHECK-STRAP, STRIDE LENGTH CONTROL STRAP)

One end is attached laterally about 5 cm (2 in) behind the hip joint. The other end is attached to the shank anteriorly about 7.6 cm (3 in) below the knee joint. The strap is installed so that it can rotate about the points of attachment. The strap serves a dual role by preventing excessive hip flexion and acting as a knee extension assist. It is designed to give the amputee a greater sense of security and a more functional, cosmetic, and relaxed gait by equalizing stride length.

ANKLE/FOOT ASSEMBLY

A SACH foot or an articulated foot may be used. A soft heel wedge or soft plantarflexion bumper is used for added stability.

ADVANTAGES

1. The socket can accommodate irregularities of body shape.
2. The molded socket transfers forces between the torso and the prosthesis comfortably.
3. The unlocked knee and hip offer a more natural looking gait than the previously described historic limbs. Little effort is required in the swing phase and a full stride is easily obtained. The amputee can stoop, squat, and sit without using manual controls.
4. The broad hip joint is durable.
5. The prosthesis is mechanically simple.
6. The socket is usually quite comfortable, due in part to the distribution of weight over a wide area.

DISADVANTAGES

1. The patient must be able to use the pelvis and lumbar spine to advance the leg. This may be a problem with elderly people.
2. It is often difficult to ascend stairs that are open or have overhangs, because the toe can catch under the step since the leg swings forward from the hip joint as it is lifted. The patient may have to assist manually.
3. In very warm climates, the enclosing socket can present hygiene and skin problems from perspiration because heat dissipation is restricted.
4. Walking speed is limited by the characteristic of the pendulum system of the leg. It is, however, greater than with the earlier prostheses.
5. The prosthesis does not allow an aesthetic gait.

ADAPTATIONS FOR THE VERY SHORT ABOVE-KNEE AMPUTATION

In the true hip disarticulation, the prosthesis must be suspended from the iliac crests. In the very short above-knee amputation, however, the greater trochanter, which projects more laterally than the iliac crest, remains. The prosthesis can then be suspended between the crests and the trochanters (the usual location for a pelvic band) rather than above the iliac crests.* The resulting socket is thus less confining. If the femur is very long, however, the socket will be unnatural in appearance, having an anterior protuberance for the flexed limb.

BIBLIOGRAPHY

Bell, JW: *Disarticulation of the hip for benign disease.* Arch Surg, 80:267–275, 1960.

Berkas, EM, Chesler, MD, and Sako, Y: *Multiple decubitus ulcer treatment by hip disarticulation and soft tissue flaps from lower limb.* Plast Reconstr Surg 27:618–619, 1961.

---

*This may be a good argument for leaving some of the femur, when surgically feasible.

BOYD, HB: *Anatomic disarticulation of the hip.* Surg Gynecol Obstet 84:346–349, 1947.

BURROWS, HJ: *Hindquarter amputation and disarticulation at the hip.* In MURDOCH, G (ED): *Prosthetic and Orthotic Practice.* Edward Arnold & Co, London, 1970, pp 277–284.

CARNES, EH: *Amputations, stumps and prostheses.* War Med 1:656–663, 1941.

FOORT, J: *Construction and fitting of the Canadian-type hip-disarticulation prosthesis.* Artificial Limbs 4:39–51, 1957.

FOORT, J: *Some experience with the Canadian-type hip-disarticulation prosthesis.* Artificial Limbs 4:52–70, 1957.

FORD, LT AND HOLDER, BK: *Disarticulation for failed surgical procedures about the hip.* South Med J 70:1293–1296, 1977.

GEORGIADE, N, PICKRELL, K, AND MAGUIRE, C: *Total thigh flaps for extensive decubitus ulcers.* Plast Reconstr Surg 17:220–225, 1956.

GHIULAMILA, RI, ET AL: *Prosthetic rehabilitation of a paraplegic with bilateral hip disarticulation and partial pelvectomy.* Arch Phys Med Rehabil 57:475–478, 1976.

GIACCONE, V AND STACK, D: *Temporary prosthesis for the hip-disarticulation amputee.* Phys Ther 57:1394–1396, 1977.

GILLIS, L: *A new prosthesis for disarticulation of the hip.* J Bone Joint Surg 50B:389–391, 1968.

HAMPTON, F: *Northwestern University suspension casting technique for hemipelvectomy and hip disarticulation.* Artificial Limbs 10:56–61, 1966.

HAMPTON, FL: *Above knee prostheses.* Orthop Clin North Am 3:359–372, 1972.

HAMPTON, FL: *Prosthetic principles in the lower extremity amputee.* Orthop Clin North Am 3:339–347, 1972.

HEPP, O AND BURGER, S: *Hip joint with automatically activated stop for the hip-disarticulated amputee.* Orth Pros Appl J 20:240–244, 1966.

HOGSHEAD, HP: *Experience with hip disarticulation and hemipelvectomy procedures.* J Bone Joint Surg 53A:1031, 1971.

HOLSCHER, EC, CURTIS, RJ, AND FARRIS, HG: *Hip-level amputation: A report of a survey of the United States military veterans.* Bull Prosthet Res 10–4:52–64, 1965.

LEE, CM, JR AND ALT, LP: *Hemipelvectomy and hip disarticulation for malignant tumors of the pelvis and lower extremity.* Ann Surg 137:704–717, 1953.

LOON, HE: *The past and present medical significance of hip disarticulation.* Artificial Limbs 4:4–21, 1957.

MAYNARD, RL: *Hip-joint disarticulations.* Trans N Engl Surg Soc 24:248–256, 1941.

MCBURNEY, C: *Direct intra-abdominal finger-compression of the common iliac artery during amputation at the hip-joint.* Ann Surg 25:610–613, 1897.

MCLAURIN, CA: *The evolution of the Canadian-type hip-disarticulation prosthesis.* Artificial Limbs 4:22–28, 1957.

MCLAURIN, CA: *The Canadian hip disarticulation prosthesis.* In MURDOCH, G (ED): *Prosthetic and Orthotic Practice.* Edward Arnold & Co, London, 1970, pp 285–304.

MCQUIRCK, AW: *The Canadian hip disarticulation prosthesis and modifications required for the hemipelvectomy.* In MURDOCH, G (ED): *Prosthetic and Orthotic Practice.* Edward Arnold & Co, London, 1970, pp 305–311.

MURDOCH, G: *Amputation surgery in the lower extremity.* Prosthet Orthot Int 1:72–83, 1977.

PACK, GT: *Major exarticulations for malignant neoplasms of the extremities: Interscapulothoracic amputation, hip-joint disarticulation, and interilio-abdominal amputation: A report of end results in 228 cases.* J Bone Joint Surg 38A:249–262, 1956.

PACK, GT AND EHRLICH, HE: *Exarticulation of the lower extremities for malignant tumors: Hip joint disarticulation (with and without deep iliac dissection) and sacro-iliac disarticulation* (hemipelvectomy). Ann Surg 123:965–985, 1946.

PACK, GT, EHRLICH, HE, AND de C GENTIL, F: *Radical amputations of the extremities in the treatment of cancer.* Surg Gynecol Obstet 84:1105–1116, 1947.

RADCLIFFE, CW: *The biomechanics of the Canadian-type hip-disarticulation prosthesis.* Artificial Limbs 4:29–38, 1957.

SALTZSTEIN, HC: *Osteogenic sarcoma of upper third of femur: Well ten years after disarticulation at the hip joint.* J Mich Med Soc 43:145–147, 1944.

SEDDON, HJ AND SCALES, JT: *A polythene substitute for the upper two-thirds of the shaft of the femur.* Lancet 2:795–796, 1949.

SMITH, BC: *Disarticulation of the hip for endothelioma (Ewing's tumor): 31-year follow-up.* Ann Surg 115:318–320, 1942.

SMITH, BC: *A 54-year follow-up report of disarticulation of the left hip for recurrent Ewing's tumor of the femur.* Surg Gynecol Obstet 118:120–122, 1964.

SOLOMONIDIS, SE, ET AL: *Biomechanics of the hip disarticulation prosthesis.* Prosthet Orthot Int 1:13–18, 1977.

SPIRA, M AND HARDY, SB: *Our experiences with high thigh amputations in paraplegics.* Plast Reconstr Surg 31:344–352, 1963.

SWEETNAM, R: *Amputation in osteosarcoma: Disarticulation of the hip or high thigh amputation for lower femoral growths?* J Bone Joint Surg 55B:189–192, 1973.

THOMPSON, RG: *Amputation in the lower extremity.* J Bone Joint Surg 45A:1723–1734, 1963.

TOSBERG, WA: *Prosthetic management of the proximal A-K amputations.* In *Prosthetics International, Proceedings of the Second International Prosthetics Course, Committee on Prostheses, Braces and Technical Aids, International Society for the Welfare of Cripples.* Copenhagen, 1960, pp 111–112.

TROUP, JB AND BICKEL, WH: *Malignant disease of the extremities treated by exarticulation: Analysis of two hundred and sixty-four consecutive cases with survival rates.* J Bone Joint Surg 42A:1041–1050, 1960.

VAN ENST, W: *Hip disarticulation in patients with paraplegia and a survey of the treatment of pressure sores and its complications.* Arch Chir Neerl 15:249–274, 1963.

WESTBURY, G: *Hindquarter and hip amputation.* Ann R Coll Surg Engl 40:226–234, 1967.

WILSON, AB, JR: *Limb prosthetics: 1970.* Artificial Limbs 14:1–52, 1970.

Workshop on Knee-Disarticulation and Hip-Disarticulation Prostheses. Subcommittee on Design and Development. Committee on Prosthetics Research and Development, Division of Engineering-National Research Council, National Academy of Sciences, National Academy of Engineering, San Francisco, Calif, 1969.

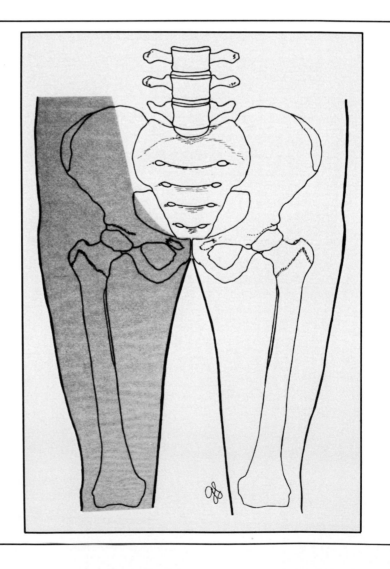

CHAPTER **14**

HEMIPELVECTOMY (HIP [HIP], COMPLETE)

(HINDQUARTER AMPUTATION, INTER-INNOMINO-ABDOMIN-AL AMPUTATION, INTERILIOSACROPUBIC AMPUTATION, SAC-ROILIAC DISARTICULATION, EXARTICULATION THROUGH THE SACROILIAC JOINT, INTERPELVI-ABDOMINAL AMPUTATION, TRANSILIAC AMPUTATION, DISARTICULATION OF THE IN-NOMINATE BONE, INTERILIOABDOMINAL AMPUTATION, LOWER QUARTERECTOMY, TRANSISCHIOSACROPUBIC DISAR-TICULATION, TRANSPELVIC AMPUTATION)

Although the first hemipelvectomy was reported in 1895 (an unsuccessful attempt by Theodor Billroth in Vienna in 1891), the occurrence of this radical surgery has been rare. Charles Girard of Berne, Switzerland, is credited with the first successful hemipelvectomy in 1895. The patient, a 17-year-old girl with osteosarcoma of the proximal femur, at first received a hip disarticulation in May 1894. The hemipelvectomy was performed in March 1895 for recurrence in the scar. The patient died from recurrence approximately 1 year following the hemipelvectomy.

Leonard Freeman of Denver is credited with having performed the first successful amputation of a leg and part of the pelvis in the United States in 1899. The anterior third of the acetabulum and the ilium were left. In 1909, Joseph Ransohoff of Cincinnati performed the first successful complete hemipelvectomy in the United States on a patient who lived for 38 days following the surgery. The operative wound was well healed, and autopsy showed that the patient died of pulmonary tuberculosis and acute toxic nephritis.

Hogarth Pringle, a British surgeon, reported three cases in 1909, all of which were treated in two stages: disarticulation at the hip or high above-knee amputation followed later by hemipelvectomy. He also listed 21 cases in all that he was able to find up to that time. In 1916, Pringle reported two more cases of his own (both of these patients received a one-stage procedure) and described the principles of the surgical procedure in detail. The estimated operative time was 55 to 60 minutes. The operative mortality was low when it is remembered that blood transfusion was not readily available in Great Britain and saline infusion was the means to combat shock. T.C. Davison of Atlanta claimed to have performed the operation successfully in 1921 on a patient who lived for 7 years, then died of pneumonia. The case was not reported in the literature at the time, however.

Gordon Gordon-Taylor, a British surgeon, first attempted this operation in 1922. In 1935, with Phillip Wise, he reported his first five cases, including his first success in 1929. By this time, the operation had been performed at least 79 times by 48 different surgeons. In 1952, with Monro, he described his technique and management in detail. By 1957, Gordon-Taylor had a personal total of 108 cases. The procedure gained wider acceptance because of his writings on the subject. He described it as "one of the most colossal mutilations practiced on the human frame." In 1942, more American cases were reported by W.E. Leighton of St. Louis (3 cases) and J.J. Morton of Rochester (4 cases without a death).

A hemipelvectomy is usually performed for malignant disease of the upper thigh, hip joint, or pelvis that cannot be extirpated by more conservative means. Hemipelvectomy amputations have even been reported in infants as young as 13 days old and in children for such massive congenital malformations as massive mixed angiomas (hemolymph angiomas). Occasionally, it is performed for osteomyelitis of the pelvis or proximal femur and for certain massive benign tumors in the pelvic region if they cannot be resected adequately by a less radical procedure. This disfiguring surgical procedure has also been performed as a palliative measure for excruciating pain when analgesia could not be obtained by pharmacologic or neurosurgical means, or when the mass is bulky, infected, and foul smelling, causing limited function. Most patients have received some unsuccessful form of treatment prior to this radical amputation.

Several cases of survival following traumatic (traffic, mine, and combine harvester accidents) hindquarter avulsion have been reported. These patients may require permanent colostomies due to irreparable damage to the anus and rectum, but urinary tract involvement is rare.

SURGICAL PROCEDURES

A catheter is placed in the bladder and the anus is closed with a purse-string suture to prevent inadvertent contamination of the massive amputation wound. The primary purpose of the amputation is eradication of the lesion. The location of the skin incision is secondary to this purpose and is dictated by the condition of the skin and the location and size of the lesion. Radiation fibrosis makes dissection more difficult.

POSTERIOR SKIN FLAP METHOD

The patient is usually placed in a semilateral position on the side opposite to the lesion. The incision consists of anterior and posterior parts. The anterior incision (Fig. 14-1) is made just above and parallel to the inguinal (Poupart's) ligament, extending posteriorly just above the iliac crest and downward (anteriorly) across the pubic tubercle into the crease between the thigh and the perineum. The posterior incision (made later in the surgery) extends from the iliac crest incision downward (Fig. 14-2). An anterior convexity is made as the incision extends anterior to the greater trochanter and comes around the posterior aspect of the upper thigh or along the gluteal fold to meet the lower end of the anterior incision at the ischial tuberosity. The biopsy scar, if present, should not be included in the flaps. The ipsilateral abdominal musculature is sectioned. The peritoneum and attached ureter are pushed medially. The pelvis is usually separated at the pubic symphysis.

Either the common or the external iliac artery is ligated and divided. This procedure preserves the superior and inferior gluteal arteries, thus ensuring a well-vascularized gluteal flap. The psoas muscle is divided along with the femoral, obturator, and lateral cutaneous nerves. The gluteus maximus is reflected with the skin flap if it or the ilium is not pathologically involved. The crest of the ilium is skeletonized (the attachments of the quadratus lumborum and other muscles are severed). The ilium is usually divided at the junction of the middle and posterior thirds of the iliac crest or at the sacroiliac joint (Fig. 14-3), depending on the location and nature of the pathology. Section can be made through the ala of the sacrum, if necessary. Shock* occasionally occurs during partition of the sacroiliac synchondrosis. A blood transfusion may be given at this time to prevent shock, especially since the gluteal and obturator arteries will soon be divided.

The sciatic nerve and sacrotuberous and sacrospinous ligaments are divided. Sharp projections of the ilium are trimmed. The longer posterior flap is tailored to fit by removing redundant skin and muscle tags. The gluteus maximus, if preserved, is sutured to the lateral or anterior abdominal musculature, and the skin is closed.

---

*Other measures that have been recommended to reduce the incidence of shock are gentle handling of tissues, careful and deliberate dissection, reduction in the number of sudden changes of the patient's position, lowering the head of the table, and injection of large nerve trunks with alcohol or procaine prior to sectioning.

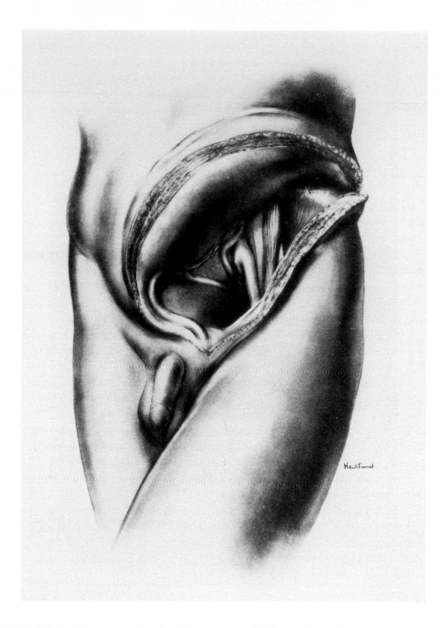

FIGURE 14-1. The anterior incision extends from just above the iliac crest downward to the crease between the thigh and perineum to expose the common iliac artery bifurcation. (From Gordon-Taylor, G and Monro, R: *The technique and management of the "hindquarter" amputation.* Br J Surg 39:537, 1952, with permission.)

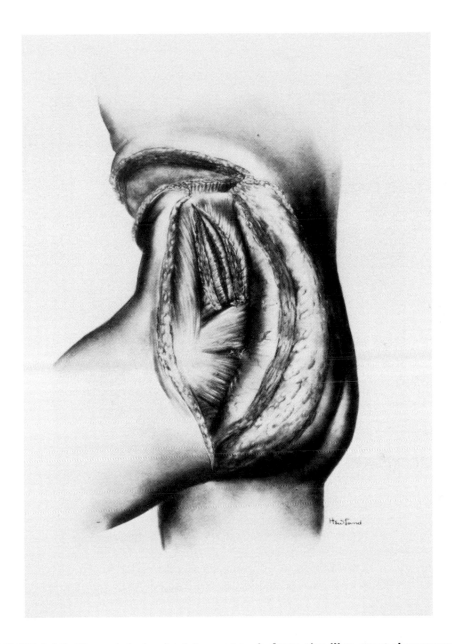

FIGURE 14-2. The posterior incision extends from the iliac crest downward, curving anterior to the greater trochanter then along or just below the gluteal fold until it medially meets the anterior incision at the ischial tuberosity. (From Gordon-Taylor, G and Monro, R: *The technique and management of the "hindquarter" amputation.* Br J Surg 39:538, 1952, with permission.)

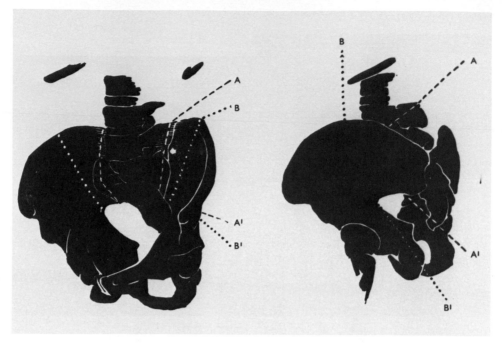

FIGURE 14-3. Posterior section of the bony pelvis may be at the sacroiliac joint (A-A') or more laterally through the ala of the ilium (B-B'). (From Gordon-Taylor, G and Monro, R: *The technique and management of the "hindquarter" amputation.* Br J Surg 39:539, 1952, with permission.)

ANTERIOR SKIN FLAP METHOD

When lesions are present in the area of the buttocks, it is necessary to use an anterior flap rather than a posterior flap. The anterior incision begins 5 cm (2 in) above the knee and extends laterally to the anterior superior iliac spine and medially to the crease between the adductor muscles and the perineum (Fig. 14-4). The femoral nerve, artery, and vein, and all of the muscles anterior to the femur are included in the large anterior flap. The incision is continued posteriorly from the anterior superior iliac spine to the midline and then inferiorly to meet the medial incision between the perineum and adductor muscles.

The oblique and transverse muscles are detached from the ilium and pubic bone. The iliac muscle is detached from the ilium, as are the inguinal ligament and all muscles attaching to the anterior superior iliac spine and pubic ramus. Osteotomies are made at or near the pubic symphysis and sacroiliac joint. The superior and inferior gluteal vessels and sciatic nerve passing through the greater sciatic notch are identified and ligated (Fig. 14-5). The obturator vessels and nerve passing through the obturator foramen are ligated and divided. The anterior flap is brought posteriorly and closed loosely (Fig. 14-5 *inset*).

Antibiotics are given preoperatively if the tumor is infected and fungating. Postoperative antibiotics are given because of the massiveness of the wound. Either the posterior or anterior skin flap operation can usually be performed in 2 to 4 hours.

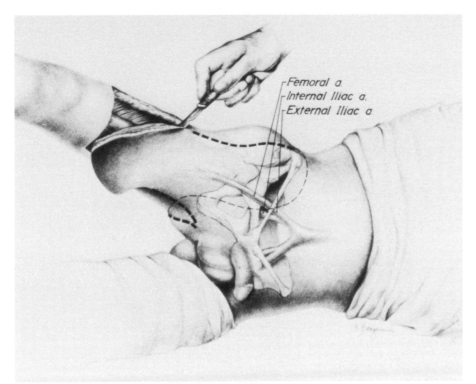

FIGURE 14-4. The anterior incision *(heavy dash line)* creates a large pedicle flap that contains the femoral artery, vein, and nerve, as well as the muscles anterior to the femur. The posterior incision *(light dash line)* continues from the anterior superior iliac spine posteriorly to the midline and then inferiorly to meet the medial anterior incision. (From Frey, C, et al: *A new technique for hemipelvectomy.* Surg Gynecol Obstet 143:754, 1976, with permission.)

OPERATIVE VARIATIONS

ABDOMINAL EXPLORATION

In certain cases (e.g., malignant melanoma), hepatic metastases may appear early. To determine the tumor's operability, a preliminary laparotomy or liver scan should be considered. If intra-abdominal metastases are present in cases of malignant tumors, then the decision can be made to terminate the amputation. Computerized axial tomography can be performed when suspicious lesions are present. Pulmonary fields are also checked clinically and roentgenologically.

SURGICAL POSITION

LATERAL

The lateral position allows exposure to both the anterior and posterior incisions and allows for a gravitational shift of viscera; therefore, retraction of the viscera is not necessary to expose the pelvic structures.

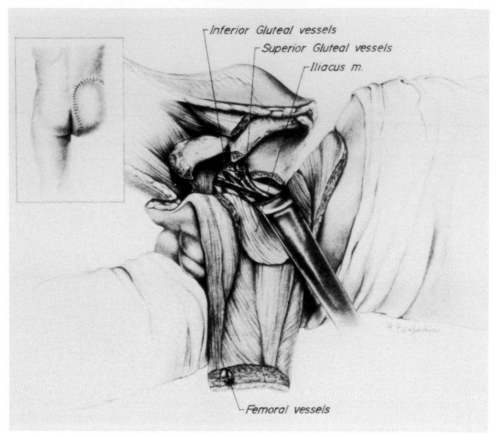

FIGURE 14-5. Following osteotomies of the pubic symphysis and posterior ilium, the superior and inferior gluteal vessels are ligated. (Inset) The anterior flap is closed posteriorly. (From Frey, C, et al: *A new technique for hemipelvectomy.* Surg Gynecol Obstet 143:755, 1976, with permission.)

SUPINE

Some surgeons prefer the supine position because it allows rapid exposure of the major vessels for preliminary ligation.

EXTENDED HEMIPELVECTOMY

Extended hemipelvectomy is the term used for the standard procedure plus excision of organs (kidney, uterus, ovaries or testes, or portions of the bowel and urinary bladder) or additional bone (wing of the ipsilateral sacrum or parts of the contralateral pubic bone and ischium). This procedure is used to eradicate a tumor that extends beyond that area circumscribed by the classical operation. If the wing of the ilium is involved in osteogenic sarcoma or chondrosarcoma, removal of the articular surface and wing of the ipsilateral sacrum has been recommended by some surgeons. In any case, the tumor-bearing bone should be removed in its entirety, and thus the ilium should not be divided lateral to the sacroiliac joint if it is involved. If a small rim of the iliac crest is retained, clothing with a waist may be worn more easily and suspension of a prosthesis will be more easily obtained. However, the remaining segment of the ilium may ride upward and cause pain at the synchondrosis. Disarticulation at the sacroiliac joint has been viewed by some as the most critical part of the operation owing to blood loss and impending shock. This point has been used as an argument to retain a portion of the ilium.

SKIN FLAPS

A thick skin flap from the anterior aspect of the extremity, without inclusion of the muscles on the anterior thigh, may be used. It is desirable that the inferior epigastric, external iliac, circumflex iliac, and other branches of the circumflex femoral vessels be left intact to provide nutrition to the anterior flap.

ANTERIOR BONE SECTION

Section through the pubic bone about 1 cm (0.4 in) lateral to the symphysis has been suggested in some cases. This retains support to the abdominal viscera by the rectus abdominis muscle. There is less chance of impairment of sexual function if the pubic bone is divided below the attachment of the corpus cavernosum. Also, bleeding from the retropubic venous plexus does not usually occur. If an osteotomy is made at the symphysis, then care must be taken not to injure the bladder or urethra. The site and extent of the tumor usually determine whether the pubic bone is disarticulated at the symphysis or divided at the rami. Experience has shown that saving the rectus attachment is not necessary for adequate support of the abdominal viscera. Section may also be made beyond the symphysis through the contralateral pubic bone if indicated by the extent of the tumor.

POSTERIOR BONE SECTION

Removal of the entire innominate bone is generally recommended in cases where malignant disease involves the bone itself. If the tumor extends to or across the sacroiliac joint, the lateral portion of the sacral segments is excised. Section through the ipsilateral ilium is more likely to be considered for benign tumors of the ilium or tumors of the proximal thigh.

PRESERVATION OF THE GLUTEUS MAXIMUS

Preservation of the gluteus maximus allows for more symmetric buttocks because it helps to fill the large defect. Its removal, however, does not result in a higher frequency of herniation of the abdominal viscera. Some surgeons suggest the removal of the gluteus maximus because of the possibility of pathologic invasion in cases of tumors and surgical damage to its blood supply from the superior gluteal artery.

REMOVAL OF THE INNOMINATE BONE WITHOUT AMPUTATION OF THE ENTIRE LOWER EXTREMITY (INTERNAL HEMIPELVECTOMY)

Kocher, in 1884, was the first to substitute resection of part or all of the innominate bone without removal of the entire lower extremity. In these early cases, the operative mortality was considerably lower and the patient was able to stand and walk. This procedure was possible only in certain limited cases. A prosthetic metal or plastic pelvic implant is individually made (Fig. 14-6). The shape and measurements are deter-

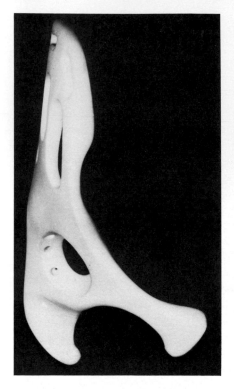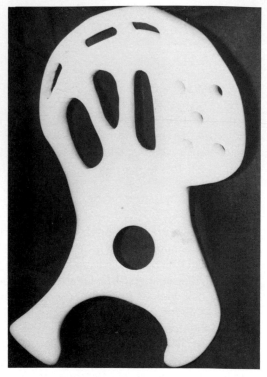

FIGURE 14-6. A pelvic implant with acetabular bed and windows for muscle attachments. (From Burri, C, et al: *Total "internal" hemipelvectomy.* Arch Orthop Trauma Surg 94:222, 1979, with permission.)

mined by external and roentgenographic measurements or, more recently, by computer tomograms. Osseous muscular origins and insertions are re-established. The implant is attached to the symphysis anteriorly by plate fixation and through the sacroiliac joint posteriorly by screws and corticocancellous grafts. A total hip replacement is necessary. Muscles are attached to the implant through windows in the implant.

BLADDER FUNCTION

Although hemipelvectomy presumably involves the pelvic plexus and pudendal nerve unilaterally, it has been determined from follow-up investigations that neurogenic bladder dysfunction does not result. These results agree with animal studies that have shown that unilateral denervation of the bladder does not result in disturbances of micturition. Control of the anal sphincter is usually maintained without difficulty.

PREGNANCY

Successful vaginal and cesarean deliveries of mature, healthy infants by women who have had a hemipelvectomy have been reported. These have included both cephalic and breech presentations. Genital prolapse was reported in one patient but was repaired successfully following two vaginal deliveries.

POSTOPERATIVE COMPLICATIONS

HEMORRHAGE AND FLAP NECROSIS

Primary sources of hemorrhage are the deep dorsal vein of the penis anteriorly during section of the symphysis and the large superior gluteal artery during section of the innominate bone posteriorly, because it is in close proximity to the sacroiliac synchondrosis. Amputation is relatively bloodless if the common rather than the external iliac artery is ligated; however, skin flap necrosis of the posterior flap is more common if the common iliac artery is ligated, especially if the flap is particularly long. If the patient is viewed as a poor operative risk, some surgeons prefer to ligate the common iliac artery and risk possible necrosis of the posterior flap rather than ligating the external iliac artery and risking operative death. In such cases, it is recommended that a thin posterior skin flap be used because the lost blood supply is essentially to the subcutaneous tissue rather than to the overlying skin. The gangrenous process originates in the subcutaneous fat with delayed or latent secondary necrosis of the skin. Thus, by the time the necrosis can be seen externally, the wound is extensively infected. A V-shaped wedge taken from the central portion of the posterior flap has been described to avoid ischemic difficulties (Fig. 14-7). This procedure leaves a T-shaped scar.

The incidence of necrosis can also be minimized by using the anterior flap method because the femoral vessels are present for vascularization of the flap. Another technique used to minimize the incidence of skin flap necrosis has been the intravenous injection of fluorescein dye just prior to closure. Visualization of the wound edges under ultraviolet light reveals the skin flap's vascularity, and revisions can be performed as indicated. Care must be taken not to use skin for the flap that has been devitalized by roentgenotherapy.

A procedure in which an atraumatic vascular clamp is temporarily placed on the common iliac artery during the amputation has also been described. In this way, blood loss is markedly reduced during surgery. Actual division of the arterial supply can be performed later in the procedure at the level of the external iliac artery. The vascular clamp on the common iliac artery is released before wound closure.

PARESIS OF THE URINARY BLADDER

Bladder paresis sometimes occurs, but it is temporary (function usually returns in 4 to 7 days). An indwelling catheter is used during surgery so that the bladder is empty and thus less likely to be injured.

URINARY FISTULA

A urinary fistula can result from injury to the ureters or bladder at the time of division of the pubic symphysis.

ABDOMINAL DISTENTION

Either trauma to the retracted abdominal contents or the division of the lumbosacral plexus might be the cause of abdominal distention. Paralytic ileus is rarely encountered if nasogastric suction is used for 24 to 48 hours postoperatively. Prostigmin (neostigmine) may also be used during the immediate postoperative period.

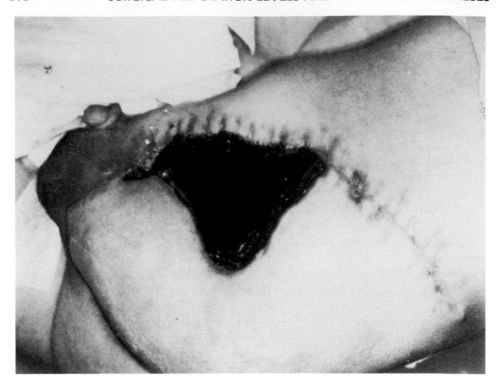

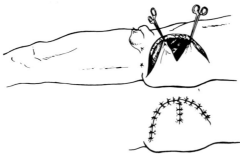

FIGURE 14-7. *(Top)* A triangular area of necrosis in the central portion of the posterior flap following ligation of the common iliac artery. *(Bottom)* A wedge-shaped excision of the posterior flap to prevent necrosis. (From Miller, TR: *Hemipelvectomy in lower extremity tumors.* Orthop Clin North Am 8:914, 1977, with permission.)

WOUND INFECTIONS

Postoperative wound infections may be due to the close proximity of the anus and genitals to the operative area, or to the state (ulcerated, necrotic, infected) of the tumor. Wound infections are minimized if prophylactic antibiotic therapy is started preoperatively and continued through the postoperative period.

WOUND DRAINAGE

Profuse wound drainage can usually be avoided by severing muscles at their insertions when possible, thus avoiding pocketing under the flaps and preventing infection.

SCOLIOSIS

This can usually be managed with a prosthetic socket.

PHANTOM PAIN

Phantom pain has been reported, but it is usually not disabling and lessens with prosthetic usage.

EPIDIDYMITIS

Interference with testicular blood supply or trauma caused by retraction of the cord may cause epididymitis.

OSTEOMYELITIS

Osteomyelitis has been encountered when the contralateral pubic arch was severed, exposing cancellous bone, rather than the pubic symphysis.

ANEMIA

Anemia, presumed to be the result of removal of so much hematopoietic bone marrow, frequently occurs within 10 days after surgery and persists for about 3 weeks. Transfusions may not control the anemia. Compensatory marrow hyperplasia does occur, however, but may be a problem in the patient who has previously received chemotherapy or radiation therapy.

HERNIATION

Herniation is rare even when the abdominal contents are supported only by the peritoneum, fascia, subcutaneous tissue, and skin. There is no need to preserve the gluteus maximus in the flap for additional strength; however, it does provide padding.

MORTALITY

Death can be due to hemorrhage and shock or to recurrence of the cancer. Although the mortality for hemipelvectomy amputation was estimated to be about 60 percent through 1935, the operation itself is now considered to be a safe procedure. Benign lesions offer the best prognosis. Of those patients resected for cure of malignant neoplasms, there is a probable cure rate of about 20 percent. Patients with chondrosarcomas have the longest survival rate. Because there is little difference in the ease of prosthetic fitting and wearing following either hip disarticulation or hemipelvectomy, some surgeons reason that in cases of tumor, sparing the ilium, ischial tuberosity, or rectus abdominis muscle attachments adds little. The advantage gained by a wide excision to eradicate the tumor may be lost if a hip disarticulation or partial hemipelvectomy is performed. Tumors such as fibrosarcoma, malignant synovioma, and malignant neurilemoma may proceed insidiously upward along fascial planes, intermuscular planes, or nerve sheaths and may recur in the residual limb even after very high, radical amputations.

HEMIPELVECTOMY OR HIP DISARTICULATION

Of primary concern to physicians in many instances is not whether an amputation should be performed, but whether to perform a hip disarticulation or a hemipelvectomy.

Hip Disarticulation:
1. The ipsilateral ischial tuberosity remains, which makes sitting easier.
2. Clothing drapes more naturally below the waist when a prosthesis is not being worn.

Hemipelvectomy:
1. For tumors of the proximal thigh, it provides a greater margin of normal tissue.
2. It is considered to be technically less difficult because fewer muscle masses are transected.

PROSTHESES

CANVAS SUPPORT

A canvas support with adjustable abdominal straps and a shoulder strap may be used for support to the amputation flap and pelvic contents in lieu of a prosthesis. This device may be of particular benefit to pregnant women (Fig. 14-8).

PROSTHETIC BODY JACKET

A body jacket made of plaster or plastic has been successfully used for patients who will not use a prosthetic leg following hemipelvectomy (e.g., paraplegic patients). Because the jacket is rigid on the side of the amputation and flexible on the contralateral side, it reduces the inevitable scoliotic curve. Postural deformity with resultant backache can also be corrected with a molded artificial buttock incorporated into a lumbosacral corset. A lightweight container socket may be desirable to support the viscera when the prosthesis is not being worn.

MODIFIED CANADIAN-TYPE
HIP-DISARTICULATION PROSTHESIS

Three levels of amputation can be fitted with the hip-disarticulation prosthesis: very short above-knee (usually above the lesser trochanter), hip disarticulation, and hemipelvectomy.

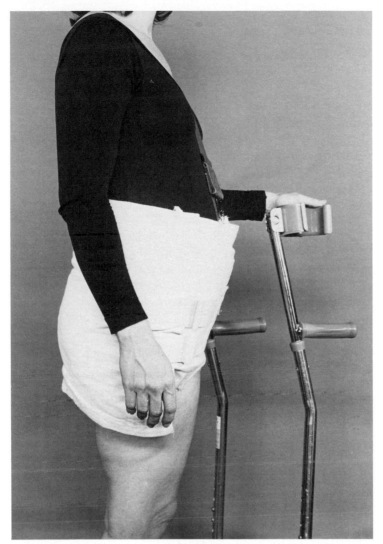

FIGURE 14-8. Anterior view of a cotton canvas sling support garment with Velcro abdominal and crotch closures. (From Stavrakas, PA and Sanders, GT: *Sling support during pregnancy after hemipelvectomy: Case report.* Arch Phys Med Rehabil 64:333, 1983, with permission.)

FUNCTION

The prosthetic limb functions in the same manner for the hemipelvectomy patient as it does for the hip-disarticulation patient. The components, principles of alignment, and mechanics are essentially the same. The major differences, and thus the problems in construction of the prosthesis, are the areas used for weight-bearing with the ipsilateral ischial tuberosity missing, and stabilization/suspension of the prosthesis with the absence of the ipsilateral iliac crest.

SOCKET

The loads imposed through the hip joint are the same as with the hip-disarticulation prosthesis, but the loads are distributed over the residual tissue in a different pattern in the hemipelvectomy prosthesis. Since the ischial tuberosity is completely removed, the only remaining areas for weight-bearing are the residual soft-tissue mass, the ribs and lower thorax, and the ischial tuberosity of the sound leg. The soft-tissue mass of the abdominal parietes, which is a large, broad, sloping surface, provides a primary weight-bearing area. Since the forces are applied obliquely (Fig. 14-9), generally 35 to 40 degrees horizontally, the shear stress is significant. Normal, full-thickness skin is needed to withstand full body weight-bearing during the stance phase. If the amputee has skin problems at the amputation site, then weight-bearing must be limited over this area. The use of alternative weight-bearing to the rib cage, as with the hemicorporectomy amputee, becomes a necessity. In most cases, weight-bearing is divided between the residual soft tissue and the lower thorax in varying proportions. If the gluteal muscles are retained and the skin is in good condition, then more pressure can be applied over the residual soft tissue and the height of the socket can be kept lower. Amputees may inspire reflexively and hold their breath during weight-bearing on the prosthesis to fill the bucket and thus offer a counterpressure.

Patients can usually only tolerate full weight-bearing supported by the ribs for short periods of time. The extended socket necessary for weight-bearing through the rib cage greatly restricts body movement and hinders heat dissipation. Because the socket is rigid and partially compresses the abdomen, the amputee may experience discomfort if large amounts of food are eaten in one sitting.

Some weight may be borne through the contralateral gluteus maximus. Utilization of the contralateral ischial tuberosity for weight-bearing has met with limited success.

The socket cast is taken under weight-bearing conditions. Foam is used to fill the cavity in the distal socket. Direct pressure on the coccyx and remaining sacrum is avoided. If part of the ipsilateral ilium or pubic bone remains, then care must be taken to provide relief for these sensitive areas. Review of appropriate roentgenograms may be necessary for adequate evaluation of the bony structure. Relief is also provided over the anterior superior iliac spine on the sound side. Although amputees who are very thin are the most difficult to fit, the degree of pistoning is greatly reduced.

The socket for the hemipelvectomy amputee extends lower on the sound side than for the hip disarticulation amputee. Since the force on the contralateral side of the socket is greater with a hemipelvectomy, the extended socket allows the force to be spread over a larger area.

SUSPENSION

With the absence of most or all of the ipsilateral iliac crest, suspension presents more of a problem following hemipelvectomy than it does following hip disarticulation. If there is any posterolateral ilium remaining on the ipsilateral side, then it may be used for suspension along with the contralateral iliac crest. A shoulder strap may be necessary for additional support, especially if the amputee is obese.

The remaining soft tissue does not provide a good horizontal weight-bearing surface as with the hip disarticulation amputation. The soft tissue displaces vertically and medially during weight-bearing, resulting in a relative (functional) shortening. During swing phase, there is a relative lengthening of the limb.

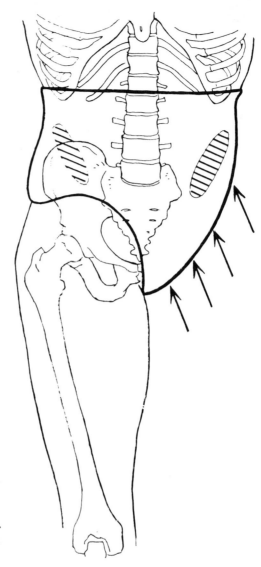

FIGURE 14-9. Hemipelvectomy socket. Arrows indicate the oblique upward forces applied by the socket to the residual semisolid abdominal mass. The shaded interior bulges aid suspension and prevent rotation. (From Hampton, F: *A hemipelvectomy prosthesis.* Artificial Limbs 8:4, 1964, with permission.)

OPENING

The opening for donning the prosthesis may be in the anterior or lateral aspect of the socket. Velcro is most often used for closure.

HIP JOINT

A flat area is built up on the anterodistal aspect of the socket for installation of the hip joint. The hip joint should be located forward enough for stability during the stance phase, lateral enough for clearance in the crotch area, and high enough so the extension stop does not impede sitting. The axis of the hip joint is essentially parallel to the floor and perpendicular to the line of progression, as is the axis of the knee joint.

FOOT

A SACH foot with a soft heel wedge, which increases stability of the prosthesis at heel-strike, is usually used.

LENGTH

Since some degree of pistoning is inevitable in the hemipelvectomy prosthesis, the overall prosthetic length is often intentionally shorter than the sound leg to facilitate clearing of the foot during swing phase. Functional telescoping is greater in the obese patient.

USE

Although the modified Canadian-type hip-disarticulation prosthesis can be satisfactorily fitted to most amputees, many amputees prefer crutches for speed and agility in ambulation and use the prosthesis for the sake of appearance on special occasions. Prosthetic use may be minimized if the skin has been damaged by radiation therapy or if skin grafting has been necessary to repair necrotic lesions of the posterior flap or skin that was invaded by a tumor.

BIBLIOGRAPHY

ARIEL, IM: *Hemipelvectomy (Interilioabdominal amputation)*. Prosthet Orthot Int 2:1–2, 1965.

ARIEL, IM AND HARK, FM: *Disarticulation of an innominate bone (hemipelvectomy) for primary and metastatic cancer*. Ann Surg 130:76–99, 1949.

ARIEL, IM AND MARGOLIS, R: *The sacroiliac twist: Inoperable chondrosarcoma rendered resectable by hemipelvectomy*. NY State J Med 62:3297–3301, 1962.

ARMOUR, JC AND LAWSON, RW: *The hindquarter amputation*. Can Med Assoc J 62:371–374, 1950.

BABCOCK, WW: *Interilio-abdominal amputation: A description of a new method, with a report of three cases*. Surg Gynecol Obstet 26:554–559, 1918.

BANKS, SW AND COLEMAN, S: *Hemipelvectomy: Surgical technique*. J Bone Joint Surg 38A:1147–1155, 1956.

BECK, NR AND BICKEL, WH: *Interinnomino-abdominal amputations: Report of 12 cases*. J Bone Joint Surg 30A:201–209, 1948.

BECKER, WF: *Sacro-iliac disarticulation (hemipelvectomy): A case report*. Va Med Monthly 78:129–131, 1951.

BEN-ADERET, N: *Pregnancy following hind-quarter amputation*. J Obstet Gynaec Brim Comm 72:306–307, 1965.

BERTELSEN, A: *On hemipelvectomy and interscapulo-thoracic amputation*. In *Prosthetics International, Proceedings of the Second International Prosthetics Course, Committee on Prostheses, Braces and Technical Aids, International Society for the Welfare of Cripples*. Copenhagen, 1960, pp 95–98.

BLOCK, GE: *Successful extended hemipelvectomy for "inoperable" chondrosarcoma of the pelvis*. Surg Clin North Am 50:985–997, 1970.

BOGRETTE, A: *Case report: A hemipelvectomy patient*. JAPTA 42:776–777, 1962.

BOWERS, RF: *Quarterectomy: Its application in malignant melanoma.* Surgery 26:523–538, 1949.

BOWERS, RF: *Observations from the use of quarterectomy.* Arch Surg 79:483–486, 1959.

BOWERS, RF: *Eleven years' experience with quarterectomy for malignant melanoma.* Arch Surg 81:752–756, 1960.

BRITTAIN, HA: *Hindquarter amputation.* J Bone Joint Surg 31B:404–409, 1949.

BROCHUNIER, A, JR: *Vaginal delivery following hemipelvectomy for malignant neoplasms of the bone and soft parts: A report of 3 deliveries in 2 patients.* Obstet Gynecol 23:67–71, 1964.

BRUNSCHWIG, A: *Hemipelvectomy in combination with partial pelvic exenteration for uncontrolled recurrent and metastatic cancer of the cervix: Five-year survival.* Surgery 52:299–304, 1962.

BUCKNER, HT, MCCONVILLE, BE, AND CALLAHAN, JJ: *Hemipelvectomy: Report of a case.* Northwest Med 49:874–875, 1950.

BURRI, C, ET AL: *Total "internal" hemipelvectomy.* Arch Orthop Trauma Surg 94:219–226, 1979.

BYRON, RL, JR, ET AL: *Interscapulothoracic amputation and sacroiliac disarticulation with adjunctive arterial chemotherapy.* Surg Gynecol Obstet 111:457–463, 1960.

CHILDS, TF AND HOLTZMAN, M: *Postoperative management and rehabilitation of the hemipelvectomized patient.* Arch Phys Med Rehabil 40:227–230, 1959.

CHURCHILL, CJ, ET AL: *Postoperative "restoration" of the hemipelvectomized patient.* J Ky Med Assoc 55:904–906, 1957.

CLEATOR, IGM AND SMITH, AN: *Hindquarter amputation by a synchronous combined approach.* J R Coll Surg Edinb 17:51–54, 1972.

CLUTTS, GR AND DEATON, WR, JR: *Hemipelvectomy: A palliative procedure.* Am Surg 24:511–514, 1958.

COLEY, BL AND HIGINBOTHAM, NL: *Management of malignant disease in neighborhood of the hip.* Surg Gynecol Obstet 99:727–732, 1954.

COLEY, BL AND HIGINBOTHAM, N: *Indications for hemipelvectomy.* Surgery 44:766–774, 1958.

COLEY, BL, HIGINBOTHAM, NL, AND ROMIEU, C: *Hemipelvectomy for tumors of bone: Report of fourteen cases.* Am J Surg 82:27–43, 1951.

COOPER, JF AND TAYLOR, GW: *Prosthesis following hemipelvectomy.* N Engl J Med 241:1047–1049, 1949.

CORYN, J: *Une indication rare de la désarticulation interilioabdominale: L'osteomyelite de la hanche.* Acta Chir Belg 49:249–252, 1950.

CREGAN, JCF AND BURSLEM, RW: *Pregnancy and successful caesarean section after hemipelvectomy for malignant disease.* Br Med J 1:1614, 1964.

DAVIS, BP, ET AL: *The problem of fitting a satisfactory prosthesis following hemipelvectomy.* Inter-Clinic Info Bull 3:5–9, 1964.

DIDOLKAR, MS, BAFFI, RR, AND BAKAMJIAN, VY: *Use of a tuber thoracoepigastric flap to cover the defect from a hindquarter amputation: Case Report.* Plast Reconstr Surg 61:112–114, 1978.

DINSDALE, SM, PETERSON, M, AND COLE, TM: *Prosthetic spinal support following hemipelvectomy in a paraplegic patient.* Arch Phys Med Rehabil 49:42–44, 1968.

DOUGLASS, HO, JR, RAZACK, M, AND HOLYOKE, ED: *Hemipelvectomy.* Arch Surg 110:82–85, 1975.

FITZGERALD, RR: *Amputation for sarcoma of the neck of the femur by the interinnomino-abdominal method.* J Bone Joint Surg 18:402–407, 1936.

FITZWILLIAMS, DCL: *Hindquarter amputation for sarcoma.* Proc R Soc Med 31:548–550, 1938.

FOX, JA AND JENKINS, H: *Hind quarter amputation.* Nurs Times 68:1058–1060, Aug 1972.

FREDELL, CH: *Hemipelvectomy for soft tissue tumor in a child.* Am J Orthop 6:39–41, 1964.

FREY, C, ET AL: *A new technique for hemipelvectomy.* Surg Gynecol Obstet 143:753–756, 1976.

FRIEDMANN, LW: *Comments and observations regarding hemipelvectomy and hemipelvectomy prosthetics.* Orthot Pros 21:271–273, 1967.

GAMBLE, HA: *Interinnomino-abdominal amputation of the lower extremity with indications for the extension of its use.* South Surg 13:248–252, 1947.

GANAPATHY, DH: *A report of traumatic hindquarter amputation.* Injury 5:51–53, 1973.

GHORMLEY, RK, HENDERSON, MS, AND LIPSCOMB, PR: *Interinnomino-abdominal amputation for chondrosarcoma and extensive chondroma: Report of two cases.* Proc Mayo Clinic 19:193–199, 1944.

GORDON-TAYLOR, G: *A further review of the interinnomino-abdominal operation: Eleven personal cases.* Br J Surg 643–650, 1940.

GORDON-TAYLOR, G AND HAND, BH: *Hindquarter amputation.* In ROB, C AND SMITH, R (EDS): *Operative Surgery.* Butterworth & Co, London, 1958, pp 5–11.

GORDON-TAYLOR, G AND MONRO, R: *The technique and management of the "hindquarter" amputation.* Br J Surg 39:536–541, 1952.

GORDON-TAYLOR, G AND PATEY, DH: *A further review of the interinnomino-abdominal operation: Based on 21 personal cases.* Br J Surg 34:61–69, 1946.

GORDON-TAYLOR, G AND WILES, PW: *Interinnomino-abdominal (hind-quarter) amputation.* Br J Surg 22:671–695, 1935.

GORDON-TAYLOR, G AND WILES, P: *Pulsating angio-endothelioma of the innominate bone treated by hindquarter amputation.* J Bone Joint Surg 31B:410–413, 1949.

GORDON-TAYLOR, G AND WILES, P: *Interinnomino-abdominal (hind-quarter) amputation.* Clin Orthop 53:3–11, 1967.

GORDON-TAYLOR, G, ET AL: *The interinnomino-abdominal operation: Observations on a series of fifty cases.* J Bone Joint Surg 34B:14–21, 1952.

HAMPTON, F: *A hemipelvectomy prosthesis.* Artificial Limbs 8:3–27, 1964.

HAMPTON, F: *Northwestern University suspension casting technique for hemipelvectomy and hip disarticulation.* Artificial Limbs 10:56–61, 1966.

HAMPTON, FL: *Above knee prostheses.* Orthop Clin North Am 3:359–372, 1972.

HAWK, JC, JR AND RICHARD, JT: *Letter: Hemipelvectomy.* Arch Surg 110:761, 1975.

HIGINBOTHAM, NL AND COLEY, BL: *Hemipelvectomy: Experience in a series of thirty-nine cases.* Cancer 9:1233–1238, 1956.

HIGINBOTHAM, NL, MARCOVE, RC, AND CASSON, P: *Hemipelvectomy: A clinical study of 100 cases with five year follow-up on 60 patients.* Surgery 59:706–708, 1966.

HILL, IM AND TODD, IP: *A case of hindquarter amputation for chondromyxosarcoma of the right thigh.* Br J Surg 33:277–279, 1946.

HOGSHEAD, HP: *Experience with hip disarticulation and hemipelvectomy procedure.* J Bone Joint Surg 53A:1031, 1971.

HOLZAEPFEL, JH: *Pregnancy and delivery post radical hemipelvectomy.* Obstet Gynecol 42:455–458, 1973.

HUDSON, OC AND JANELLI, DE: *Emergency hemipelvectomy.* Am J Surg 88:340–342, 1954.

INMON, WB AND BLEDSOE, JW: *Surgical repair of genital prolapse after hemipelvectomy.* Am J Obstet Gynecol 123:766–769, 1975.

IWAKURA, H, ET AL: *Locomotion of the hemipelvectomy amputee.* Prosthet Orthot Int 3:111–114, 1979.

JABOULAY, PM: *La désarticulation interilio-abdominale.* Lyons Med 75:507–510, 1894.

JACOBS, JT AND WOODRUFF, R: *Inter-innomino-abdominal amputation.* Rocky Mt Med J 45:564–566, 1948.

JOHANSSON, H AND OLERUD, S: *Traumatic hemipelvectomy in a ten-year-old boy.* J Bone Joint Surg 53A:170–172, 1971.

JONES, P: *Hindquarter amputations: Review of a personal series.* Aust NZ J Surg 44:1–11, 1974.

JUDIN, SS: *Ilio-abdominal amputation in a case of sarcoma: Recovery, pregnancy and birth of a living child.* Surg Gynecol Obstet 43:668–676, 1926.

KEEN, WW AND DACOSTA, JC: *A case of interilio-abdominal amputation for sarcoma of the ilium, and a synopsis of previously recorded cases.* Internat Clin Phil 4:127–147, 1904.

KING, D AND STEELQUIST, J: *Transiliac amputation.* J Bone Joint Surg 25:351–367, 1943.

KONZEN, CM AND KOEPKE, GH: *Hemipelvectomy following trauma.* Arch Phys Med Rehabil 53:530–532, 1972.

KOSKINEN, EVS: *Hemipelvectomy for malignant tumours of bone: A study with preoperative arteriographic examination of the growth.* Ann Chir Gynaecol 56:9–17, 1967.

LANE, D: *Hind-quarter amputation for advanced malignant melanoma of the lower limb.* Med J Aust 49:709–710, 1962.

LAZZARI, JH AND RACK, FJ: *Method of hemipelvectomy with abdominal exploration and temporary ligation of the common iliac artery.* Ann Surg 133:267–269, 1951.

LEE, CM, JR AND ALT, LP: *Hemipelvectomy and hip disarticulation for malignant tumors of the pelvis and lower extremity.* Ann Surg 137:704–717, 1953.

LEIGHTON, WE: *Interpelvi abdominal amputation. Report of three cases.* Arch Surg 45:913–925, 1942.

LEIGHTON, WE: *Hindquarter amputation: Report of ten cases.* Arch Surg 65:195–200, 1952.

LE QUESNE, LP: *Hind-quarter amputation.* Postgrad Med J 25B:433–442, 1949.

LEWIS, RC, JR AND BICKEL, WH: *Hemipelvectomy for malignant disease.* JAMA 165:8–12, 1957.

LYQUIST, E: *Canadian-type plastic socket for a hemipelvectomy.* Artificial Limbs 5:130–132, 1958.

LYQUIST, E: *Fitting the plastic socket for a hemipelvectomy.* In *Prosthetics International, Proceedings of the Second International Prosthetics Course, Committee on Prostheses, Braces and Technical Aids, International Society for the Welfare of Cripples.* Copenhagen, 1960, pp 99–101.

MARX, HW: *Some experience in hemipelvectomy prosthetics.* Orthot Pros 21:259–270, 1967.

McLEAN, EM: *Avulsion of the hindquarter.* J Bone Joint Surg 44B:384–385, 1962.

McPHERSON, JHT, JR: *Traumatic hind-quarter amputation.* J Med Assoc Ga 49:494–495, 1960.

McQUIRK, AW: *The Canadian hip disarticulation prosthesis and modifications required for the hemipelvectomy.* In MURDOCH, G (ED): *Prosthetic and Orthotic Practice.* Edward Arnold & Co, London, 1970, pp 305–311.

MEESTER, GL AND MYERLEY, WH: *Traumatic hemipelvectomy: Case report and literature review.* J Trauma 15:541–545, 1975.

MILLER, TR: *Interilio-abdominal amputation: A report of 32 cases.* Acta Radiol (Suppl) 188:173–189, 1959.

MILLER, TR: *Hemipelvectomy in the treatment of advanced cancer.* Am J Roentgenol Radium Ther Nucl Med 87:531–535, 1962.

MILLER, TR: *Extended interscapulothoracic amputation and hemipelvectomy.* Cancer 23:325–326, 1970.

MILLER, TR: *100 cases of hemipelvectomy: A personal experience.* Surg Clin North Am 54:905–913, 1974.

MILLER, TR: *Hemipelvectomy in lower extremity tumors.* Orthop Clin North Am 8:903–919, 1977.

MNAYMNEH, W AND TEMPLE, W: *Modified hemipelvectomy utilizing a long vascular myocutaneous thigh flap: Case report.* J Bone Joint Surg 62A:1013–1015, 1980.

MONAHAN, DT: *Hemipelvectomy for fibrosarcoma.* Ann Surg 148:189–191, 1958.

MORRIN, FJ: *Interinnomino-abdominal (hind-quarter) amputation.* Ir J Med Sci 6:21–26, 1952.

MORTON, JJ: *Interinnomino-abdominal (hindquarter) amputation.* Ann Surg 115:628–646, 1942.

MURDOCH, G: *Amputation surgery in the lower extremity.* Prosthet Orthot Int 1:72–83, 1977.

NIELSEN, ML, ET AL: *Bladder function after hemipelvectomy.* Acta Orthop Scand 48:181–185, 1977.

NILSONNE, U, HJELMSTEDT, Å, AND HAKELIUS, A: *Surgical problems in hemipelvectomy.* Acta Orthop Scand 39:161–170, 1968.

NUSS, RC AND LEE, JH, JR: *Pregnancy following hemipelvectomy: Report of a case.* Obstet Gynecol 29:789–791, 1967.

OGILVIE, WH: *Hind-quarter amputation.* Trans Med Soc Lond 60:139, 1937.

ORCUTT, TW, ET AL: *Reconstruction and rehabilitation following traumatic hemipelvectomy and brachial plexus injury.* J Trauma 14:695–704, 1974.

PACK, GT: *Major exarticulations for malignant neoplasms of the extremities: Interscapulothoracic amputation, hip-joint disarticulation, and interilio-abdominal amputation: A report of end results in 228 cases.* J Bone Joint Surg 38A:249–262, 1956.

PACK, GT AND ARIEL, IM: *Sacroiliac disarticulation (hemipelvectomy).* In *Tumors Of The Soft Somatic Tissues.* Paul B. Hoeber, New York, 1958, pp 105–122.

PACK, GT AND EHRLICH, HE: *Exarticulation of the lower extremities for malignant tumors: Hip-joint disarticulation (with and without deep iliac dissection) and sacro-iliac disarticulation (hemipelvectomy).* Ann Surg 123:965–985, 1946.

PACK, GT AND EHRLICH, HE: *Exarticulation of the lower extremities for malignant tumors: Hip-joint disarticulation (with and without deep iliac dissection) and sacro-iliac disarticulation (hemipelvectomy). I. Sacro-iliac disarticulation (hemipelvectomy).* Ann Surg 124:1–27, 1946.

PACK, GT, EHRLICH, HE, AND GENTIL, F DE C: *Radical amputations of the extremities in the treatment of cancer.* Surg Gynecol Obstet 84:1105–1116, 1947.

PACK, GT AND MILLER, TR: *Exarticulation of the innominate bone and corresponding lower extremity (hemipelvectomy) for primary and metastatic cancer: A report of one hundred and one cases with analysis of the end results.* J Bone Joint Surg 46A:91–95, 1964.

PACK, GT AND MILLER, TR: *Exarticulation of the innominate bone for primary and metastatic cancer: An experience with 201 cases.* In ARIEL, IM (ED): *Progress in Clinical Cancer,* ed 2. Grune & Stratton, New York, 1966, pp 98–106.

PACK, GT, MILLER, TR, AND ARIEL, IM: *Hemipelvectomy (interilioabdominal amputation).* In PACK, GT AND ARIEL, IM (EDS): *Treatment of Cancer and Allied Diseases, Vol VIII, Tumors of the Soft Somatic Tissues and Bone.* Hoeber Medical Division, Harper & Row, New York, 1964, pp 284–302.

PAINTER, CW AND VON WERSSOWETZ, OF: *Prosthetic training of a hemipelvectomy patient.* Phys Ther Rev 33:10–16, 1953.

PALUMBO, LT: *Hemipelvectomy in the treatment of osteogenic sarcoma of the ilium.* J Iowa State Med Soc 37:190–196, 1947.

PALUMBO, LT: *Hemipelvectomy in treatment of osteogenic sarcoma of the ilium.* Am J Surg 77:654–660, 1949.

PARKER, G: *Letter: Traumatic hindquarter amputation.* Br Med J 4:290, 1974.

PAUL, M: *The interinnomino-abdominal operation.* Aust NZ J Surg 20:311–312, 1951.

PHELAN, JT, GRACE, JT, JR, AND MOORE, GE: *Hemipelvectomy for management for soft tissue tumors of lower extremity.* Am J Surg 107:604–607, 1964.

PHELAN, JT, AND NADLER, SH: *A technique of hemipelvectomy.* Surg Gynecol Obstet 119:311–318, 1964.

PRINGLE, JH: *Some notes on the interpelvi-abdominal amputation: With a report of three cases.* Lancet 1:530–533, 1909.

PRINGLE, JH: *The interpelvi-abdominal amputation: With notes on two cases.* Br J Surg 4:283–296, 1916.

RANDLE, APH, WILSON, JN, AND TUCK, WH: *Rehabilitation after hindquarter amputation.* Br Med J 5336:1001–1002, 1963.

RANSOHOFF, J: *Interilio-abdominal amputation: With report of a case.* Ann Surg 50:925–935, 1909.

RAVITCH, MM: *Hemipelvectomy.* Surgery 26:199–214, 1949.

RAVITCH, MM: *Radical treatment of massive mixed angiomas (hemolymph angiomas) in infants and children: With report of hemipelvectomy in a 13-day-old infant.* Ann Surg 134:228–243, 1951.

RAVITCH, MM AND WILSON, TC: *Long-term results of hemipelvectomy.* Ann Surg 159:667–682, 1964.

ROBINSON, RA: *Interinnomino-abdominal (hindquarter) amputation.* J Bone Joint Surg 32A:446–448, 1950.

SAINT, JH: *The hindquarter (interinnomino-abdominal) amputation.* Am J Surg 80:142–160, 1950.

SALERNO, DJ: *Forequarter and hindquarter amputation.* J Am Osteopath Assoc 61:15–21, 1961.

SCALES, JT, DUFF-BARCLAY, I, AND BURROWS, HJ: *Some engineering and medical problems associated with massive bone replacement.* In KENEDI, RM (ED): *Biomechanical and Related Bio-Engineering Topics.* Pergamon Press, London, 1965, pp 205–239.

SELIG, S: *Interinnomino-abdominal (hind-quarter) amputation.* J Bone Joint Surg 23:929–934, 1941.

SHARMA, BC, PAONASKAR, V, AND WOSORNU, L: *Osteosarcoma and emergency hind-quarter amputation: A case report.* Med J Zambia 12:104–106, 1978.

SHERMAN, CD, JR AND DUTHIE, RB: *Modified hemipelvectomy.* Cancer 13:51–54, 1960.

SPEED, K: *Hemipelvectomy.* Ann Surg 95:167–173, 1932.

STAVRAKAS, PA AND SANDERS, GT: *Sling support during pregnancy after hemipelvectomy: Case report.* Arch Phys Med Rehabil 64:331–333, 1983.

STENER, B: *Transthoracosacral amputation in case of large retroperitoneal pelvic chondrosarcoma: Greater omentum used for closing the abdomen after vast excision of the abdominal wall.* Clin Orthop 62:124–132, 1969.

SUGARBAKER, ED AND ACKERMAN, LV: *Disarticulation of the innominate bone for malignant tumors of the pelvic parietes and upper thigh.* Surg Gynecol Obstet 81:36–52, 1945.

TAYLOR, GW AND ROGERS, WP, JR: *Hindquarter amputation: Experience with eighteen cases.* N Engl J Med 249:963–969, 1953.

THOMPSON, RG: *Amputation in the lower extremity.* J Bone Joint Surg 45A:1723–1734, 1963.

TROUP, JB AND BICKEL, WH: *Malignant disease of the extremities treated by exarticulation: Analysis of two hundred and sixty-four consecutive cases with survival rates.* J Bone Joint Surg 42A:1041–1050, 1960.

VON WERSSOWETZ, OF AND PAINTER, CW: *Physical rehabilitation of a hemipelvectomy amputee.* Ann Surg 137:395–398, 1953.

WADE, FV AND MACKSOOD, WA: *Traumatic hemipelvectomy: Report of two cases with rectal involvement.* J Trauma 5:554–562, 1965.

WATKINS, AL: *Rehabilitation after hemipelvectomy.* JAMA 181:793–794, 1962.

WATKINS, AL: *Prosthetic rehabilitation after hemipelvectomy.* Ortho Pros Appl J 17:173–174, 1963.

WERNE, S: *Two cases of hindquarter-amputation.* Acta Orthop Scand 22:90–99, 1953.

WESTBURY, G: *Hindquarter and hip amputation.* Ann R Coll Surg Engl 40:226–234, 1967.

WHITTAKER, AH: *Inter-innomino-abdominal amputation.* Indus Med 2:1–3, 1942.

WHITTAKER, AH AND SOBIN, DJ: *Interinnomino-abdominal amputation: Case report.* Ann Surg 115:435–440, 1942.

WILSON, AB, JR: *Limb prosthetics: 1970.* Artificial Limbs 14:1–52, 1970.

WISE, RA: *Control of the common iliac artery during sacroiliac disarticulation (hemipelvectomy).* Ann Surg 128:993–998, 1948.

WISE, RA: *A successful prosthesis for sacro-iliac disarticulation (hemipelvectomy).* J Bone Joint Surg 31A:426–427, 1949.

WISE, RA: *Hemipelvectomy for malignant tumors of the bony pelvis and upper part of the thigh.* Arch Surg 58:867–874, 1949.

WU, KK, ET AL: *The surgical technique for hindquarter amputation: A report of 19 cases.* Acta Orthop Scand 48:479–486, 1977.

WYNDHAM, N: *Hindquarter amputation for sarcoma of the femur.* Med J Aust 44:466–467, 1957.

YANCEY, AG, JOHNSTON, GA, AND GREEN, JE, JR: *Some surgical principles in hemipelvectomy.* J Natl Med Assoc 42:210–213, 1950.

YOUNG, EL AND BARNES, WA: *Hemipelvectomy: The most radical of all amputations.* Am J Nurs 58:361–364, Mar, 1958.

YUE, SJ AND GOLDSTINE, CR: *An improved prosthesis for hemipelvectomy.* Arch Phys Med Rehabil 38:781–784, 1957.

ZALEWSKI, N, GERONEMUS, D, AND SIEGEL, H: *Hemipelvectomy: The triumph of Ms. A.* Am J Nurs 73:2073–2077, Dec, 1973.

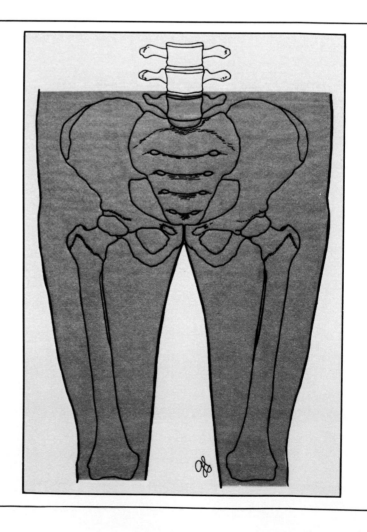

CHAPTER 15

HEMICORPORECTOMY
(PELVIC [Pel], COMPLETE)

(PARACORPORECTOMY; LUMBOSACRAL, TRANSLUMBAR,
TRANSVERTEBRAL AMPUTATION)

SURGICAL PROCEDURE

POSTOPERATIVE
CONCERNS

MORTALITY

PROSTHESIS

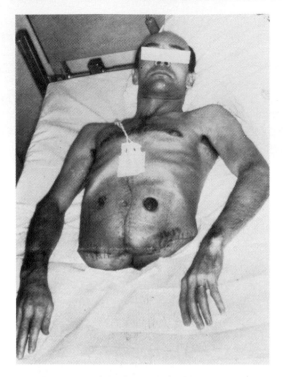

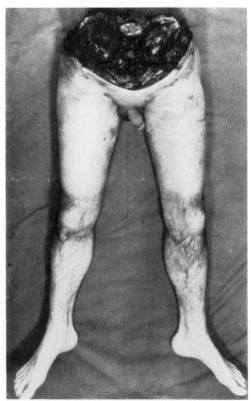

FIGURE 15-1. *(Top)* A patient 10 days postoperative. *(Bottom)* Gross specimen. (From Miller, TR, et al: *Hemicorporectomy.* Surgery 59:992, 1966, with permission.)

The first translumbar amputation was performed in 1960, but the patient died of pulmonary complications, presumably because of overtransfusions. The first successful lumbosacral amputation was reported by Drs. Bradley Aust and Karel Absolon at the University of Minnesota in 1962. Since that time, the number of case reports indicates that a hemicorporectomy is technically feasible. This drastic procedure, in which the lower half of the body is removed (Fig. 15-1), is performed most often for extensive recurrent and nonresectable cancer of the bladder (Fig. 15-2), cancer of the rectum that implicates the entire pelvis where there is no evidence of spread of the tumor beyond the pelvis, or intractable pelvic decubiti (Table 15-1). The biologic nature of the tumor should be compatible with prolonged survival following the amputation. Many patients also have intractable pain, infection, or hemorrhage.

SURGICAL PROCEDURE

A careful exploratory laparotomy is usually performed initially to determine if the tumor is limited to the pelvis and can be removed by translumbar amputation. If the

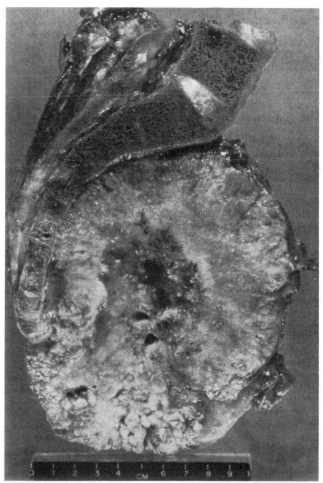

FIGURE 15-2. Recurrent bladder tumor invading the sacrum, showing the level of amputation between the fourth and fifth lumbar vertebrae. (From Miller, TR, et al: *Hemicorporectomy.* Surgery 59:990, 1966, with permission.)

TABLE 15-1. INDICATIONS FOR HEMICORPORECTOMY

1. Carcinomas of the anus, rectum, perineum, or pelvic structures with local invasion but no known distant metastases
   (a) squamous cell carcinoma that developed in a large sacral decubitus ulcer in a paraplegic meningomyelocele
   (b) squamous cell carcinoma of the cervix with vesicovaginal and rectovaginal fistulas
   (c) extensive recurrent epidermoid carcinoma of the bladder
   (d) epidermoid carcinoma, grade II with perineal urethral fistula following bilateral below-knee amputations, excisions of the ischial tuberosities, and removal of a hip plate from a previous fracture in a patient with paraplegia secondary to a spinal cord tumor
   (e) a large, fungating, recurrent tumor mass in the perineal area following colectomy for adenocarcinoma
   (f) squamous cell carcinoma in a large perineum decubitus ulcer in a paraplegic
   (g) chondrosarcoma in the pelvis following a hemipelvectomy for the same diagnosis
2. Complications of paraplegia
   (a) pelvic osteomyelitis
   (b) intractable pelvic decubiti
3. Trauma: completely crushed pelvis, avulsion of bladder and rectum

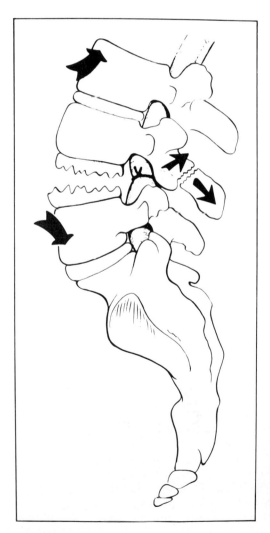

FIGURE 15-3. Diagram depicting transection between L-4 and L-5 and cauda equina ligation. (From Pearlman, NW, et al: *Hemicorporectomy for intractable decubitus ulcers.* Arch Surg 111:1141, 1976, with permission.)

disease cannot be encompassed by a lesser resection and the tumor is limited to the pelvis, the patient and surgeon will sometimes decide on a hemicorporectomy amputation. A colostomy and an ileostomy are usually performed prior to the amputation. The amputation begins with a low transverse, suprapubic, abdominal incision. Next, the common external and internal iliac arteries and veins are ligated and transected. Transection of the iliopsoas muscles is performed at the level of the iliac wings. The vertebral column is usually transected between L-4 and L-5 (Fig. 15-3) or L-5 and S-1. The spinous processes are tailored as necessary to enhance closing and to avoid potential pressure points. The cauda equina and filum terminale are ligated. The peritoneum, fascia of the anterior abdominal wall muscles, and the lumbodorsal fascia are sutured together. Skin closure is made without tension.

POSTOPERATIVE CONCERNS

The emotional impact of this amputation on the patient, the family, and supporting hospital personnel, as well as on the surgeon, is an important early concern. The proce-

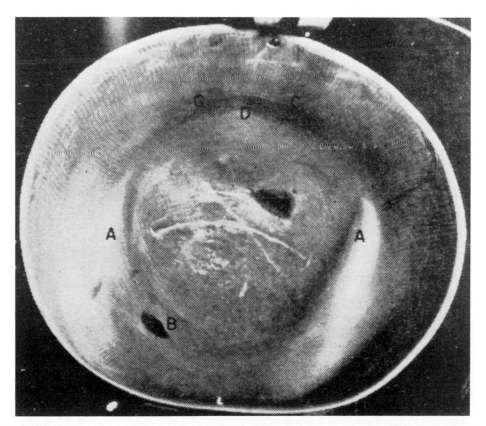

FIGURE 15-4. Prosthetic socket viewed from above showing *(A)* subcostal shelves, *(B)* opening for stoma of ileal loop bladder, *(C)* paravertebral ridges, and *(D)* relief for the inferior tip of the spinal column. (From DeLateur, BJ, et al: *Rehabilitation of the patient after hemicorporectomy.* Arch Phys Med Rehabil 50:13, 1969, with permission.)

dure should only be performed when it is viewed as a humane and compassionate approach given the circumstances. Considering the nature of the procedure, psychological counseling of the patient and family should be initiated early and should be intense.

The most frequent postoperative complications are bronchopneumonia, atelectasis, jaundice, and pulmonary edema caused by overtransfusion. Postoperative pulmonary edema can be complicated by several factors: because the abdominal muscles no longer have a fixed distal attachment, forced expiration, as in coughing, is compromised; since body volume is reduced, the amputee's absorptive capacity for intravenous fluids is altered; and the peritoneal cavity volume is reduced by 40 percent. Fluid and electrolyte therapy should be based on the reduced body weight. Wound closing problems are usually minor. A "failure to thrive" secondary to gonad loss may appear in the second and third weeks. Androgen, as well as estrogen, withdrawal may be characterized by severe flushing and sweating. Replacement of androgen or estrogen at physiologic levels is necessary. Phantom pain is not usually a problem. When it is present, it usually coincides with the presence of a urinary tract infection or wound infection.

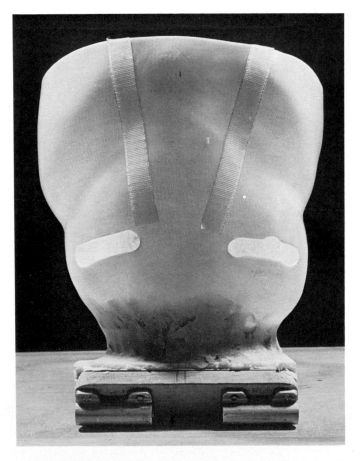

FIGURE 15-5. Anterior view of the socket. Note "mail-slot" openings, subcostal indentations, and Velcro fastenings for the suspension straps. (From DeLateur, BJ, et al: *Rehabilitation of the patient after hemicorporectomy.* Arch Phys Med Rehabil 50:14, 1969, with permission.)

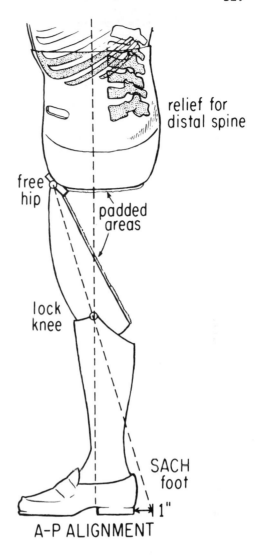

relief for
distal spine

free
hip

padded
areas

lock
knee

SACH
foot

1"

A-P ALIGNMENT

FIGURE 15-6. Anteroposterior alignment. The weight-bearing line falls
considerably posterior to the prosthetic hip joints, through the knee
joints, and anterior to the ankles.
(From Simons, BC, et al: *Prosthetic
management of hemicorporectomy.*
Orthotics and Prosthetics 22:66,
1968, with permission.)

MORTALITY

Although four of the first nine reported cases died in the immediate postoperative
period, a later (1976) estimate of the risk of death was 10 percent. The alteration in this
statistic reflects the following: (1) the realization of fluid overload in the earlier cases
and subsequent careful management; and (2) expansion of the procedure to include
patients with decubiti as well as those with pelvic malignancies. Most patients who
undergo hemicorporectomy for malignancy eventually die of metastases, while those
who receive an amputation for decubiti survive for a long term.

The benefits of this type of surgery for paraplegics may exceed those for patients
with pelvic malignancy. Factors that should be considered include:

1. Many paraplegics have no other serious disease, so removal of the infected pelvis returns them to relatively normal health. In contrast, people with tumors large enough to warrant a hemicorporectomy usually have distant metastases, with survival time generally being 6 to 24 months.
2. In the paraplegic patient, the lower half of the body is deformed and functionally useless. The psychological impact of its removal and the altered functional ability, especially when the amputee is performing transfers, may be unchanged or improved. The ambulatory patient with a malignancy, however, loses mobility and encounters a more drastic body image alteration.

PROSTHESIS

The hemicorporectomy prosthesis should provide a socket that enables independent transfer into and out of the prosthesis. It should also enable sufficient trunk stability to allow upright posture in a wheelchair, thus providing the amputee with free use of the upper extremities for propelling the wheelchair and for performing activities of daily living and recreational activities. In the standing position, it should allow the amputee to use crutches. The socket should provide sufficient strategic distribution of weight to prevent pressure sores, allowing at least two 4-hour weight-bearing periods per day. Adequate space should be allowed for chest expansion during respiration. The socket should also provide adequate abdominal pressure distribution or relief to prevent ab-

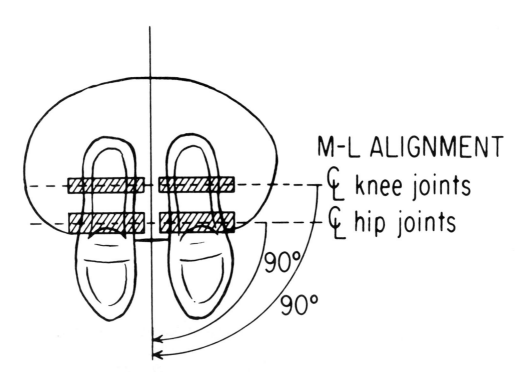

FIGURE 15-7. Mediolateral alignment. The prosthetic hip joints are located anterior to the knee joints, and both are at 90-degree angles to the line of progression. (From Simons, BC, et al: *Prosthetic management of hemicorporectomy.* Orthotics and Prosthetics 22:66, 1968, with permission.)

dominal pain, nausea, and eversion of colostomy and ileal bladder stoma. Adequate openings for easy access to the colostomy and ileal bladder receptacles should be provided. Reliefs over susceptible bony areas are necessary so that sternal, rib, and distal lumbar pressure and pain are avoided when leaning forward or backward in the prosthesis. The prosthesis should be cosmetic in appearance. The socket surface that comes in contact with the body should be easy to clean.

The initial prosthesis usually consists of a plaster sitting socket, which is later replaced by a permanent sitting prosthesis of laminated plastic. The sitting socket is preflexed and attached to a platform to provide stability for upright posture in the wheelchair. Too much tilt in the prosthesis may cause pressure at the tip of the spine and thus must be avoided. Insufficient flexion reduces sitting balance.

The prosthesis has large areas of soft-tissue support but does not offer distal weight-bearing. The main weight-bearing area is usually provided by a definitive subcostal indentation.

Reliefs over the lumbar spine and ribs are necessary. Openings are made in the plastic socket for placement of colostomy and ileostomy receptacles, for heat release, and for reducing the weight of the prosthesis (Fig. 15-4). "Mail-slot" openings are designed to prevent eversion of the stoma yet allow free drainage of feces and urine (Fig. 15-5).

The prosthesis reaches the xiphoid process anteriorly and just below the scapulae posteriorly. Total contact is desirable. Shoulder straps maintain the suspension necessary for transfer and ambulation. A foam rubber lining of 1.3 cm (½ in) is used inside the socket to distribute weight more evenly and reduce pressure at vulnerable points. For ambulation, the prosthetic legs consist of the following: either single-axis hip and knee joints with manual hip and knee locks that permit only a swing-through gait; Canadian-type hip joints with a stride-length control strap, hip locks that are controlled by a cable in a housing and shoulder strap that permit either a four-point reciprocal or swing-through gait; or free-swinging hip joints and locked knee joints for a reciprocal gait. SACH feet are usually used. The thigh and leg sections are shortened to lower the center of gravity, thus improving balance. Anteroposterior alignment (Fig. 15-6) is similar to the Canadian hip prosthesis. The hip and knee joints are perpendicular to the line of progression (Fig. 15-7).

BIBLIOGRAPHY

Aust, JB and Absolon, KB: *A successful lumbosacral amputation: Hemicorporectomy.* Surgery 52:756–759, 1962.

Baker, TC, et al: *Hemicorporectomy.* Br J Surg 57:471–476, 1970.

Davis, SW, Chu, DS, and Yang, CJ: *Translumbar amputation for non neoplastic cause: Rehabilitation and follow-up.* Arch Phys Med Rehabil 56:359–362, 1975.

DeLateur, BJ, et al: *Rehabilitation of the patient after hemicorporectomy.* Arch Phys Med Rehabil 50:11–16, 1969.

Easton, JKM, et al: *Fitting of a prosthesis on a patient after hemicorporectomy.* Arch Phys Med Rehabil 44:335–337, 1963.

Eskridge, C, Jr: *New from the waist down.* Rehabil Rec 9:5–7, 1968.

Frieden, FH, et al: *Rehabilitation after hemicorporectomy.* Arch Phys Med Rehabil 50:259–263, 1969.

Grimby, G and Stener, B: *Physical performance and cardiorespiratory function after hemicorporectomy.* Scand J Rehabil Med 5:124–129, 1973.

KENNEDY, CS, ET AL: *Lumbar amputation or hemicorporectomy for advanced malignancy of the lower half of the body.* Surgery 48:357–365, 1960.

LAMIS, PA, JR, RICHARDS, AJ, JR, AND WEIDNER, MG, JR: *Hemicorporectomy: Hemodynamic and metabolic problems.* Am Surg 33:443–448, 1967.

LEICHTENTRITT, KG: *Rehabilitation after hemicorporectomy.* Am J Proctol 23:408–413, 1972.

MACKENZIE, AR, MILLER, TR, AND RANDALL, HT: *Translumbar amputation for advanced leiomyosarcoma of the prostate.* J Urol 97:133–136, 1967.

MILLER, TR: *Translumbar amputation for advanced cancer.* Cancer 19:36–39, 1969.

MILLER, TR, MACKENZIE, AR, AND KARASEWICH, EG: *Translumbar amputation for carcinoma of the vagina.* Arch Surg 93:502–506, 1966.

MILLER, TR, MACKENZIE, AR, AND RANDALL, HT: *Translumbar amputation for advanced cancer: Indications and physiologic alterations in four cases.* Ann Surg 164:514–519, 1966.

MILLER, TR, ET AL: *Hemicorporectomy.* Surgery 59:988–993, 1966.

NORRIS, JEC, ET AL: *Hemicorporectomy: A case report.* Am Surg 39:344–348, 1973.

PEARLMAN, NW, ET AL: *Hemicorporectomy for intractable decubitus ulcers.* Arch Surg 111:1139–1143, 1976.

SIMONS, BC, ET AL: *Prosthetic management of hemicorporectomy.* Orthot Pros 22:63–68, 1968.

WILLIAMS, RD AND FISH, JC: *Translumbar amputation.* Cancer 23:416–418, 1969.

YANCEY, AG, RYAN, HF, AND BLASINGAME, JT: *An experience with hemicorporectomy.* J Natl Med Assoc 56:323–325, 1964.

UNIT 3
REHABILITATION PHASE

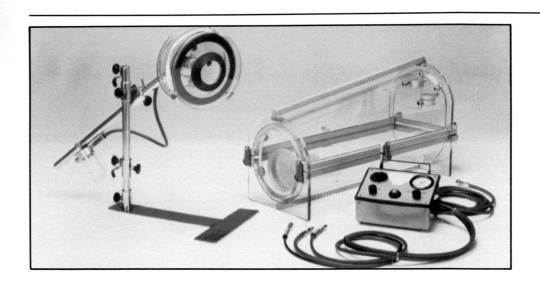

CHAPTER **16**

PREOPERATIVE MANAGEMENT

BELLA J. MAY, Ed.D., R.P.T.

Most amputations for peripheral vascular diseases are elective in that the patient has received treatment for circulatory deficiencies for a considerable time. Many individuals undergo a variety of surgical procedures to increase the circulation of the lower limb; some will be referred to physical therapy, and many will avoid the complications that lead to amputation. Ideally, individuals with peripheral vascular disease should be seen by a physical therapist early in the course of the disease for preventive management; unfortunately, this does not happen very often. The need for physician education is great; if each physical therapist who is involved in the management of patients with peripheral vascular diseases could convince one vascular surgeon of the benefits of early referral, the number of such referrals would increase dramatically. In support of this concept, preoperative management will be considered in two sections: general care of individuals with dysvascularities, and immediate pre-amputation care.

THE PERSON WITH PERIPHERAL VASCULAR DISEASE

Many diseases may affect the arteries and veins; most are systemic and develop slowly. These diseases will be the only ones considered in this section. A holistic approach to treatment that intimately involves the person in goal setting and management activities holds the greatest potential for success. People must learn to live and function with their diseases; they must understand the physiologic and psychological effects and must assume responsibility for themselves and their care. In this chapter, general concepts will be presented; however, it must be remembered that each individual is unique and that general concepts must be adapted to the needs of each person.

EVALUATION

All programs of care flow from a data base that is obtained through careful evaluation. The evaluation of an individual with peripheral vascular disease does not differ widely from the evaluation of any individual who is in need of physical therapy. The following information will be useful in planning treatment programs:

1. Gross upper and lower extremity strength.
2. Active and passive range of motion of major joints.
3. Ambulatory status.
4. Sensory status of both lower extremities.
5. General medical status, including any other systemic problems.
6. Previous surgical procedures.
7. Self-care capabilities.
8. Cardiopulmonary status, if indicated.
9. Diet and diabetes control, if appropriate.

Specific information on the vascular status of both lower extremities, including the presence or absence of edema, is vital. Evaluation may include observation of the lower extremities for evidence of dysvascularity, such as loss of hair, skin calluses, dry or shiny skin, dependent rubor, and changes in the thickness of toenails. Feet are inspected for abrasions, fissures, cuts, or evidence of undue pressure. The presence or absence of pedal pulses and the lower extremity skin temperature are noted. Doppler recordings, if available, are noted. If an ulcer is present, its size and condition (e.g., infected, purulent, clean) are described. If edema is present, the type and extent are noted (e.g., pitting, toes only). Circumferential measurements of the lower limbs may be useful for assessing changes in edema over time.

Persons with diabetes may have sensory changes secondary to involvement of one or more nerve roots. A careful and complete sensory evaluation will provide valuable information for future patient education as well as being a guide to treatment. An individual with diminished sensation may not be aware of a shoe that is too tight or a bruised foot. The presence or absence of pain, when it occurs, and its duration are carefully noted. Excessive pain is debilitating, and pain management is often difficult.

A careful interview will elicit information on the person's lifestyle, work, and family activities, as well as the person's understanding of and attitude toward the disease. The availability of transportation to and from the clinic influences the physical therapy program, as does the therapist's determination of the extent to which the person is prepared to assume responsibility for the management of the disease process. Information on the person's perceptions of the symptoms can be correlated with the results of evaluative tests for a more complete analysis of the problems. The interview is a vital part of the evaluation process; it must be thorough and ongoing.

GOALS OF PHYSICAL THERAPY

There are four major goals in the physical therapy care of individuals with peripheral vascular disease:

1. to help the person understand the disease process and its management
2. to enhance the development of collateral circulation
3. to prevent or help heal ulcers if present
4. to guide the individual toward the maintenance or resumption of a functional lifestyle.

TREATMENT PROGRAMS

PATIENT EDUCATION

The patient must understand the physiologic and functional implications of the disease and available alternatives. The patient must be guided to assume responsibility for his or her own care. The educational program must be meaningful and individually relevant and may include the following:

1. Discussion of the disease itself.
2. Explanation of the physiologic effects as related to the symptoms being experienced.
3. Discussion of the benefits of exercises, lower extremity cleanliness, proper foot care, and correct shoe fitting.
4. The importance of weight control and good nutrition.
5. Methods of edema control.
6. The use of exercises in the development of collateral circulation.

Supplemental handouts and descriptions that the person can use at home reinforce the discussion that took place in the physical therapy department.

The application of educational theories can improve patient education programs. Several sessions are often needed since only one major concept can effectively be introduced at one time. The individual needs time to think about the ideas and ask questions. Frequent reiteration of major concepts over time helps retention. Instructions must be relevant and must be perceived by the patient as being necessary. Concepts can be reinforced by practice and handouts. Ask the person to tell you how he or she will implement parts of the program at home. Support adaptation of ideas to meet unique needs. Provide opportunities for feedback and clarification, and relate new ideas to those already learned. Therapy time spent on careful and relevant patient education is effective treatment time.

COLLATERAL CIRCULATION

Most therapists have treated individuals who have severe arterial disease and have maintained viable lower extremities for many years. As major vessels slowly become occluded, collateral vessels develop and increase in size to provide necessary nutrients to the tissues. It is believed that the development of collateral circulation is in response to local tissue need and is a valuable mechanism for maintaining tissue viability in areas where major circulation is no longer adequate. There is some question about the role of exercise in the process and about the benefits of Buerger-Allen exercises in particular. Regardless, the value of active exercises in the total management of the dysvascular patient has been well documented. Walking is probably one of the best exercises for the lower extremities, and implementation of a specific walking program will aid the development of collateral circulation. The dimensions of the walking program are dictated by the person's particular condition.

If a walking program is precluded because of ulcerations, claudication, or other factors, less strenuous active exercises can be used. The exercise bicycle provides an excellent medium for controlled active exercises of both legs within a limited amount of time. Resistance is graded to the person's tolerance and circulatory status.

Edema is a major deterrent to the development of collateral circulation. Edema may occlude the small vessels that form the collateral system. Initially, edema may be controlled by elevation of the lower extremities; as the edema progresses, however, it becomes more difficult to control since the swelling stretches tissues, thus reducing the elasticity that usually controls fluid accumulation.

Active exercises may help control edema in patients with mild to moderate arterial disease. If impaired, the venous system, which is responsible for returning fluid from the extremities toward the heart, may not be able to cope with the increased circulation that results from exercise. Patients with edema should spend some time each day with their legs elevated to heart level. Prolonged sitting increases edema and should be avoided. Elastic stockings can help control edema; individually measured stockings are more effective than the ready-made ones that are found in many drug stores. Elderly individuals may have difficulty donning and removing the stockings; elastic bandages can be substituted, but the patient must learn to use overlapping figure-of-8 turns to avoid the possibility of creating a tourniquet. The patient must also understand the importance of frequent rewrapping to avoid excessive pressure on the skin.

Some women like to wear individual leg hose suspended with an elastic garter just above the knee or rolled just above the knee then twisted in a knot. Either method can create a tourniquet and severely compromise circulation of the distal limb segment. Dysvascular patients must avoid such methods of hose suspension and must be warned of the consequences. The person must either suspend the hose with a garter belt or wear pantyhose. Edema may be more successfully reduced through the regular application of an intermittent compression unit in combination with external elastic support.

SKIN CONDITIONS

Frequently, the patient with vascular disease will only be referred to physical therapy after an ulcer has developed. At that point, healing the ulcer becomes the major focus of treatment. Increasing circulation to the ulcerated area, preventing or eliminating infection, and reducing edema will all enhance healing. Specific treatment is determined by the size of the ulcer, the presence of infection, and the patient's general condition. A complete evaluation will provide the necessary data for developing the treatment plan.

HYDROTHERAPY

Hydrotherapy, usually whirlpool, is a frequently used modality in ulcer care. The whirlpool can cleanse and débride the wound as well as stimulate local circulation. Antibacterial agents can be added to the water to reduce infection. A major disadvantage of the whirlpool is that it places the limb in a dependent position, which may increase edema. A Loboy or Hubbard tank eliminates the problem of the dependent position but may not be advisable in the presence of cardiovascular or pulmonary disease. In selecting hydrotherapy to treat an ulcer, consideration must be given to the severity of the ulcer, the presence of infection, and the patient's general physiologic condition, sensory status, and propensity for edema development. In some instances, other means of ulcer care may be more effective.

DRESSINGS

Various types of dressings have been used with some success, including wet to dry dressings, acetic acid, and more recently, Unna's paste boot. The Unna's paste boot is a semirigid dressing that is easily applied, provides support for the extremity, and helps control edema. It consists of a gauze dressing that is impregnated with Unna's paste and can be purchased in ready-to-apply rolls. It is wrapped as any dressing from the toes to just below the popliteal area for foot or lower leg problems. Pressure is even throughout, and care must be taken over bony prominences and the peroneal nerve. It takes approximately 12 hours to dry and is then lightweight and semirigid. Since it is not bulky, the patient can wear a shoe. The boot is total contact in nature and must be reapplied if it loosens. It is water soluble, so contact with water must be avoided. Once applied, it can stay on for an extended time.

HYPERBARIC OXYGEN CHAMBERS

Hyperbaric oxygen chambers (Fig. 16-1) have been used to enhance healing, with considerable success. The chamber was developed from research that indicated that

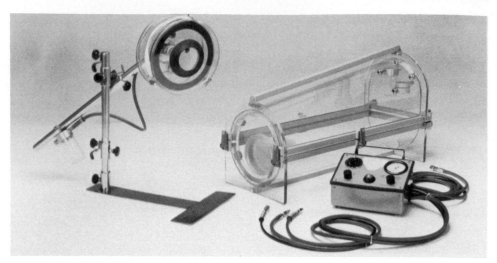

FIGURE 16-1. A hyperbaric oxygen chamber. (From Topox Corporation, Jersey City, New Jersey, with permission.)

saturating tissues with oxygen under pressure promotes healing and deters bacterial growth. Single-extremity portable chambers are available for use in physical therapy departments.

OTHER TREATMENTS

A variety of other modalities have been used to treat ulcers, including Dynawave and cold quartz; the effectiveness of any of these approaches has not been well documented. Proper foot care and reducing or eliminating weight-bearing are important adjuncts to ulcer treatment. It may be beneficial to have the patient walk non–weight-bearing with crutches to reduce trauma to the ulcer, particularly if the ulcer is on the plantar surface of the foot. Elderly individuals may have difficulty learning to use crutches and may spend considerable time sitting. While such reduced activity may help the ulcer, it does not help the development of collateral circulation. The elderly sedentary individual needs to be encouraged to maintain some degree of physical activity during the healing process. A balance must be achieved and consideration given to the total physical and physiologic needs of the individual. A program of active range-of-motion exercises may deter the development of lower extremity contractures in the more sedentary individual.

The best treatment is prevention, and proper foot care is an important part of the program. Unfortunately, it is often difficult to obtain good foot and nail care, and the therapist may have to provide necessary instruction. Good foot care is based on common sense. The foot must be kept clean and dry. Excessive pressure from poorly fitting shoes must be avoided. Barefoot walking is not advisable. The skin should be kept soft and pliable. Therapists must often overcome the patient's belief in "home cures." Many patients faithfully soak their feet in all sorts of solutions because of erroneous advertising or poor "friendly" advice.

Foot care for the person with diabetes is further complicated by the disease process. Diabetes is a systemic disease that may cause, among other problems, neurologic changes that lead to decreased or lost sensation in the foot and lower extremity. Sensory and motor loss can be along single or multiple nerve roots and will usually follow a distal to proximal pattern initially involving the intrinsic muscles of the foot or hand. The person with diabetes also has a greater problem with dry skin because systemic involvement of the autonomic nervous system leads to a decrease in perspiration and a loss of normal skin moisture. Excessive pressure on fragile skin may enhance callus formation or skin breakdown, with resulting infection. Even without excessive pressure, lack of skin moisture may cause spontaneous breaks followed by infection. It is important for the patient to understand the disease process, to learn to maintain adequate skin moisture through the use of appropriate lotions and creams, and to learn to recognize a potential area of breakdown quickly. Many authors recommend that the person with diabetes obtain professional foot care for routine nail clipping. Unfortunately, that is often difficult to find and may be financially beyond the person's means. Most individuals can be properly trained to manage their own feet, particularly if instruction is given before the nails become deformed from dysvascularities.

Proper shoes are necessary for all patients with peripheral vascular disease. Pressure is the enemy, and shoes must provide adequate support without exerting undue pressure on any part of the foot. The person with sensory loss must be taught to watch for any sign of pressure since he or she cannot depend on the sensation of pressure. A good shoe provides support for the patient's weight, allows normal motion through each phase of gait, and contains the foot without undue pressure in any area. The shoe must also protect the foot from external trauma; shoes with open toes or heels are not recommended for individuals with dysvascularities.

FUNCTIONAL LIFESTYLE

Peripheral vascular disease is not curable, and the person must develop patterns of living that will limit the negative effects while enhancing the quality of life. It is a wise therapist who recognizes the importance of one's pattern of living and who helps the person incorporate the therapeutic program into that pattern. Information about the patient's lifestyle can be gathered formally during the initial evaluation and informally during treatment. The more obvious information needed includes—but is not limited to—the following:

1. Where and how the person lives (e.g., rural or urban setting; house or apartment).
2. Employment situation.
3. Preferred leisure-time activities.
4. Exercise patterns, if any, and attitudes toward exercise. Often, asking the person about leisure-time activities will elicit a great deal of data on the person's attitude toward exercise. A person with a positive attitude toward the benefits of exercise will more likely maintain a home program, while a person whose major exercise is going from the television to the refrigerator will most likely "forget" to do the home program.
5. Financial status may influence the person's ability to obtain necessary supplies and to purchase well-fitting shoes. Information on living arrangements will give insights into the constraints placed upon the person by everyday life. Are there numerous small children to be cared for? Does the person live with the family of a grown child? Does the person live with a sick spouse?
6. Educational level in itself is not a direct predictor of the person's ability to understand the home program, but it does provide the therapist with guidelines for the education program.

7. The cultural heritage and religious preference of the individual, if freely shared.
8. The person's self-perception, while sometimes difficult to determine, provides the therapist with a better awareness of the person's value system. Such awareness increases the therapist's ability to involve the patient in his or her own rehabilitation program.

Most patients come to physical therapy because of an acute problem, which then becomes the focus of treatment. It is important to recognize the patient's own priorities in selecting treatment activities. Many people enter the health care system expecting to be told what to do. Once home, however, they respond to the pressures of everyday life, and their compliance may be rather low. Compliance with a self-imposed program is usually higher. Involving the patient may not be easy because many people prefer to place the responsibility on the therapist or the doctor. Patience and an understanding of human motivation are necessary ingredients if such an approach is to succeed.

Many people with long-standing vascular disease are older. An understanding of the physical, physiologic, and psychological aspects of aging helps one realize that each elderly person is an individual with unique needs, wants, and aspirations. While some goals may change and the focus of life may be different with aging, many goals remain the same. Most older people want to maintain their independence both physically and psychologically. Some older people may be a little less adaptable and may have more difficulty coping with stress, while others actually become more open to change as they age. Care must be taken when interpreting physical changes. Decreased vision is not necessarily accompanied by decreased hearing, and decreased hearing is not necessarily accompanied by decreased mental ability. The apparently confused individual who cannot follow a series of hurriedly stated instructions is probably quite capable of following a home program that is slowly and carefully discussed. Most older people know their own capabilities and usually have a good idea of what they can achieve. Many will fear that the disability may lead to a loss of independence. It is helpful to provide the person with an opportunity to voice fears and concerns and to listen to him or her.

PREOPERATIVE PROGRAM

On occasion, the therapist will have the opportunity to treat a person scheduled for amputation prior to the surgery. The goals of treatment are to help prepare the person physically and psychologically for (1) the stress of the surgery, and (2) life as an amputee. Frequently, treatment is initiated when the patient has developed such severe necrosis, ulceration, or other problem that amputation is inevitable but the surgeon is waiting for a line of demarcation to develop or for infection to be brought under control. The person may be on complete bed rest and may be allowed only limited activities.

The evaluation focuses on the patient's general physical and mental state and the gross strength and range of motion of the upper extremities and uninvolved lower extremity. Exercising the involved lower extremity is often contraindicated. While all of the items mentioned earlier in this chapter under evaluation are valuable at this time, the extent of the evaluation will be determined by the patient's physical and mental state.

The treatment program is also limited by the patient's condition. General strengthening and range-of-motion exercises for the upper extremities and uninvolved lower extremity are beneficial. If the patient's condition allows, transfer activities can be taught. Positioning the patient properly in bed is important. The postoperative treatment program can also be explained at this time.

PSYCHOLOGICAL CONSIDERATIONS

The loss of a limb, regardless of its condition, is a traumatic and mutilating process. Anticipation may create anxiety, fear, anger, or depression. Accurate information and emotional support will help the patient cope with the coming trauma. Without making promises, the therapist can help the patient understand both the process of amputation itself and the postoperative rehabilitation program. A visit to the department where other amputees are being treated and the opportunity to talk with other amputees may relieve some fears. If the anticipated level of amputation is known, the patient can be shown one or more prostheses, and a general explanation of function can be given. Care should be taken not to overwhelm the person with too much information at one time. A useful guide is to let the person ask questions and respond to those questions. Patients will usually ask for information they are prepared to receive and will avoid areas they have yet to face. The patient may voice realistic concerns about social, sexual, and financial problems; the therapist can help by listening.

In some situations, the patient's status will be such that prosthetic replacement is not planned. It may be that the person is essentially bedridden or that a previous amputation will mitigate against fitting. In that instance, the preoperative program will focus on helping the patient plan and prepare for the highest possible potential level of postoperative independence.

As with all treatment programs, preoperative activities must be individualized and developed to meet postoperative goals. An understanding of prosthetic fitting and mechanics will help the therapist develop relevant preoperative programs.

BIBLIOGRAPHY

ALBERT, SF AND JAHNIGEN, DW: *Treating common foot disorders in older patients.* Geriatrics 38(6):42–52, 1983.

CEDERBERG, PA, PRITCHARD, DJ, AND JOYCE, JW: *Doppler-determined segmental pressures and wound-healing in amputations for vascular disease.* J Bone Joint Surg 65A:363–365, 1983.

FISCHER, BH: *Topical hyperbaric oxygen treatment of pressure sores and skin ulcers.* Lancet 2:405–409, 1969.

FISCHER, BH: *Treatment of ulcers on legs with hyperbaric oxygen.* J Dermatol Surg 1(3):55–58, 1975.

Hyperbaric oxygenation therapy now making "careful comeback." JAMA 246:1057–1066, 1981.

JOHNSTON, KW: *The roles of the vascular surgeon in the management of peripheral arterial occlusive disease: Diagnosis, selections, operations.* In KOSTUIK, JP (ED): *Amputation Surgery and Rehabilitation.* Churchill-Livingstone, New York, 1981.

MOORE, WS AND BLAISDELL, FW: *Diagnosis and management of arterial occlusive disease.* In *Current Problems in Surgery.* Yearbook Medical Publishers, Chicago, 1973.

GRIEF
DENIAL
ANGER
INSOMNIA
HOPELESSNESS
Fear of
IMPOTENCE and STERILITY
projection
MOURNING
DISBELIEF
DEPRESSION
Social
Withdrawal

CHAPTER 17

PSYCHOLOGICAL CONSIDERATIONS

REACTIONS TO AMPUTATION

INITIAL REACTIONS

The initial reactions to the loss of a limb are usually grief and depression. The experience may be similar to the death of a loved one: A part of the body has been irrevocably lost, and the person may feel incomplete and mourn for the lost extremity. If the amputation was traumatic, the immediate reactions may include disbelief. The person may experience insomnia and restlessness and may have difficulty concentrating. Some individuals may actually mourn for the possible loss of a job or the ability to participate in a favorite sport or other activity rather than mourning for the lost limb per se.

Some studies suggest that the lack of a formal burial or ritual of mourning may prevent individuals from expressing their grief or sense of loss, believing that such expressions would not be socially acceptable. The individuals may wonder what happened to their limbs and may feel some unease at not knowing their disposition. Repression of normal expressions of grief and loss may actually interfere with eventual acceptance of the amputation.

In the early stages, the amputee's grief may alternate with feelings of hopelessness, despondency, bitterness, and anger. The person may experience feelings of internal loss and mutilation. Some people state that they would prefer to be dead and wonder why the amputation has happened to them. Amputees may be jealous of others who have not suffered as they have; they may blame themselves or their surgeon for the loss. Socially, they may feel lonely and isolated. They may also feel as though they are the object of pity or horror.

Some of the amputee's reactions will be determined by concern about the future. The amputees may be concerned about how they will look and how family and friends will respond. Some may be worried about employment, particularly if they are the sole support of the family. Some amputees wonder if they will ever walk again or be attractive to a member of the opposite sex. Realistic concerns about the future will affect the person's emotional state.

LONG-TERM REACTIONS

Long-term adjustment to amputation depends to a great extent on the individual's basic personality structure, sense of accomplishment, and place in the family, community, and world. In general, many amputees make a satisfactory adjustment to the loss and are reintegrated into a full and active lifestyle. In achieving final acceptance, the individual may go through a number of stages, including denial, anger, euphoria, and social withdrawal.

Some amputees may try to avoid distressing thoughts of the lost limb through conscious self-control or by avoiding situations or people that remind them of the lost limb. Some may display temper tantrums or irrational resentment. Some may revert to childlike states of helplessness and dependence.

Many amputees are not fully aware of the consequences of amputation and may fear other physical limitations as a result of the surgery. Fear of impotence or sterility may lead some men to make grandiose statements or to display reckless behavior to mask the fear. Thorough explanations of the amputation process and its implications by the surgeon or other health care worker may alleviate many of these fears.

Amputees may use projection as a defense mechanism, viewing healthy people as amputees or feeling that amputees are not appreciated by other people. They may express bitterness, accusing the doctor of incompetence and insensitivity when it may not be justified. Some amputees resent offers of assistance and emphasize their independence. Their ostentatious defiance may be a protective mechanism against fear of the future. Some people have a compulsive need to convince themselves and others that they are not incapacitated.

Some amputees are cheerful and easygoing by nature and will make an easy adjustment to the loss. For others, joking and laughing may be a mechanism for self-deception, hiding fears about the possible incapacitating effects of the amputation. They may choose jobs or try to perform activities that they are not physically able to do.

The severity of the reaction is thought to be related to the level of amputation. Prosthetic, social, occupational, and financial factors can either soften or intensify the degree of reaction.

Generally, amputees dream of themselves as not being amputated. This image may be so vivid that they fall when they get up at night and attempt to walk to the bathroom without a prosthesis or crutches. Individuals who have lost the leg through injury may dream about the battle or accident in which they were injured. Such reenactments may lead to insomnia, trembling fits, speech impediments, and difficulty with concentration.

An amputee's emotional state can sometimes be assessed by certain psychological tests. Psychological testing may be helpful with patients who exhibit chronic difficulty in adjustment.

In the Draw-a-Person test, the individual is asked to draw a person. Almost all amputees show some alterations in drawing the extremities. Persons who are adapting poorly often accentuate the amputated limb or draw it larger. Persons who are adapting satisfactorily omit the amputated limb or draw it smaller.

In the Rorschach test, amputees who use functioning prostheses show greater self-control than those who use a prosthetic device for cosmetic purposes only. Amputees who name body parts in a great many of their responses are considered to have difficulty relinquishing body image integration.

Soldiers who become amputees show an unusually high incidence of anxiety of the so-called free-floating type. This is thought to represent anxiety and uncertainty about emotional demands of future life and the ability to adjust to the environment. No correlation has been found between reaction to injury, educational level, and length of military service.

The Bender Gestalt is another psychological test that is used with amputees. A score on the Bender Gestalt that usually indicates brain damage is thought to indicate poor total adjustment when made by the amputee.

PSYCHOLOGICAL SUPPORT

The amputee needs to receive reassurance and understanding from the entire rehabilitation team. Each amputee should be regarded as a unique individual. The staff should create an open and receptive environment and should be willing to listen. The amputee should know what to expect during the entire process. The steps of rehabilitation and the expectations should be carefully explained by the surgeon and therapists. Audio-visual media, such as films or slides, may be helpful in orienting the amputee.

Other amputees who have made satisfactory adjustments in their lives and have successfully completed rehabilitation may provide support and encouragement to the new amputee in private or group sessions. Professionals who are skilled in group dynamics should be present, especially for medical or technical advice regarding such issues as diabetes, medications, or peripheral vascular disease. Family and friends are often invited to attend. The atmosphere should be non-threatening so that patients can express their feelings and frustrations. As rehabilitation proceeds, other amputees who are receiving treatment can arouse a fraternal feeling and a friendly, competitive spirit.

Patients, in general, have a way of finding other patients who are, in their opinion, worse off than they. This helps amputees put their own problems in perspective and offers them the opportunity to talk with others who are experiencing misfortune. For these reasons, it is usually desirable to conduct as much of the rehabilitation as possible in open areas rather than isolating the amputee from other patients. This does not mean, however, that the amputee's privacy should be violated.

Amputees have various attitudes toward the prosthesis. Some are particularly concerned about its appearance, hoping that it will conceal their disability and give the illusion of an intact body. Others claim to be concerned primarily with the restoration of function. When the artificial limb is fitted, the amputee must face the fact that the natural limb has been lost irrevocably. If amputees have been told that the prosthesis will replace their own limb, then they may have unrealistic expectations that appearance and function will be as good as in the amputated leg. Realistic adjustment will be necessary as the amputee learns to use the artificial substitute. Good predictors of adjustment to the prosthesis are motivation to master the prosthesis and motivation for gainful employment.

When the amputee returns home, acts of kindness and consideration are appreciated. That does not mean that the amputee wants to be fussed over or to become the center of attention. The reaction of family and friends may vary from feelings of over-protection to repulsion.

Mutual assistance and interactions help provide amputees with the feeling that they are not alone. There are various organizations for amputees across the United States and in other parts of the world (see Table 22-1). These groups also help to fulfill the amputee's social needs.

SPECIAL AGE GROUPS

INFANTS AND YOUNG CHILDREN

Shock is the usual parental reaction to the birth of a child with a congenital anomaly or to an amputation owing to injury or tumor. Parents may go through periods of denial and anger and may experience feelings of guilt and shame before accepting their child's amputation. In some cases, parents may be overwhelmed and inconsolable; others may not fully appreciate the implications of disability. Parents of children with acquired amputations may accept the deficit more easily than parents of children with congenital amputations because of the genetic implication. Rehabilitation team members should be concerned with parental adjustment since parental acceptance of the amputation and the prosthesis will likely correlate with the child's adjustment.

Lower limb child amputees are fitted early, as soon as they are mature enough to stand, partly in an effort to integrate the prosthesis into their body image. Children usually incorporate into their body image amputations performed under the age of 2. If children sustain an amputation after they have acquired a body image, then they experience an insult to a previously intact body image. Thus, in cases of congenital deformity, it is generally recommended that surgery be performed during the first year of life, if practical. Surgery and associated hospitalization during the second or third year of life may disrupt the child's attachment to the parents. It has been suggested that surgery during the fourth to sixth years of life, when the child is developing a sense of sexual differences, may result in anxieties or phobias in later life because the surgery is interpreted as a castration.

It is important for physicians, therapists, and family to touch the residual limb to indicate acceptance. Examples have been given of the use of a transitional object, such as a special prosthesis doll, in the psychological rehabilitation of very young children. It is especially recommended for children who have regressed to behaviors such as loss of toilet training, return of thumb sucking, and repressed verbalization. Through simulation, the doll, which represents the self, can provide an opportunity for the child to cope with the painful reality of the amputation and future developments such as a prosthesis. The "like me–not me" doll is constructed to undergo the same medical and surgical procedures as the child. Some contend that these play activities, if used indiscriminately, could have a countertherapeutic effect and suggest an alternative, such as storytelling.

OLDER CHILDREN AND ADOLESCENTS

Regardless of age, the child's emotional reactions must be considered by the rehabilitation team. Too often, detailed discussions about the amputation and postoperative care are conducted with the parents, and the child is overlooked. The physician should talk with the child before and after surgery to explain what will happen. The child should be aware of what to expect during anesthesia, surgery, and the recovery period. Misinformation or distortions should be detected and corrected.

Mourning is a normal process for the child as well as for the adult. When depressed, children are likely to regress to a more infantile level of behavior and must be given the opportunity to express their feelings through play or talk. The early adolescent may grieve over the loss of self-image, while the adolescent may be afraid of rejection and social ostracization. Adolescence is a dynamic phase during which profound changes lead people to feel sexually attractive and capable of reproduction. Self-esteem is very vulnerable at this time. The adolescent may feel inadequate after amputation and needs reassurance from significant others. Contact with other young amputees may be quite constructive.

The reaction to the loss of a limb will be affected by the child's previous experiences and the reaction of family members. Parental reaction profoundly influences the way the child copes.

THE ELDERLY

Elderly people's immediate reactions to amputation depend in part on the severity of preoperative pain and the extent of attempts to save the limb. Individuals who had suffered considerable pain may be grateful that the pain has ended. Patients who underwent extensive medical and surgical procedures to save the limb may have a sense of failure because the efforts were not successful.

In general, the reactions of an elderly amputee will be similar to those of any adult amputee. Some may feel a sense of hopelessness and despair, and they may have a preoccupation with impending death. Some may have insomnia and anorexia and may be withdrawn. Some elderly individuals may experience a loss of self-esteem and may be afraid of becoming dependent. In some instances, the amputees may express the feeling that they have nothing to live for and desire death. Occasionally, suicide may be attempted. Elderly people seldom use denial since the functional and anatomic deficit is obvious. Elderly amputees are more likely to dream that the amputation has taken place than younger individuals. The elderly person may view the amputation as impending death because the rest of the body is vulnerable.

If preoperative attitudes are unrealistically hopeful, then postoperative disturbances may be more severe. The elderly amputee should not be misled into expecting a total cure. Learning to use an artificial limb may be a slow and discouraging ordeal, and the patient may not express distress or depression in front of the optimism of others. Sharing and support from other elderly amputees can be quite helpful, as can a realistic attitude by rehabilitation team members.

SUMMARY

Complete rehabilitation includes not only preparation of the amputee physically and psychologically for the community, but preparation of the community for the amputee. Public education media can be used to inform people of the potentials of amputees in society and employment. Amputees, as others, need to be accepted and integrated into the community because of their abilities—not their disabilities.

BIBLIOGRAPHY

ABRAM, HS, ET AL: A multidisciplinary computerized approach to the study of adjustment of the lower limb amputation. South Med J 62:1072–1076, 1969.

BROWN, J: The theory and the practice: Patients' reactions to amputation of a lower limb. Nurs Times 19:639–640, 1966.

CAINE, D: Psychological considerations affecting rehabilitation after amputation. Med J Aust 2:818–821, 1973.

CAPLAN, LM AND HACKETT, TP: Emotional effects of lower-limb amputation in the aged. N Engl J Med 269:1166–1171, 1963.

CHAIKLIN, H AND WARFIELD, M: Stigma management and amputee rehabilitation. Rehabil Lit 34:162–166, 1973.

CHILVERS, AS AND BROWSE, NL: The social fate of the amputee. Lancet 2:1192–1193, 1971.

EARLE, EM: The psychological effects of mutilating surgery in children and adolescents. Psychoanal Study Child 34:527–546, 1979.

FISCHER, WG AND SAMELSON, CF: Group psychotherapy for selected patients with lower extremity amputations. Arch Phys Med Rehabil 52:79, 1971.

FOORT, J: *How amputees feel about amputation.* In *Selected Readings: A Review of Orthotics and Prosthetics.* American Orthotics and Prosthetics Association, Washington, DC, 1980, pp 12–20.

FRANK, JL: *The amputee war casualty in a military hospital: Observations on psychological management.* Psychiatry Med 4:1–16, 1973.

FRANK, JL AND HERNDON, JH: *Psychiatric-orthopedic liaison in the hospital management of the amputee war casualty.* Int J Psychiatry Med 5:105–114, 1974.

FREEMAN, AM, III AND APPLEGATE, WR: *Psychiatric consultation to a rehabilitation program for amputees.* Hosp Community Psychiatry 27:40–42, 1976.

FRIEDMANN, LW: *The quality of hope for the amputee.* Arch Surg 110:760, 1975.

HABER, WB: *Effects of loss of limb on sensory functions.* J Psychol 40:115–123, 1955.

HABER, WB: *Reactions to loss of limb: Physiological and psychological aspects.* Ann NY Acad Sci 73:14–24, 1958.

HADDAN, CC: *Psycho-social implications of the geriatric amputee.* Ortho Pros Appl J 16:32–36, 1962.

HEALY, MH AND HANSEN, H: *Psychiatric management of limb amputation in a preschool child: The illusion of "like me–not me."* J Am Acad Child Psychiatry 16:684–692, 1977.

KERSTEIN, MD: *Group rehabilitation for the vascular-disease amputee.* J Am Geriatr Soc 28:40–41, 1980.

KESSLER, HH: *Psychological preparation of the amputee.* Indus Med Surg 20:107–108, 1951.

KOLB, LC: *The psychology of the amputee: A study of phantom phenomena, body image and pain.* Collected Papers of the Mayo Clinic 44:586–590, 1952.

KYLLONEN, RR: *Body image and reactions to amputations.* Conn Med 28:19–23, 1964.

LANE, HJ: *Working with problems of assault to self-image and life-style.* Soc Work Health Care 1:191–198, 1975–1976.

LIPP, MR AND MALONE, ST: *Group rehabilitation of vascular surgery patients.* Arch Phys Med Rehabil 57:180–183, 1976.

MACBRIDE, A, ET AL: *Psychosocial factors in the rehabilitation of elderly amputees.* Psychosomatics 21:258–261, 1980.

MAY, CH, MCPHEE, MC, AND PRITCHARD, DJ: *An amputee visitor program as an adjunct to rehabilitation of the lower limb amputee.* Mayo Clin Proc 54:774–778, 1979.

NOBLE, D, PRICE, DB, AND GILDER, R, JR: *Psychiatric disturbances following amputation.* Am J Psychiatry 110:609–613, 1954.

PARKES, CM: *Components of the reaction to loss of a limb, spouse or home.* J Psychosom Res 16:343–349, 1972.

PARKES, CM: *Psycho-social transitions: Comparison between reactions to loss of a limb and loss of a spouse.* Br J Psychiatry 127:204–210, 1975.

PARKES, CM AND NAPIER, MM: *Psychiatric sequelae of amputation.* In SILVERSTONE, T AND BARRACLOUGH, B (EDS): *Contemporary Psychiatry.* Headley Brothers, Ashford, England, 1975, pp 440–446.

PFEFFERBAUM, B AND PASNAU, RO: *Post-amputation grief.* Nurs Clin North Am 11:687–690, 1976.

PLANK, EN AND HORWOOD, C: *Leg amputation in a four-year-old: Reactions of the child, her family, and the staff.* Psychoanal Study Child 16:405–422, 1961.

RANDALL, GC, EWALT, JR, AND BLAIR, H: *Psychiatric reaction to amputation.* JAMA 128:645–652, 1945.

ROGERS, J, ET AL: *The use of groups in the rehabilitation of amputees.* Int J Psychiatry Med 8:243–255, 1978.

ROSEN, VH: *The role of denial in acute postoperative affective reactions following removal of body parts.* Psychosom Med 12:356–361, 1950.

SHAW, M, ET AL: *Traumatic triple amputation: Psycho-social problems in rehabilitation.* Arch Phys Med Rehabil 58:460–462, 1977.

SIMPSON, EB AND ALBRONDA, HF: *Psychologic aspects of amputation of a lower limb.* Lancet 87:429–431, 1967.

STUART, E: *Amputation for osteogenic sarcoma.* Nurs Times 68:1453–1454, Nov 1972.

TAYLOR, IW: *Psychologic needs of the handicapped child.* Inter-Clinic Info Bull 9:9–17, 1970.

WEISS, SA: *The body image as related to phantom sensation: A hypothetical conceptualization of seemingly isolated findings.* Ann NY Acad Sci 74:25–29, 1958.

WEISS, SA, FISHMAN, S, AND KRAUSE, F: *Symbolic impulsivity: The Bender-Gestalt test and prosthetic adjustment in amputees.* Arch Phys Med 51:152–158, 1970.

WITTKOWER, ME: *Rehabilitation of the limbless: A joint surgical and psychologic study.* J Occup Med 3:20–44, 1947.

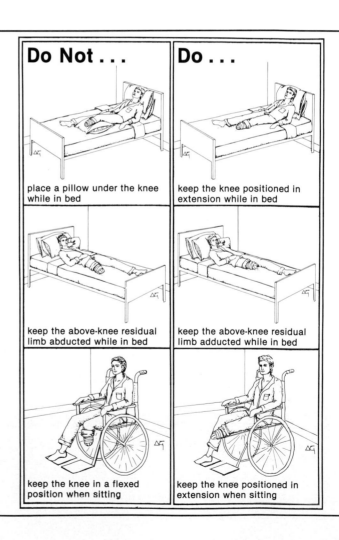

Do Not . . .

place a pillow under the knee while in bed

keep the above-knee residual limb abducted while in bed

keep the knee in a flexed position when sitting

Do . . .

keep the knee positioned in extension while in bed

keep the above-knee residual limb adducted while in bed

keep the knee positioned in extension when sitting

CHAPTER **18**

POSTOPERATIVE MANAGEMENT

BELLA J. MAY, Ed.D., R.P.T.

The earlier the onset of a rehabilitation program after amputation surgery, the greater the potential for success. The longer the delay, the more likely the development of secondary complications such as joint contractures, general debilitation, and a depressed psychological state. The postoperative program can be arbitrarily divided into two phases: the early phase, which encompasses the first few days after surgery; and the preprosthetic phase, which includes the rest of the time until fitting with a definitive prosthesis or until a decision not to fit. In some places, the two phases are combined and called the preprosthetic period.

The long-term goal of the total rehabilitation program is to help the patient regain the preoperative level of function. For some patients, it will mean a return to gainful employment with an active recreational life. For others, it will mean independence in the home and community. For still others, it may mean living in the sheltered environment of a retirement center or nursing home. If the amputation resulted from a chronic disease, the goal may be to help the person function at a higher level than immediately before surgery.

CLINIC TEAM

The majority of amputations today are performed by vascular surgeons, who may or may not be knowledgeable about prosthetic rehabilitation. Referral to the clinic team or to physical therapy may be delayed until healing has taken place and the sutures have been removed. Such delays are undesirable and may limit the eventual level of rehabilitation. Ideally, the clinic team should become involved before surgery, or at least immediately afterward. Unfortunately, many amputations are performed in hospitals that do not have the services of an amputee clinic or a well-trained team that can develop and supervise the program. The physical therapist may be the only person with competence in prosthetic rehabilitation. It is desirable for the physical therapist to work closely with the vascular surgeon to increase the likelihood of early referrals.

MEMBERS

The amputee clinic team plans and implements comprehensive rehabilitation programs that are designed to meet the physical, psychological, and economic needs of the amputee. Most amputee clinic teams are located in rehabilitation facilities or university health centers. The team generally includes a physician, a physical therapist, an occupational therapist, a prosthetist, a social worker, and a vocational counselor. Other health professionals who often contribute to the team are the nurse, dietician, psychologist, and possibly, the administrative coordinator.

FUNCTIONS

The physician should be an individual with firsthand knowledge of the process of amputation surgery, the scope of comprehensive rehabilitation programs, and the biomechanics and engineering principles of prosthetic components. The orthopedic surgeon has the skill to construct a residual limb designed to obtain the most effective control of the prosthesis and the most satisfactory person-machine interface. Orthopedic surgeons learn basic prosthetic and engineering principles as well as comprehensive rehabilitation as part of their training and are thus often clinic chiefs. However, any physician with interest and competence in the areas listed can serve as clinic chief. Each member of the team is dependent on the skills of the other members, as no one person can meet all of the patient's needs. An effective team functions as a team and not as a group of different health professionals.

The prosthetist recommends prosthetic components, fabricates the appliance, provides information on new engineering developments, suggests adaptations to standard components to meet unique needs, and works closely with the therapist and the patient to ensure optimum fit and alignment of the prosthesis. As an essential member of the team, the prosthetist regularly attends the clinic.

The physical therapist is involved in all aspects of the rehabilitation program and often serves as clinic coordinator. Information gathered during the preprosthetic phase influences the team's decisions. The physical therapist becomes well acquainted with the patient and the family and shares insights regarding the patient's home situation and lifestyle. The physical therapist can help the patient and family members learn how to live with an amputation and adjust emotionally to the loss.

The occupational therapist is generally involved in the management of upper extremity amputees. The occupational therapist evaluates and prepares the upper extremity amputee for a prosthesis, makes recommendations to the team about components, and trains the individual in the use of the appliances. The functions of the physical therapist and occupational therapist overlap to some degree. When both are members of the team, they develop a mutually cooperative relationship that enhances the utilization of resources and the quality of care.

In many centers, the social worker has become the team's financial advisor and general troubleshooter. The complexities of insurance coverages, governmental programs, covered benefits, and increasing costs have altered their traditional role, and many of their activities are centered on the economic problems that are engendered by severe chronic disability.

The vocational counselor is involved primarily with amputees of working age. The major function of the vocational counselor is to help the individual return to gainful employment. Support may be financial (such as providing funds for prosthetic replacement and training), educational (such as preparing an individual for some employment), or both. In many teams, the vocational counselor is a consultant who is called upon as needed.

Other individuals who may be members of a clinic team include the nurse, dietician, psychologist, and the administrative coordinator. The nurse has a very important role during the hospitalization phase. By spending considerable time with the patient and family, the nurse can provide valuable information to the team. The nurse can enhance the physical restoration program by ensuring that proper positioning, bandaging, and bed exercises are carried out throughout the day and night. The nurse will also help educate the patient regarding continued care of the skin and the residual limb. It is vital for the nurse and physical therapist to work closely together to ensure a well-integrated program.

The dietician teaches the diabetic amputee about proper diet. Together, the dietician and physical therapist can help the amputee to develop proper dietary habits to meet the physiologic demands of the program and to maintain an appropriate weight level. A clinical psychologist may be called upon to help individuals who are having difficulty making satisfactory emotional adjustment. Finally, in some centers, a coordinator may be employed to manage the operations of the clinic: maintaining records, arranging appointments, and coordinating the distribution of information to all members of the team.

The amputee clinic team meets frequently, as dictated by the case load. Patients are seen regularly, and decisions are made using input from all team members. A screening clinic held by the physical and occupational therapists prior to the actual amputee clinic allows for the careful evaluation of each person to be seen and improves the effectiveness of the clinic function.

EARLY POSTOPERATIVE MANAGEMENT

The major goals of the early postoperative phase are to:

1. deter edema development and enhance healing of the residual limb
2. prevent contractures and other secondary complications
3. maintain or regain strength in the affected lower extremity
4. begin adjustment to the loss of a body part
5. begin to regain independence in mobility and self-care
6. begin to learn proper care of the other extremity.

To some extent, the success of the rehabilitation program is determined by the individual's psychophysiologic status and by the physical characteristics of the residual limb. The longer the residual limb, the better potential for successful prosthetic ambulation regardless of level of amputation. A well-healed, cylindrical limb with a nonadherent scar is easier to fit than one that is conical or has redundant tissue distally or laterally. The vascular status of the remaining extremity will affect the rehabilitation program, as will the physiologic age of the individual. The presence of conditions such as diabetes, cardiovascular disease, visual impairment, limitation of joint motion, and muscle weakness may affect the eventual level of function. From the onset of treatment, it is important to consider the individual as an integrated being and to develop a comprehensive plan of action.

EVALUATION

Patient assessment is an integral part of each phase of treatment; data regarding the condition of the residual limb, strength of the affected extremity, joint range of motion, condition of the other extremity, and the patient's feelings about the amputation are used in establishing treatment activities and in setting priorities and terminal expectations. The availability of some of this data will depend in part on the surgeon's treatment of the residual limb.

RESIDUAL LIMB CARE

Surgeons today have several options regarding the postoperative dressing, including: (1) immediate postoperative fitting or rigid dressing, (2) semirigid dressing, (3) controlled environment, or (4) soft dressing. Regardless of the type of dressing used, the limb must not be allowed to remain uncovered for any length of time between dressing changes or edema will increase. Excessive edema in the residual limb can compromise healing and cause pain.

RIGID DRESSING

In the early 1960s, orthopedic surgeons in the United States started experimenting with a technique, developed in Europe, that consisted of fitting the amputee with a plaster of Paris socket made in the configuration of the definitive prosthesis. In some instances, a foot and pylon were attached and the patient was allowed to walk with limited weight-bearing within 48 hours of surgery. Application techniques varied to some extent. In some centers, the dressing was brought above the knee to prevent possible movement between the residual limb and the socket; in another center, the dressing was wrapped below the knee, with the knee joint temporarily immobilized by a soft dressing. Regardless of the method of suspension, the immediate postoperative prosthesis that is applied in the operating room provides several advantages over the more traditional soft dressing.

Advantages:
1. Greatly limits the development of postoperative edema in the residual limb, thereby reducing postoperative pain and enhancing wound healing.
2. Allows for earlier ambulation with the attachment of a pylon and foot.
3. Allows for earlier fitting of the definitive prosthesis by reducing the length of time needed for shrinking the residual limb.
4. It is configured to each individual residual limb.

Disadvantages:
1. Requires careful application by individuals knowledgeable about prosthetic principles.
2. Requires close supervision during the healing stage.
3. Does not allow for daily wound inspection and dressing changes.

After several years, research indicated that early ambulation did not influence wound healing positively and, in fact, might interfere with healing if the patient could not control the amount of weight borne on the amputated extremity. Since then, the immediate postoperative prosthesis has generally given way to the molded rigid dressing that is applied in the operating room. In addition to the surgeon, the prosthetist, physical therapist, nurse, or cast technician can, after training, apply the rigid dressing. The dressing consists of a total-contact plaster of Paris socket that is padded over bony prominences and suspended so as to prevent any motion between the skin and the cast. Individuals who are interested in learning casting techniques should attend a course given for that purpose because an improperly applied dressing can lead to skin abrasions and delayed healing.

Like the postoperative prosthesis, the rigid dressing limits the development of postoperative edema, thereby decreasing postoperative pain and improving the environment for healing. Studies indicated that even in limbs without circulation through the major vessels, healing takes place if there is good bleeding through the skin flaps at the time of surgery. The absence of edema allows for good skin circulation in the surgical site, thereby allowing surgeons to perform more amputations at below-knee levels. The rigid dressing is considered to be the most effective postoperative treatment available today.

SEMIRIGID DRESSINGS

Semirigid dressings include the Unna paste, the air splint, and the controlled environment treatment (CET).

UNNA'S PASTE

Unna's paste is a compound of zinc oxide, gelatin, glycerin, and calamine. It is applied in the operating room in a manner similar to that described in Chapter 16. Once dry, it is light and semirigid and controls postoperative edema. Depending on the length of the residual limb, the dressing may be applied to mid-thigh or to just below the knee for a below-knee amputation. The above-knee dressing may include a hip spica, if necessary, for suspension.

> *Advantages:*
> 1. Good control of postoperative edema.
> 2. Self-suspension without additional straps.
> 3. Can be changed easily if there is much wound exudate.
> 4. Allows freedom of motion in the proximal joint of long residual limbs.
> 5. Conforms to the shape of the residual limb.
>
> *Disadvantages:*
> 1. It may loosen before being fully dry, thus allowing edema to develop.
> 2. Because it is less rigid than the plaster of Paris dressing, it does not protect the residual limb as well.
> 3. It needs more frequent changing than the plaster of Paris dressing.

The Unna paste dressing has, on some occasions, been used with a temporary prosthesis as a covering for the residual limb.

AIR SPLINT

Little, in 1970, first reported the use of an air splint to control postoperative edema as well as to aid in early ambulation. The air splint (Fig. 18-1) is a plastic double-wall bag that is pumped to the desired level of rigidity. It has a zipper and encases the entire extremity, which is covered with an appropriate postsurgical dressing.

> *Advantages:*
> 1. Provides better edema control than the soft dressing, but not as effective as the rigid dressing.
> 2. Availability of incision for inspection.
> 3. Bipedal support for the patient in the upright position.
> 4. Relatively inexpensive because it can be reused.
> 5. Can be applied by most health care personnel with minimal training.
>
> *Disadvantages:*
> 1. The pressure, once applied, is constant and does not intimately conform to the shape of the residual limb.
> 2. The environment of the plastic is hot and humid, requiring frequent cleaning.
> 3. The thickness of the inflated walls encourages hip abduction.

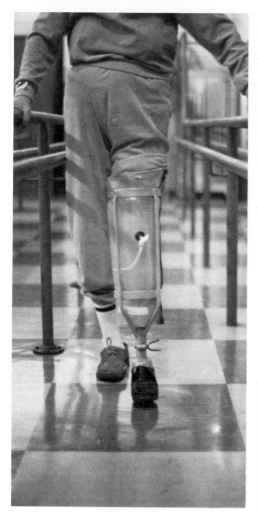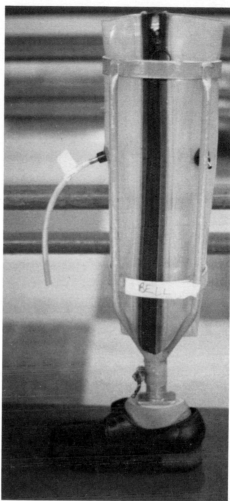

FIGURE 18-1. Air splint.

Pressure is measured in millimeters of mercury and can be varied. The system appears to be more effective with below-knee than with above-knee amputees because of the difficulty in suspending the appliance with the shorter residual limb.

CONTROLLED ENVIRONMENT TREATMENT (CET)

The CET was developed at the National Biomechanical Research and Development Unit of Roehampton, England, and has been used in some centers in the United States. It is composed of a console that controls pressure, temperature, and humidity and sterilizes the air in the unit, and a polyvinyl transparent bag that encases the residual limb. Bags are available in a variety of sizes and can be used with long above-knee limbs as well as with below-knee and Syme's amputations.

Kegel, in a preliminary report on 20 patients, indicated that the CET decreased postoperative edema and pain and appeared to improve circulation to the wound as a result of the cyclical pressure changes. The bag's flexibility allowed active exercises of the involved extremity as well as standing at the bedside. The hose connecting the bag to the console made ambulation somewhat difficult. Kegel indicated that in addition to the advantages of the rigid dressing for control of edema and pain, the CET allowed some 60 degrees of active knee motion and gave the therapist and nursing staff an excellent opportunity to observe the condition of the wound. On the negative side, the size of the equipment kept the patient in the hospital room, and the bag interfered with lying prone, so that a definitive program of hip extension had to be undertaken. In addition, the nursing staff had to pay particular attention to skin care because the individual spent more time in bed than other amputees.

SOFT DRESSINGS

The soft dressing is the oldest method of postoperative management of the residual limb.

> *Advantages:*
> 1. Relatively inexpensive.
> 2. Lightweight and readily available.
> 3. Can be laundered.
>
> *Disadvantages:*
> 1. Relatively poor control of edema.
> 2. Requires skill in proper application.
> 3. Needs frequent reapplication.
> 4. Can slip and form a tourniquet.

A dressing is applied to the incision, followed by some form of gauze pad, then the compression wrap. The soft dressing is indicated in cases of local infection but is not the treatment of choice for the majority of individuals. The amputee should learn to apply the wrap as soon as possible after wound care is no longer necessary. Many elderly above-knee amputees do not have the necessary balance and coordination to wrap effectively.

There are many methods of wrapping the residual limb, and most therapists will adapt a method to their own needs. Patients tend to wrap their own residual limb in a circular manner, often creating a tourniquet, which may compromise healing and will foster the development of a bulbous end. While the below-knee residual limb can be effectively wrapped in a sitting position, it is difficult to properly wrap and anchor the above-knee limb while sitting. Elderly patients often cannot balance themselves in the standing position while wrapping.

An effective bandage will be smooth and wrinkle-free, will emphasize angular turns, will provide pressure distally, and will encourage proximal joint extension. The ends of bandages should be fastened with tape, safety pins, or Velcro rather than with clips, which can cut the skin and do not anchor well. A wrapping system that uses mostly angular or figure-of-8 turns was developed specifically to meet the needs of the elderly and has been in use for the past 20 years. Figures 18-2 and 18-3 illustrate the techniques.

BELOW-KNEE BANDAGE

Two 4-inch elastic bandages will usually be enough to wrap most below-knee residual limbs. Very large residual limbs may require three bandages. The below-knee bandages should not be sewed together, so that the weave of each bandage can be brought in

BELOW—KNEE STUMP BANDAGING

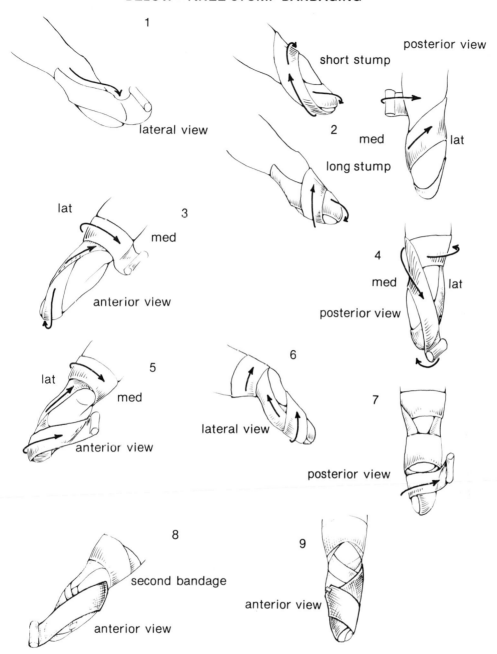

FIGURE 18-2. Below-knee residual limb wrapping.

contraposition to the other to provide more support. Although an elastic wrap does not provide as much pressure as a rigid dressing, it still must help to deter the development of postoperative edema as much as possible; therefore, a firm, even pressure against all soft tissues is desirable. If the incision is placed anteriorly, then an attempt should be made to bring the bandages from posterior to anterior over the distal end.

ABOVE-KNEE STUMP BANDAGING

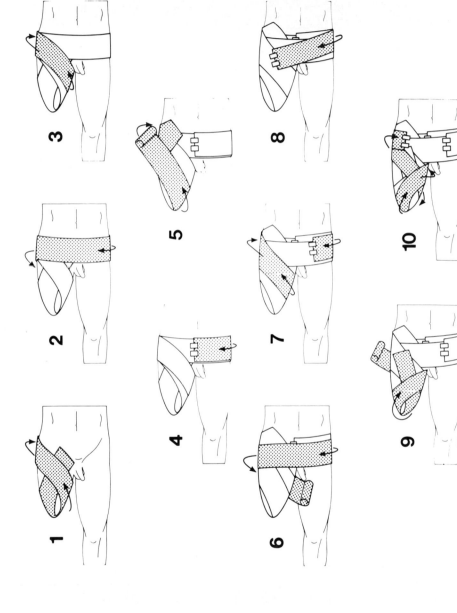

FIGURE 18-3. Above-knee residual limb wrapping.

The first bandage is started at either the medial or lateral tibial condyle and is brought diagonally over the anterior surface of the limb to the distal end. One edge of the bandage should just cover the midline of the incision in an anterior-posterior plane. The bandage is continued diagonally over the posterior surface then back over the beginning turn as an anchor. At this point, there is a choice: the bandage may be brought directly over the beginning point, as indicated in Figure 18-2, or it may be brought across the front of the residual limb in an "X" design. The latter is particularly useful with long residual limbs and aids in bandage suspension. An anchoring turn over the distal thigh is made, making sure that the wrap is clear of the patella and is not tight around the distal thigh.

After a single anchoring turn above the knee, the bandage is brought back around the opposite tibial condyle and down to the distal end of the limb. One edge of the bandage should overlap the midline of the incision and the other wrap by at least 1.3 cm (1/2 in) to ensure adequate distal end support. The figure-of-8 pattern is continued as depicted in Figure 18-2 until the bandage is used up. Care should be taken to completely cover the residual limb with a firm, even pressure. Semicircular turns are made posteriorly to bring the bandage in line to cross the anterior surface in an angular line. This maneuver provides greater pressure on the posterior soft tissue while distributing pressure anteriorly where the bone is close to the skin. Each turn should partially overlap other turns so that the whole residual limb is well covered. The pattern is usually from proximal to distal and back to proximal, starting at the tibial condyles and covering both condyles as well as the patellar tendon. Usually, the patella is left free to aid in knee motion; however, with extremely short residual limbs, it may be necessary to cover the patella for better suspension.

The second bandage is wrapped like the first except that it is started at the opposite tibial condyle from the first bandage. Bringing the weave of each bandage in contraposition exerts a more even pressure. With both bandages, an effort is made to bring the angular turns across each other rather than in the same direction.

ABOVE-KNEE BANDAGE

For most residual limbs, two 6-inch bandages and one 4-inch bandage will adequately cover the limb. The two 6-inch bandages can be sewed together end to end, taking care not to create a heavy seam; the 4-inch bandage is used by itself. The patient is depicted side-lying in Figure 18-3, which allows a family member or therapist easy access to the residual limb. Patients can bandage themselves in the standing position if they have good balance on the remaining limb, but it is difficult for them to self-bandage correctly in the sitting position.

The 6-inch bandages are used first. The first bandage is started at the groin and is brought diagonally over the anterior surface to the distal lateral corner, around the end of the residual limb, and diagonally up the posterior side to the iliac crest and around the hips in a spica. The bandage is started medially so that the hip wrap will encourage extension. After the turn around the hips, the bandage is wrapped around the proximal portion of the residual limb high in the groin, then back around the hips. While this is a proximal circular turn, it does not create a tourniquet as long as it is continued around the hips. Going around the medial portion of the residual limb high in the groin ensures coverage of the soft tissue in the adductor area and reduces the possibility of an adductor roll, a complication that can seriously interfere with comfortable prosthetic wear. In most instances, the first bandage ends in the second spica and is anchored with tape or a pin.

The second 6-inch bandage is wrapped like the first but is started a bit more laterally. Any areas not covered by the first bandage must be covered at this time. The second bandage is also anchored in a hip spica after the first figure-of-8 and after the second turn high in the groin. While more of the first two bandages are used to cover the proximal residual limb, care must be taken that no tourniquet is created. Bringing the bandage directly from the proximal-medial area into a hip spica helps keep the adductor tissue covered and prevents rolling of the bandage to some degree.

The 4-inch bandage is used to exert the greatest amount of pressure over mid and distal areas of the residual limb. It is usually not necessary to anchor this bandage around the hips because friction with the already applied bandages and good figure-of-8 turns provide adequate suspension. The 4-inch bandage is generally started laterally to bring the weave across the weave of previous bandages. Regular figure-of-8 turns in varied patterns to cover all of the residual limb are the most effective.

Bandages are applied with firm pressure from the outset. Elastic bandages can be wrapped directly over a soft postoperative dressing so that bandaging can begin immediately after surgery. The elastic wrap controls edema more effectively if minimal gauze coverage is used over the residual limb. Several gauze pads placed just over the incision are usually adequate protection without compromising the effect of the wrap. Care must be taken to avoid any wrinkles or folds, which can cause excessive skin pressure, particularly over a soft dressing.

One of the major drawbacks of the elastic wrap is that it needs frequent rewrapping. Movement of the residual limb against the bedclothes, bending and extending the proximal joints, and general body movements will cause slippage and, thus, changes in pressure. Covering the finished wrap with a stockinet helps to reduce some of the wrinkling. However, careful and frequent rewrapping is the only effective way to prevent complications. Along with the therapy staff, the nursing staff, family members, and the patient need to assume responsibility for frequent inspection and rewrapping of the residual limb.

Some surgeons prefer to delay the elastic wrap until the incision has healed and the sutures have been removed. Leaving the residual limb without any pressure wrap allows for full development of postoperative edema, which may be quite uncomfortable and which may interfere with circulation in the many small vessels in the skin and soft tissue, thereby potentially compromising healing. The therapist can discuss the benefits of early wrapping if no other form of rigid dressing is used.

SHRINKERS

Shrinkers are sock-like garments that are knitted of rubber-reinforced cotton; they are conical and come in a variety of sizes. Shrinkers are an alternative to the elastic wrap and can be used to control edema of the residual limb. A shrinker of appropriate size is rolled over the residual limb to mid-thigh for below-knee amputations and to the proximal thigh for above-knee amputations. The shrinker is suspended with garters, a waist belt, or occasionally, a shoulder harness. Care must be taken to ensure that the patient understands the importance of proper suspension, as any rolling of the edges or slipping of the shrinker can create a tourniquet around the proximal part of the residual limb. Although shrinkers are easier to apply than the elastic wrap, there is some controversy regarding their effectiveness. A recent study reported shrinkers to be more effective than an elastic wrap for decreasing limb volume in below-knee residual limbs; however, others have not shared this experience. The shrinker is easier to use with below-knee amputees. Like the elastic wrap, it is difficult to suspend in the above-knee residual limb. Any rolling or slipping will enhance the development of an adductor roll. Shrinkers are more expensive to use than elastic wrap; the initial cost is greater, and new shrinkers of smaller sizes must be purchased as the limb volume decreases.

TREATMENT PROGRAM

POSITIONING

One of the major goals of the early postoperative program is to prevent secondary complications such as contractures of adjacent joints. Contractures can develop as a result of muscle imbalance or fascial tightness, from a protective withdrawal reflex into hip and knee flexion, from loss of plantar stimulation in extension, or as a result of faulty positioning (Fig. 18-4) such as prolonged sitting. The patient should understand the importance of proper positioning and regular exercises in preparing for eventual prosthetic fit and ambulation.

The below-knee amputee needs full range of motion in the hips and knee, particularly in extension. While sitting, the patient can keep the knee extended by using a posterior splint or a board attached to the wheelchair. The above-knee amputee needs full range of motion in the hip, particularly in extension and adduction. Prolonged sitting is to be avoided, especially for individuals who have difficulty walking on crutches. Some time each day should be spent in the prone position. Elevation of the residual limb on a pillow, while beneficial for edema control, can lead to the development of hip flexion contractures and should be avoided. The early postoperative period is critical for establishing positive patterns of activity that will aid the patient throughout the rehabilitation period. Taking the time to teach the patient to assume responsibility for his or her own care can reap later benefits.

EXERCISES

Mild active range-of-motion exercises are indicated for the joint immediately proximal to the incision, which needs to be protected until healing has occurred. If the immediate postoperative dressing limits joint motion, isometric contractions can be initiated. Isometric quadriceps and gluteal muscle exercises can be taught prior to surgery and started early after amputation. An understanding of the function of muscles involved in prosthetic ambulation helps the therapist emphasize appropriate strengthening activities.

Active and resistive exercises for the uninvolved lower extremity, the trunk, and the upper extremities are initiated immediately after surgery. There are a variety of approaches that can be used to help the patient regain strength and coordination. Proprioceptive neuromuscular facilitation techniques are particularly valuable because they use combination movements and total body involvement in appropriate patterns. Such exercises can be started to the patient's tolerance early in the program as long as care is taken to prevent stress or trauma to the involved limb.

MOBILITY

Early mobility is an important adjunct to total physiologic recovery. The amputee needs to resume the upright position and develop new patterns of balance and mobility as soon as feasible. This is particularly important for the elderly individual, who may have

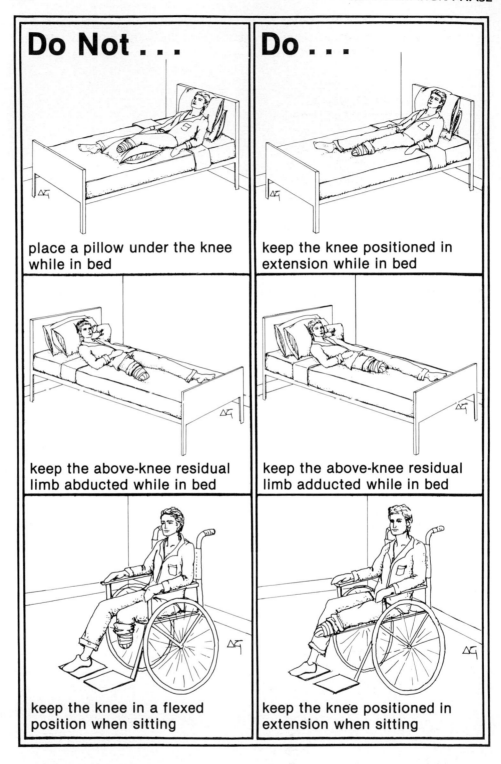

FIGURE 18-4. Correct and incorrect positioning for the below- and above-knee amputee.

more difficulty adapting to a changed body alignment. Bed movements and wheelchair transfers are preliminary to crutch ambulation. Use of the tilt table and standing in the parallel bars may be indicated in some instances.

EMOTIONAL ADJUSTMENT

The loss of a limb, no matter how long anticipated, is a severe emotional blow. The psychological considerations were discussed in some detail in Chapter 17. Members of the clinic team need to be sensitive to the patient's feelings and give the patient time to grieve the loss. Health professionals are frequently pressed for time, and some therapists believe that time spent listening rather than in active treatment is wasted. Actually, listening can be very helpful and supportive. Each person reacts individually to the loss of the limb; the astute health professional recognizes the individual's emotional state and provides a comfortable environment that encourages the person to express feelings of anger, frustration, or denial. While an understanding of the rehabilitation process is important, the patient may not be ready to hear all about the wonders of modern prostheses in the early postoperative period. Such information is better received in small doses as the patient becomes ready to listen.

Most patients benefit from interaction with others who have sustained a similar loss. It may be helpful to have the patient come to the physical therapy department for treatment in order to see other amputees in various stages of rehabilitation. Let the person examine an artificial limb, but guard against giving too much technical information too fast.

Loss of a limb often affects the personhood of the individual. Both men and women may feel that they are no longer valued sexual beings; some elderly individuals may feel that their usefulness is now over and may fear becoming a burden on family members. Other people may believe that the care of the family is due them and will subconsciously be reluctant to achieve a complete level of independence. Awareness and understanding of the person's feelings and a sensitive, caring approach provide support for each individual.

PREPROSTHETIC PROGRAM

EVALUATION

Careful assessment of each individual is an integral part of the management of the amputee. Evaluation data are obtained continuously throughout this period as the incision heals and the person's tolerance improves.

RANGE OF MOTION

Gross range-of-motion estimations are adequate for assessment of the uninvolved extremity, but specific goniometric measurements are necessary for the amputated side. Hip flexion/extension, abduction/adduction measurements are taken early in the postoperative phase of the below-knee amputee. Measurements of knee flexion and extension are taken, if the dressing allows, after some incisional healing has occurred. Hip flexion/extension and abduction/adduction range-of-motion measurements are taken several days after surgery, when the dressing allows, in the above-knee amputee. Measurements of internal and external hip rotation are difficult to obtain and are unnecessary if no gross abnormality or pathology is evident. Joint range of motion is monitored throughout the preprosthetic period.

MUSCLE STRENGTH

Gross manual muscle testing of the upper extremities and uninvolved lower extremity is performed early in the postoperative period. Manual muscle testing of the involved lower extremity must usually wait until most of the healing has occurred. The below-knee amputee needs good strength in the hip extensors and abductors, as well as in the knee extensors and flexors, for satisfactory prosthetic ambulation. The above-knee amputee uses the hip extensors and abductors to a great extent. The strength of these muscles should be monitored throughout the preprosthetic program.

RESIDUAL LIMB

Circumferential measurements of the residual limb are taken as soon as the dressing will allow, then regularly throughout the preprosthetic period. Measurements are made at regular intervals over the length of the residual limb. Circumferential measurements of the below-knee or Syme residual limb are started at the medial tibial plateau and are taken every 5 to 8 cm (2 to 3.2 in), depending on the length of the limb. The length is measured from the medial tibial plateau to the end of the bone. Circumferential measurements of the above-knee or through-knee residual limb are started at the ischial tuberosity or the greater trochanter, whichever is most palpable, and are taken every 8 to 10 cm (3.2 to 4 in). Length is measured from the ischial tuberosity or the greater trochanter to the end of the bone. In all instances, if there is considerable excess tissue distal to the end of the bone, then length measurements are taken to both the end of the bone and the incision line. For accuracy of repeat measurements, exact landmarks are carefully noted. If the ischial tuberosity is used in above-knee measurement, hip joint position is noted as well.

Other information gathered about the residual limb includes the shape (conical, bulbous, redundant tissue), skin condition, incisional condition, location of incision, skin sensation, and joint proprioception.

OTHER DATA

The vascular status of the uninvolved lower extremity is determined; data gathered include condition of the skin, presence of pulses, sensation, temperature, edema, pain on exercise or at rest, presence of wounds, ulceration, or other abnormalities.

Activities of daily living, including transfer and ambulatory status, are evaluated and documented. Information on the patient's home situation, including any constraints or special needs, is valuable in establishing an individually relevant treatment program. Data regarding preoperative activity level and the person's own long-range goals are obtained through interview.

The presence or absence of phantom sensation or pain is noted, as is the person's apparent emotional status and degree of adjustment. Exploration of the patient's suitability and desire for a prosthesis is begun and continues throughout the preprosthetic period. Any other problems that may affect the rehabilitation program and goals are assessed and documented. Table 18-1 illustrates an evaluation guide.

TABLE 18-1. GUIDE FOR PREPROSTHETIC EVALUATION

Skin	1. Scar (location; healed, unhealed; adherent, mobile; invaginated, flat, thickened, keloid; from other surgery or a burn) 2. Open lesions (size, shape, exudate) 3. Moisture (moist, dry, crusting) 4. Sensation (absent, diminished, hypersensitive to touch or pressure) 5. Grafts (location, type, degree of healing) 6. Dermatologic lesions (psoriasis, eczema, acne vulgaris, dermatitis, boils, epidermoid cysts)
Length	(Bone length; soft tissue, redundant tissue length; the length of the below-knee limb is usually measured from the medial tibial plateau, and the above-knee limb from the ischial tuberosity or the greater trochanter)
Shape	(Cylindrical, conical, hourglass, "dog-ears," bulbous, above-knee adductor roll)
Vascularity (Both limbs if cause of amputation is vascular disease)	1. Pulses (femoral, popliteal, dorsalis pedis, posterior tibial) 2. Color (cyanotic, redness) 3. Temperature (cool, warm) 4. Edema (circumference measurements, water displacement measurement, diameter measurement using calipers) 5. Pain (in dependent position, throbbing, claudication) 6. Tropic changes (shininess, dryness, loss of hair)
Range of motion (ROM)	1. Hips (flexion, abduction, or external rotation contracture) 2. Knee (flexion, extension contracture) 3. Ankle (plantarflexion contracture)
Strength	Major muscle groups, adaptation must be made for shortened lever arm
Neurologic	1. Neuroma (location, tenderness) 2. Phantom (sensation; pain; description: throbbing, burning, electrical; duration) 3. Diabetic neuropathy (touch, joint proprioception, nerve conduction velocity, electromyogram) 4. Mental status (alert, senile; intelligent, limited ability to understand)
Activities of Daily Living	1. Transfers (bed to wheelchair, to toilet, to tub, to automobile; independent, dependent) 2. Ambulatory status (with crutches, walker; type of gait; independent, dependent) 3. Home (architectural barriers, safety rails; stairs; other hazards, such as small rugs, unsturdy rails) 4. Self-care (independent, dependent; includes residual limb care)
Psychological	1. Emotional status (depression, denial, cooperativeness, enthusiasm, motivation) 2. Family situation (interest, support, level of understanding, ability to help) 3. Work situation (job opportunity) 4. Prosthetic goals (desire for a prosthesis, anticipated activity level and lifestyle)
Medical Status	1. Cause of amputation (disease, tumor, trauma, congenital) 2. Associated diseases/symptoms (neuropathy, visual disturbances, cardiopulmonary disease, renal disease, congenital anomalies) 3. Medications
Prior prosthesis	(Type, components, problems, gait deviations)

TREATMENT PROGRAM

The goals of the preprosthetic treatment program are to:

1. help the individual regain or maintain functional strength and joint range of motion in all extremities
2. promote healing of the incision and shrinking of the residual limb
3. help the individual regain independence in mobility and self-care
4. determine the individual's physical and emotional suitability for prosthetic replacement
5. help the individual adjust physically and mentally to the loss of a limb
6. maintain the viability of the uninvolved lower extremity.

EXERCISES

The exercise program is individually designed and includes strengthening and coordination activities. The postoperative dressing, degree of postoperative pain, and healing of the incision will determine when resistive exercises for the involved extremity can be started. The postoperative exercise program can take many forms, and a home program is desirable. The hip extensors and abductors and the knee extensors and flexors are particularly important for prosthetic ambulation. A general strengthening program that includes the trunk and all extremities is often indicated, particularly for the elderly person who may have been quite sedentary prior to surgery.

An exercise program that emphasizes coordinated activities between parts of the body and muscle groups is more effective than one that works only individual muscles. Eisert and Tester published a program of dynamic exercises that emphasized coordinated action between the residual limb and the rest of the body. The exercises help the individual adjust to the changed body alignment and balance. Proprioceptive neuromuscular exercise routines are also beneficial in amputee rehabilitation programs.

The younger, more active, traumatic amputee does not usually lose a great deal of muscle strength. Many elderly individuals, however, are relatively sedentary after surgery and need encouragement to develop good strength, coordination, and cardiopulmonary endurance for later ambulation.

Some individuals will present with hip or knee flexion contractures. Mild contractures may respond to manual mobilization and active exercises, but it is almost impossible to reduce moderate to severe contractures by manual stretching, especially hip flexion contractures. There are some who advocate holding the extremity in a stretched position with weights for a considerable length of time. There is little evidence that this traditional approach is successful. Active stretching techniques are more effective than passive stretching; hold-contract and resisted motion of antagonist muscles may increase range of motion, particularly of the knee. One of the more effective ways of reducing a knee flexion contracture is to fit the patient with a patellar-tendon-bearing (PTB) prosthesis aligned in a manner that places the hamstring muscles on stretch with each step. Such prosthetic alignment provides an active stretch that is quite effective. Hip flexion contractures are more frequently found in above-knee amputees. It is difficult to walk out a hip flexion contracture with the above-knee prosthesis. In some instances, depending on the severity of the contracture and the length of the residual limb, the contracture can be accommodated in the alignment of the prosthesis. A hip or knee flexion contracture of less than 15 degrees is not usually a problem. Prevention, however, continues to be the best treatment for contractures.

MOBILITY

Gait training can start early in the postoperative phase. The unilateral lower extremity amputee can become quite independent by using a swing-through gait on crutches. However, many elderly individuals have difficulty learning to walk on crutches; some are afraid, some lack the necessary balance and coordination, and some lack endurance. Some studies have indicated that walking with crutches without a prosthesis requires a greater expenditure of energy than walking with a prosthesis.

Independence in crutch walking is a goal worthy of considerable therapy time. The individual who can ambulate with crutches will develop a greater degree of general fitness than the person who spends most of the time in a wheelchair. Crutch walking is good preparation for prosthetic ambulation, and the person who can learn to use crutches will not have difficulty learning to use a prosthesis. However, the individual who cannot learn to walk independently with crutches may still become a very functional prosthetic user. It may take considerable time for an elderly person to learn to use crutches, but the benefits are worth the efforts. Even if the individual can only use crutches in the sheltered environment of the home, such ambulation should be encouraged.

There are advantages and disadvantages to using a walker for support during the preprosthetic period. Certainly, walking with a walker is physiologically and psychologically more beneficial than sitting in a wheelchair, but it should be used only if the person cannot learn to walk with crutches. A walker is sturdier than crutches but cannot be used on stairs and is difficult to use on curbs. It is sometimes difficult for the person who has used a walker during the preprosthetic period to switch to one crutch or a cane when fitted with a prosthesis, yet the gait pattern used with a walker is not appropriate with a prosthesis.

All amputees need to learn some form of mobility without a prosthesis for use at night or when the prosthesis is not worn for some reason. Some patients, forgetting that they do not have a leg, try to stand up in the middle of the night; they fall and may injure themselves. Teach the patient some method of moving about without a prosthesis, or recommend the use of a bedside commode at night.

TEMPORARY PROSTHESES
(INTERMEDIATE, PROVISIONAL, OR PREPARATORY)

Many amputees are not fitted with any type of prosthetic appliance until the residual limb is free from edema and much of the soft tissue has shrunk, a process that can take many months of conscientious limb wrapping and exercises. During this period, the patient is limited to a wheelchair or to ambulation with crutches or a walker. Most amputees cannot return to work or fully participate in activities of daily living while waiting for the residual limb to mature. Once fitted with a definitive prosthesis, the residual limb continues to change in size; a second prosthesis is often required within the first year. Early fitting with a temporary prosthesis can greatly enhance the postoperative rehabilitation program.

A temporary prosthesis includes a socket that is designed and constructed according to regular prosthetic principles and is attached to some form of pylon, a foot, and some type of suspension strap. A temporary prosthesis can be fitted as soon as the wound has healed.

Advantages:
1. It shrinks the residual limb more effectively than the elastic wrap.

2. It allows early bipedal ambulation.
3. Many elderly people can walk safely with a temporary prosthesis and crutches who otherwise would not be ambulatory during the preprosthetic period.
4. Some individuals can return to work.
5. It provides a means of evaluating the rehabilitation potential of individuals with a questionable prognosis.
6. It is a positively motivating factor because it provides a replacement for the missing part of the body.
7. It reduces the need for a complex exercise program since many people can return to a full, active daily life.
8. It can be used by individuals who may have difficulty paying for a definitive prosthesis.

The temporary socket for the below-knee amputee should be easy to fabricate to allow for prompt replacement as limb volume changes. In the early days, temporary sockets were made of plaster of Paris with a wooden crutch extension and tip for support. The narrow tip did not adequately distribute the forces transmitted from the floor to the end of the residual limb and is now contraindicated, particularly for the dysvascular person. The temporary socket can still be made of plaster of Paris, but a regular prosthetic foot of the proper size should be attached to the end of the socket by a lightweight aluminum pylon, which is readily available from manufacturers of prosthetic components. The foot and pipe can be used with several sockets until the definitive prosthesis is fabricated. In many instances, the foot can also be used with the definitive prosthesis. Many temporary sockets today are made of lightweight thermoplastic materials that can be formed over a positive cast of the residual limb; some are constructed of a fiberglass material that can be formed directly over the residual limb. The prosthesis is usually suspended by a supracondylar cuff to which a waist belt can be added if necessary. The prosthesis is worn with a wool sock of appropriate thickness; when the residual limb has shrunk so that three heavy wool socks are needed to maintain socket fit, a new socket needs to be constructed. The socket can be fabricated by a therapist, prosthetist, or physician, or by any individual who understands the application of prosthetic principles and socket design. Prosthetic components such as feet of various sizes, suspension straps, knee joints, and pylons must be available.

It is easier to fabricate a below-knee socket, but the use of a temporary prosthesis is very important in the rehabilitation of the above-knee amputee. A training leg that has an adjustable canvas socket with a pipe and crutch tip for support is commercially available. Although it allows bipedal activities, this pylon does not fit well enough to aid in shrinking the residual limb, it does not allow for good distribution of weight-bearing forces, and it encourages the development of an awkward, energy-consuming, stiff-legged gait. The temporary prosthesis for an above-knee amputee should incorporate the regular quadrilateral socket, an articulated knee joint, a foot, and a pylon. Suspension may be by Silesian bandage or a pelvic band.

Temporary prostheses are of great value in the rehabilitation of the bilateral below-knee amputee. Temporary prostheses are used to evaluate ambulatory potential and to aid in balance and transfer activities. If the individual was initially fitted as a unilateral amputee, the temporary prosthesis will allow some resumption of ambulation. The ambulatory potential of the bilateral above-knee amputee is uncertain, particularly among the elderly.

Bilateral above-knee amputees can be fitted with shortened prostheses called "stubbies." Stubby prostheses have quadrilateral sockets, no articulated knee joints or shank, and modified rocker bottoms turned backward to prevent the amputee from falling backward. Because the patient's center of gravity is much lower to the ground and the prostheses are nonarticulated, they are relatively easy to use. Stubbies allow the bilateral above-knee amputee to acquire erect balance and to participate in ambulatory activities quickly and with only moderate energy expenditure. Patient acceptance of stubbies, however, is quite variable; some amputees like to use them for activities of daily living in the home but rely on a wheelchair outside of the home. Although prescribed rather rarely, they are most effective for individuals with short residual limbs or for those who would not be able to ambulate with regular prostheses.

Temporary prostheses of different heights can be used to determine the ambulatory potential of the bilateral amputee, but care must be taken to ensure that the temporary limbs are constructed well enough to tolerate the stresses generated by walking. The problems of fitting and training the bilateral amputee are discussed in greater detail in Chapter 19.

The use of a temporary prosthesis is sometimes curtailed because of cost; however, the temporary prosthesis hastens the attainment of rehabilitation goals and shortens the period of disability. It is of great value with the elderly who frequently cannot be ambulatory on the one remaining extremity. A temporary prosthesis increases the longevity of the first definitive limb since a majority of residual limb maturation can be achieved in the temporary socket. A temporary prosthesis is indicated for all amputees who might be considered candidates for permanent prosthetic fitting, which constitute the majority of amputees. The temporary prosthesis is contraindicated only for those individuals whose physical or psychological status precludes ambulation.

RESIDUAL LIMB CARE

Individuals who are not fitted with a rigid dressing or a temporary prosthesis use elastic wrap or shrinkers to reduce the size of the residual limb. Either the patient or a family member applies the bandage, which is worn 24 hours a day, except when bathing.

Recently, a removable rigid dressing for use with below-knee amputees was described. The dressing was more effective in shrinking the residual limb than the elastic wrap. Unfortunately, there are fewer alternatives for the above-knee amputee; rigid dressings and inexpensive temporary prostheses are more difficult to fabricate, and elastic wraps or shrinkers are only minimally effective. It may be advisable to fit the above-knee amputee with a definitive prosthesis early rather than adjusting for shrinkage by using additional socks or a liner.

Many amputees have difficulty controlling edema in the residual limb owing to complications of diabetes, cardiovascular disease, or hypertension. Therapeutically, an intermittent compression unit can be used to reduce edema on a temporary basis. Above- and below-knee sleeves are commercially available.

Proper hygiene and skin care are important. Once the incision is healed and the sutures are removed, the person can bathe normally. The residual limb is treated as any other part of the body; it is kept clean and dry. Individuals with dry skin may use a good skin lotion. Care must be taken to avoid abrasions, cuts, and other skin problems. Friction massage, in which layers of skin, subcutaneous tissue, and muscle are moved over the respective underlying tissue, can be used to prevent or mobilize adherent scar tissue. The massage is done gently, after the wound has healed and when no infection is present. Patients can learn to properly perform a gentle friction massage to mobilize the scar tissue and help decrease hypersensitivity of the residual limb to touch and pressure. Early handling of the residual limb by the patient is an aid to acceptance and is encouraged, particularly for individuals who may be repulsed by the limb.

The amputee is taught to inspect the residual limb with a mirror each night to make sure there are no sores or impending problems, especially in areas that are not readily visible. If the person has diminished sensation, careful inspection is particularly important. Since the residual limb tends to become a bit edematous after bathing as a reaction to the warm water, bathing at night is recommended, particularly once a prosthesis has been fitted. The elastic bandage, shrinker, or removable rigid dressing is reapplied after bathing. If the person has been fitted with a temporary prosthesis, the residual limb is wrapped at night and any time the prosthesis is not worn. Sometimes, individuals who were fitted with a rigid dressing in surgery and were then immediately transferred into a temporary prosthesis do not know how to bandage and encounter difficulties with edema after they remove the prosthesis at night. Learning proper bandaging is part of the therapy program for all amputees because most people need to wrap the limb at one time or another.

Patients have been known to apply a variety of "home and folk remedies" to the residual limb. Historically, it was believed that the skin had to be toughened for prosthetic wear by beating it with a towel-wrapped bottle. Various ointments and lotions have been applied. Residual limbs have been immersed in substances such as vinegar, salt water, and gasoline to harden the skin. While the skin does need to adjust to the pressures of wearing an artificial limb, there is no evidence to indicate that "toughening" techniques are beneficial. Such methods may actually be deleterious, as research indicates that soft, pliable skin is better able to cope with stress than tough, dry skin. Patient education on proper skin care can reduce the use of home remedies.

The skin of the residual limb may be affected by a variety of dermatologic problems, such as eczema, psoriasis, or radiation burns. Some of these conditions may mitigate against fitting or wrapping. Treatment may include ultraviolet irradiation, whirlpool, reflex heating, hyperbaric oxygen, or medication. Care must be taken in using ultraviolet irradiation or heat with the dysvascular amputee. The whirlpool may not be the treatment of choice because it increases circulation and edema in the part being treated. The advantages of the whirlpool as a cleansing agent for skin problems, infected wounds, or delayed healing must be balanced against its disadvantages before its effectiveness can be determined for any individual amputee.

PHANTOM LIMB

The majority of amputees over the age of 6 will encounter a phantom limb. In its simplest form, the phantom is the sensation of the limb that is no longer there. The phantom, which usually occurs initially immediately after surgery, is often described as a tingling, pressure sensation, sometimes a numbness. The distal part of the extremity is most frequently felt, although on occasion, the person will feel the whole extremity. The sensation is responsive to external stimuli such as bandaging or a rigid dressing. It may dissipate over time, or the person may have the sensation throughout life. Phantom sensation is painless and usually does not interfere with prosthetic rehabilitation. It is important that the patient be told early that the phantom is a normal occurrence.

Phantom pain, on the other hand, occurs less frequently and is usually characterized as either a cramping or squeezing sensation, a shooting-type pain, or a burning-like pain. Some patients report all three. The pain may be localized or diffuse; it may be continuous or intermittent and triggered by some external stimuli. It may diminish over time or may become a permanent and often disabling condition. There is little agreement among psychologists about the cause of either phantom sensation or pain, and the literature is replete with studies of the phenomena. While phantom sensation rarely interferes with prosthetic rehabilitation, phantom pain frequently does.

It is important to carefully examine the residual limb to differentiate phantom pain from any other condition such as a neuroma. Sometimes, wearing a prosthesis will ease the phantom pain. Noninvasive treatments such as ultrasound, icing, TENS, or hand massage have been used with varying success. Mild non-narcotic analgesics have been of limited value with some individuals, and no particular narcotic analgesic has proven effective. On occasion, in the presence of trigger points, injection with steroids or a local anesthetic has reduced the pain temporarily. A variety of surgical procedures, such as cordotomy, rhizotomy, and peripheral neurectomy, have been tried with limited success. In some instances, hypnosis has been useful in carefully selected patients. The treatment of phantom pain can be very frustrating for the clinic team and the patient. Treatment is individualized and includes psychotherapy on an ongoing basis.

PATIENT EDUCATION

Patient education is an integral and ongoing part of the rehabilitation program. Information on the care of the residual limb, proper care of the uninvolved extremity, positioning, exercises, and diet if the patient is a diabetic is necessary for the patient to be a full participant in the rehabilitation program.

Many individuals with vascular disease who lose one leg will be concerned about the other leg and thus will be receptive to learning proper care. The care of the unamputated extremity follows the guidelines outlined in Chapter 16. Edema, pain, and changes in skin color or temperature may indicate impending problems. If the person is ambulatory on the remaining extremity, the symptoms may indicate too much stress; if the person spends considerable time sitting with the leg in a dependent position, it may be necessary to elevate the extremity. Cramping during activity is an indication of a need to rest. The endurance of the remaining extremity is developed slowly through a progressive program of exercises and ambulation. It is important to remember that too little activity may be as harmful as too much.

The educational program is individually developed to meet specific needs. Care must be taken not to overwhelm the patient with too much information at one time, as information overload results in noncompliance. It is more effective to prioritize the information and ask the person to remember one new thing each session rather than to try to teach a complex program at one time. The same approach can be used for the home exercise program. Once the patient is discharged, weekly visits throughout the preprosthetic phase provide a check on home activities and on the condition of the residual limb, and are supportive to the patient and family.

BILATERAL AMPUTEES

The preprosthetic program for the bilateral lower extremity amputee is similar to the program developed for the unilateral amputee except, possibly, for ambulation. If the individual was fitted and ambulated as a unilateral amputee, the prosthesis is useful for transfer activities and limited ambulation in parallel bars. Occasionally, the individual may be able to use the prosthesis with external support to get around the house more easily, particularly for bathroom activities. Fitting with a temporary prosthesis, as previously mentioned, is advisable, particularly if the amputations are at below-knee levels. The higher the initial level of amputation, the more difficult ambulation becomes.

All bilateral amputees need a wheelchair on a permanent basis. The chair should be as narrow as possible with removable desk arms and removable leg rests. Amputee wheelchairs with offset rear wheels and no leg rests are not recommended unless the therapist is sure that the person will never be fitted with a prosthesis, even cosmetically. It is easier to add antitipping devices to the rear of the wheelchair or to attach small weights to the front uprights for use when the footrests are removed.

The preprosthetic program includes mat activities that are designed to help the person regain a sense of body position and balance, upper extremity and residual limb strengthening exercises, wheelchair transfers, and regular range-of-motion exercises. Bilateral amputees spend considerable time sitting and are therefore more prone to develop flexion contractures, particularly around the hip joint. The patient should be encouraged to sleep prone if possible, or at least to spend some time in the prone position each day. The therapy program also emphasizes range of motion of the residual limb. Some people move about their homes on their knees, on the ends of the residual limbs, or on their buttocks. Kneepads made of heavy rubber, like those used by field workers, are effective protectors for the residual limbs. Protectors can also be fabricated of foam or felt.

NONPROSTHETIC MANAGEMENT

The preprosthetic period is designed to determine the individual's suitability for prosthetic replacement. Not all amputees are candidates for a prosthesis regardless of personal desire. The cost of the prosthesis and the energy requirements of prosthetic training require that the clinic team use some judgment in selecting individuals for fitting.

There is no general rule that can safely be applied to all lower extremity amputees in making the decision to fit or not to fit. Although the patient is part of the decision-making process, the fact that the individual wants a prosthesis is not enough. Many people are not aware of the physiologic demands of prosthetic ambulation, particularly at above-knee levels. The development of lightweight prostheses, safety knees, and hydraulic mechanisms has made it possible to successfully fit many more individuals than in the past; however, some consideration for nonfitting is necessary.

BELOW-KNEE LEVELS

Most individuals amputated at any below-knee level can be successfully fitted with a prosthesis. Flexion contractures, scars, poorly shaped residual limbs, and adherent skin are not necessarily contraindications for fitting, even though such problems will create difficulty with socket fit. Circulatory problems in the nonamputated extremity, unless so severe as to preclude any ambulation, are indications for fitting at the earliest possible time since bipedal ambulation reduces stress on the remaining extremity. Additionally, the individual who has learned to ambulate as a unilateral amputee is more likely to be able to ambulate as a bilateral amputee. There are few contraindications to fitting a below-knee amputee other than the contraindications to ambulation itself. Individuals who were not ambulatory prior to amputation for reasons other than the problems leading to the amputation will probably not be ambulatory as amputees. However, individuals who were nonambulatory and debilitated because of infection, loss of diabetes control, or ulcers will probably regain the necessary strength and coordination for ambulation after the diseased limb has been removed. Generally, individuals who require nursing or custodial care will not be able to use a prosthesis; often, equipment sent to a nursing home becomes lost, and fitting such individuals may thus be a waste of limited resources.

ABOVE-KNEE LEVELS

The vast majority of unilateral above-knee amputees can become relatively functional prosthetic users with or without external support. The physiologic demands of walking with an above-knee prosthesis are considerably higher than walking with a below-knee prosthesis, and not all individuals have the necessary balance, strength, and energy reserves. Severe hip flexion contractures, weakness or paralysis of hip musculature, or poor balance and coordination may mitigate against successful ambulation. The person's level of activity and participation in the preprosthetic program help in determining the potential for prosthetic ambulation. A temporary prosthesis is a good evaluative tool.

Most individuals amputated at hip levels are younger and learn to use a prosthesis relatively easily. While early fitting is physically and psychologically beneficial, active involvement in chemotherapy or radiation therapy will delay fitting. Radiation therapy often burns the skin, making fitting impossible until the skin has healed. Patients undergoing chemotherapy are often ill, lose weight, and usually do not have the energy to participate in a prosthetic training program. The preprosthetic program is individually adjusted and supportive until the therapy is complete. If the person has lost considerable weight, fitting may have to be delayed because it is difficult to adjust a prosthesis for increases in weight.

BILATERAL AMPUTEES

Fitting or not fitting a bilateral amputee is a difficult decision. Young, agile individuals are generally good candidates for prosthetic fitting. Most bilateral below-knee amputees can become quite functional with prostheses. Most bilateral above-knee amputees have considerable difficulty learning to use two prostheses. Patients with one above-knee and one below-knee amputation generally can learn to use two prostheses if the first amputation was at the above-knee level and if the person successfully used an above-knee prosthesis before losing the other leg.

The bilateral amputee will need more strength, better coordination, better balance, and greater cardiorespiratory reserves than the unilateral amputee. The decision to fit or not to fit is made after careful individualized evaluation of the person's total potential and needs.

TREATMENT PROGRAM

Individuals who are not fitted with a prosthesis need to become as independent as possible in a wheelchair. The therapy program includes transfers and activities of daily living and education in the proper care of the residual limb. Wrapping the residual limb is no longer necessary unless the person is more comfortable with the limb covered. The program emphasizes sitting balance, moving safely in and out of the wheelchair, and other activities to support as independent a lifestyle as the person's physical and psychological conditions allow.

BIBLIOGRAPHY

BEEKMAN, C AND HUNT, AJ: *Change in function and equipment use in lower extremity amputees discharged to nursing homes.* Phys Ther 59:1374–1377, 1979.

BERGER, SM: *Conservative management of phantom-limb and amputation stump pain.* Ann R Coll Surg Engl 62:102–105, 1980.

BURGESS, EM: *Wound healing after amputation: Effect of controlled environment treatment, a preliminary study.* J Bone Joint Surg 60A:245–246, 1978.

BURGESS, EM: *Post operative management.* In *Atlas of Limb Prosthetics.* CV Mosby, St. Louis, 1981, pp 19–23.

BURGESS, EM: *Amputations of the lower extremities.* In NICKEL, VL: *Orthopedic Rehabilitation.* Churchill-Livingstone, New York, 1982, p 377.

BURGESS, EM AND PEDEGANZA, LR: *Controlled environment treatment for limb surgery and trauma.* Bull Prosthet Res Dev 10–28:16–57, 1977.

BURGESS, EM, ROMANO, RL, AND ZETTLE, JH: *The management of lower extremity amputations.* U.S. Government Printing Service, Veterans Administration Report 10-6, New York, 1969.

EISERT, O AND TESTER, OW: *Dynamic exercises for lower extremity amputees.* Arch Phys Med Rehabil 35:695–704, 1954.

GHIULAMILA, RI: *Semirigid dressing for post operative fitting of below knee prosthesis.* Arch Phys Med Rehabil 53:186, 1972.

HABER, WB: *Observation on phantom limb phenomena.* Arch Neurol Psychiat 75:624–636, 1956.

HABER, WB: *Reaction to loss of limb: Physiological and psychological aspects.* Ann NY Acad Sci 74:14–24, 1958.

KAPLOW, M, ET AL: *The dysvascular amputee: Multidisciplinary management.* Can J Surg 26:368–369, 1983.

KAY, HW: *Wound dressings: Soft, rigid or semirigid?* Orth Prosth 25:59–68, 1975.

KAY, HW AND NEWMAN, JD: *Relative incidents of new amputations.* Orth Prosth 29:3–16, 1975.

KEGEL, B: *Controlled environment treatment (CET) for patients with below-knee amputations.* Phys Ther 56:1366–1371, 1976.

KOSTUIK, FP: *Amputation Surgery and Rehabilitation.* Churchill-Livingstone, New York, 1981.

LITTLE, JM: *The use of air splints as immediate prosthesis after below-knee amputation for vascular insufficiency.* Med J Aust 2:870–872, 1970.

LITTLE, JM: *A pneumatic weight bearing prosthesis for below-knee amputees.* Lancet 1:271–273, 1971.

MANELLA, KJ: *Comparing the effectiveness of elastic bandages and shrinker socks for lower extremity amputees.* Phys Ther 61:334–337, 1981.

MAY, BJ: *Stump bandaging of the lower extremity amputee.* Phys Ther 44:808–814, 1964.

MAY, BJ: *A statewide amputee rehabilitation programme.* Prosthet Orthot Int 2:24–26, 1978.

MAY, BJ: *Residual Limb Bandaging,* a videotape. Division of Biomedical Communications, Medical College of Georgia, Augusta, Georgia, 1981.

MELZACK, R AND WALL, PD: *The Challenge of Pain.* Basic Books, New York, 1983.

MUELLER, MJ: *Comparison of removable rigid dressing and elastic bandages in preprosthetic management of patients with below knee amputations.* Phys Ther 62:1438–1441, 1982.

PAGLIARULO, MA, WATERS, R, AND HISLOP, HJ: *Energy cost of walking of below knee amputees having no vascular disease.* Phys Ther 59:538–542, 1979.

REDHEAD, RG AND SNOWDON, C: *A new approach to the management of wounds of the extremities: Controlled Environment Treatment and its derivatives.* Prosthet Orthot Int 2:148–156, 1978.

RIZZO, N: *Physical therapy management of diabetics undergoing lower extremity amputations.* Diabetes Educator 8:24–28, 1983.

SARMIENTO, A, ET AL: *Lower-extremity amputation: The impact of immediate post surgical prosthetic fitting.* Clin Orthop 68:22–31, 1970.

SCHNELL, MD AND BUNCH, WH: *Management of pain in the amputee.* In *Atlas of Limb Prosthetics.* CV Mosby, St Louis, 1981, pp 464–482.

SIMMEL, ML: *On phantom limbs.* Arch Neurol Psychiat 75:637–647, 1956.

TROUP, IM: *Controlled Environment Treatment (CET).* Prosthet Orthot Int 4:15–28, 1980.

WATERS, RL, ET AL: *Energy cost of walking of amputees: The influence of level of amputation.* J Bone Joint Surg 58:42–46, 1976.

WU, Y, ET AL: *An innovative removable rigid dressing technique for below-the-knee amputations.* J Bone Joint Surg 61:724–729, 1979.

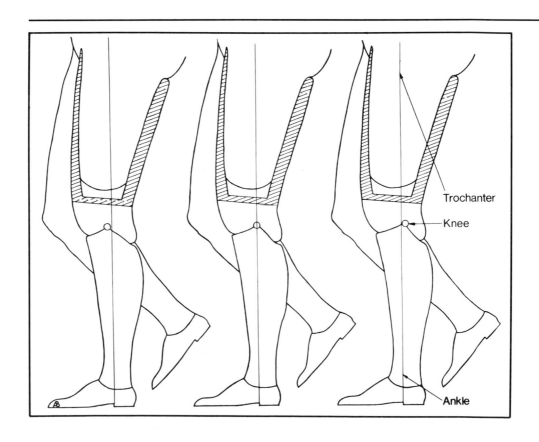

PROSTHETIC PRESCRIPTION

PELVIC BELT
SILESIAN BANDAGE OR BELT
SHOULDER SUSPENDER

KNEE MECHANISMS

CONSIDERATIONS

ALIGNMENT
  VOLUNTARY KNEE CONTROL
  INTERMEDIATE
  KNEE CONTROL
  INVOLUNTARY
  KNEE CONTROL
EXTENSION AIDS
ACTIVITY LEVEL
WEIGHT
ENERGY EXPENDITURE
LIMB CONDITION
COST
COSMETIC APPEARANCE

PRESCRIPTIONS

SHORT RESIDUAL LIMBS
MEDIUM LENGTH
RESIDUAL LIMBS
LONG RESIDUAL LIMBS

UNRESTRICTED KNEE MECHANISMS

MANUAL LOCK

SWING PHASE CONTROL

CONSTANT FRICTION
VARIABLE FRICTION
VARIABLE, CADENCE
RESPONSIVE
  HYDRA-CADENCE UNIT

SWING AND STANCE CONTROL

SWING: CONSTANT
ADJUSTABLE FRICTION;
STANCE: FRICTION
UNDER WEIGHT-BEARING
SWING: VARIABLE FRICTION;
STANCE: FRICTION
UNDER WEIGHT-BEARING
OR POLYCENTRIC
(POSTERIOR DISPLACEMENT
OF CENTER OF ROTATION)
  FRICTION UNDER
  WEIGHT-BEARING
  POLYCENTRIC
SWING: VARIABLE, CADENCE
RESPONSIVE; STANCE:
FLUID CONTROL

BILATERAL AMPUTEES

PROSTHETIC FIT
(MODIFICATIONS
AND ALIGNMENT)
BILATERAL BELOW-KNEE
AMPUTATIONS
BILATERAL ABOVE-KNEE
AMPUTATIONS
  STUBBY PROSTHESES
  STANDARD PROSTHESES
  WITH ARTICULATED KNEES
BILATERAL
HIP-DISARTICULATION
AMPUTATIONS

MODULAR SYSTEMS

ADVANTAGES
DISADVANTAGE

Because no one type of prosthesis serves amputees of a particular level equally well, many things must be considered in prosthetic prescription.

PATIENT FACTORS

Age, vascular supply to the limbs, general health conditions, motivation, intelligence, strength, balance, coordination, ability to set realistic goals, and social and vocational situations are patient variables that influence the end result.

RESIDUAL LIMB FACTORS

The length, shape, skin condition, circulation, range of motion, and maturation of the residual limb influence the type of prosthesis that is prescribed. Invaginated scars and poorly placed thick or adherent incisions can affect the choice of suspension device and socket shape.

PROSTHETIC FACTORS

If the prosthesis is poorly made or improperly aligned, it will not function satisfactorily. Other prosthetic factors that influence the functional result are the degree of socket comfort, cosmetic appearance, durability, and type of suspension or knee unit. Also, prior prosthetic use may influence the type of prosthesis prescribed and, in the case of a bilateral amputee, the success in ambulation.

TREATMENT PROCESS

The expertise of the surgeon, therapists, and other clinical personnel is a significant factor. The methods used for preamputation management, the surgical technique, the postoperative management, as well as instructions in limb hygiene, prosthetic application and removal, and proper gait by experienced therapists, all influence the outcome.

COST

The cost of the prosthetic appliance is usually far outweighed by the costs of hospitalization, medical and surgical services, and therapy. Reducing the number of hospital days is recommended to save money, rather than cutting costs by compromising the desired prosthetic function, durability, or reliability. The proximity of the amputee to the prosthetic and treatment facilities may also affect the type of prosthesis prescribed, as well as the proficiency of its use.

ENERGY EXPENDITURE

Energy expenditure is about the same for the various prostheses when they are properly fitted and aligned. The choice of type then should be based on other factors, such as the gait characteristics that are possible, appearance, cost, weight, and convenience for special activities.

Contraindications for a prosthesis of any type include severe disability, Class IV cardiac function, or severe neurologic disease. The amputee must be able to maintain balance in the erect position. Adequate tolerance for exertion must also be present.

The basic requirements for a prosthesis are that it is comfortable and functional and that the static appearance is cosmetic, as well as its having an acceptable appearance during use. For the lower extremity, comfort, function, and appearance during use are generally more important than cosmetic appearance.

ANKLE/FOOT MECHANISMS

SINGLE-AXIS ANKLE

Indications
1. With soft plantarflexion bumper and stiff dorsiflexion bumper for amputees with short or tender limbs who depend on alignment stability.

   For bilateral and geriatric amputees, since it allows quick foot-flat for knee stability.

2. With stiff plantarflexion bumper for amputees with a long limb and tolerant skin.

Contraindications
1. The active walker or those with skin problems at or near the top of the socket, since it does not allow inversion, eversion, or rotary motion of the foot.

2. When optimum cosmetic appearance is desired, since it is not as cosmetic as some of the other ankle/foot mechanisms.

3. It often is not durable enough for children.

4. Amputees who live in remote areas, since maintenance problems are encountered.

5. Amputees who want to avoid or minimize noise complications.

6. For amputees who wear the patellar-tendon-bearing (PTB) prosthesis.

MULTIPLE-AXIS (FUNCTIONAL) ANKLE

ARTICULATED ASSEMBLIES

Indications
1. The extremely active amputee who participates in sports and other advanced activities.

2. When a suction socket is used, since there is less rotation between the residual limb and the socket.

3. Amputees who have skin problems at or near the top of the socket.

4. Amputees who frequently walk on uneven ground for extensive periods.

Contraindications
1. The amputee who walks very little and on level surfaces only.

2. When optimum cosmetic appearance is desired, since they are not as cosmetic as the nonarticulated assemblies.

3. Amputees who live in remote areas, since maintenance problems are encountered.

4. Amputees who want to avoid or minimize noise complications.

TABLE 19-1. SACH FOOT HEEL STIFFNESS FOR BODY WEIGHT

Type of Amputation	Body Weight (lb)	Recommended Stiffness
Above-knee	>180	Firm
	<180	Medium
Below-knee	>140	Firm
	<140	Medium

NONARTICULATED ASSEMBLIES (SACH FOOT)

Indications

1. Most lower extremity prostheses.

2. Adult amputees with outdoor occupations or avocations, as well as child amputees, since the SACH foot can withstand dampness.

3. Generally, softer heel wedges for above-knee prostheses and firmer wedges for below-knee prostheses. The heel is usually one grade softer for above-knee amputees than for below-knee amputees of the same weight (Table 19-1).

4. Amputees who want to wear high-heeled shoes.

5. Amputees who live in remote areas, since it is relatively maintenance-free.

6. When a lightweight ankle/foot mechanism is desired.

7. When a cosmetic appearance is desired.

Contraindications

1. Soft heels for the high bilateral amputee.

2. Bilateral amputees who frequently walk up inclines, or unilateral amputees who require more dorsiflexion and plantarflexion motion.

ROTATORS

Indications

1. Amputees who are very active or who participate in sports.

2. Amputees who have skin ulcerations from residual limb/socket interface rotation.

Contraindications

1. Amputees with poor stability.

2. Amputees who live in remote areas, since maintenance problems are encountered.

3. When the added weight would compromise function.

HISTORIC BELOW-KNEE PROSTHESIS

Indications

1. None.

   When the skin on the critical areas of the residual limb is inadequate (e.g., burn scars) for weight-bearing in the usual areas with the PTB prosthesis, a modified PTB prosthesis is used.

Contraindications

1. When sensation is intact.

2. When mediolateral stability is present at the knee.

3. When the skin on the critical areas of the residual limb will tolerate weight-bearing.

4. When a normally appearing gait is desired.

5. When a more cosmetic appearance is desired.

6. When the additional weight would compromise function.

7. In hot, humid climates where the corset would present hygienic problems.

8. Amputees who want to avoid or minimize noise complications.

PTB PROSTHESIS

Indications

1. Any below-knee amputee who is a candidate for prosthetic fitting who does not have any of the contraindications.

2. The juvenile amputee. (The PTB prosthesis does not seem to adversely affect the epiphysis.)

3. Slightly limited or normal knee range of motion.

Contraindications

1. When there is inadequate leverage (the limb is too short) to control the prosthesis. Usually at least 5 cm (2 in) of tibia below the tibial tubercle are needed.

2. Paralysis of the remaining limb musculature or severe weakness. (Generalized weakness is not a contraindication. Prosthetic use will strengthen the weak musculature.)

3. If there is an irreversible knee flexion contracture greater than 35 to 40 degrees.

SOCKETS

HARD (UNLINED)

Indication

1. For most below-knee amputees.

Contraindications

1. Extremely sensitive limbs.

2. Severe skin problems, such as skin grafts.

3. An anesthetic residual limb.

SOFT (LINED)

Indications
1. Extremely sensitive limbs.

2. Severe skin problems, such as skin grafts in critical areas.

3. An anesthetic residual limb.

Contraindication
1. If a hard socket can be worn.

SUSPENSION

CUFF

Indications
1. Mediolateral stability at the knee.

2. The femur and knee can be loaded.

3. Amputees with vascular insufficiency.

4. The residual limb must have adequate length to remain in the socket during knee flexion.

5. No excessive tenderness in the areas of contact.

Contraindications
1. Extreme mediolateral instability at the knee.

2. If the limb cannot be loaded because of femoral osteoporosis or fracture.

3. For vascular insufficiency, only if improperly constructed, giving constriction proximally.

4. It may be inadequate for short residual limbs, which are forced out of the socket during flexion.

5. Should be prescribed cautiously for heavy individuals.

6. Excessive tenderness in the areas of contact.

7. Excessively arthritic knee or other serious knee pathology.

SUPRACONDYLAR/SUPRAPATELLAR

Indications
1. For short limbs, especially when the anatomic knee is unstable.

2. When the difference between the diameter of the leg at the widest point of the knee and just above the adductor tubercle is 2.5 cm (1 in) or less.

Contraindications
1. Limbs with very heavy subcutaneous tissue.

2. A significant knee extension contracture that limits adequate active flexion to apply the prosthesis.

3. Amputees who need rotary stability at the knee.

3. If an excessive irreversible knee flexion contracture exists.

4. For bilateral below-knee amputees, since the high brim augments support and they usually maintain slight knee flexion, anyway.

4. A prominent rectus femoris tendon.

5. If full knee extension is desired.

6. A very long residual limb.

SUPRACONDYLAR MEDIAL WEDGE

Indications

1. An amputee who could not comfortably wear a supracondylar/suprapatellar brim because of a prominent rectus femoris tendon.

2. A former prosthetic wearer who desires complete, unrestricted knee extension.

3. When some mediolateral stability is needed at the knee.

Contraindications

1. For extremely short or obese residual limbs.

2. If hand dexterity is inadequate to remove and apply the wedge, unless it can be applied if attached to a soft insert.

SUPRACONDYLAR MEDIAL WEDGE WITH DETACHABLE MEDIAL BRIM

Indications

1. In cases when the supracondylar circumference is smaller than the circumference at the patellar tendon.

2. When some mediolateral stability is needed at the knee.

Contraindications

1. If a supracondylar medial wedge or supracondylar/suprapatellar suspension device can be used.

2. If hand strength and dexterity are inadequate to remove and reapply the detachable medial brim.

INVERTED Y STRAP TO A WAIST BELT

Indications

1. With a temporary PTB prosthesis for readily adjustable suspension during the period of rapid change in residual limb shape.

2. With a definitive prosthesis in cases of mental confusion when the amputee has difficulty with other forms of suspension.

Contraindication

1. When another form of suspension can be successfully used.

THIGH-LACER AND METAL SIDE JOINTS

Indications

1. Extreme mediolateral instability at the knee.

Contraindications

1. New amputee, if other factors warrant supracondylar or cuff suspension.

2. Amputee preference. If the amputee has worn the corset type successfully for years.

3. A heavy manual laborer, or for work that requires frequent bending and lifting of the prosthesis, such as driving a tractor or truck, at least for the work situation.

4. For a very short residual limb that cannot be suspended by a PTS.

5. For residual limbs that break down intermittently, if a PTB prosthesis with a special insert or socket is impractical because of lack of expertise on the part of the prosthetist, or if the amputee lives very far from the prosthetic shop.

6. Excessive tenderness in the weight-bearing areas.

7. Lack of sensation in the residual limb.

8. Excessively arthritic knee.

2. When the amputee's occupation does not require prosthetic use under heavy-duty conditions.

3. When the amputee, especially the bilateral amputee, does not need stabilization against rotation.

4. Limbs longer than 7.6 cm (3 in) can usually be fitted without a thigh-lacer.

5. If a PTB prosthesis with another suspension mechanism can be worn.

6. No palpable tenderness in the weight-bearing areas.

7. Normal sensation in the residual limb.

8. No knee pathology.

BENT-KNEE PROSTHESIS

Indications

1. Amputees with an irreducible knee flexion contracture in whom surgical revision is contraindicated.

2. In areas without modern prosthetic resources.

3. Extremely short residual limbs.

Contraindication

1. Amputees with a reducible knee flexion contracture (by exercise or surgery).

ABOVE-KNEE PROSTHESIS

If the above-knee amputee has a considerable hip flexion contracture (30 degrees or more), it may not be possible to fit a prosthesis at all. The amount of hip flexion that can be accommodated in the prosthesis is greater the more proximal the amputation. In cases of existing hip flexion contractures before surgery, the surgeon may choose to amputate the limb more proximal than the pathology would suggest to make limb fitting a possibility. If the hip flexion contracture cannot be accommodated for by setting the limb in initial flexion within the socket, then there will be a strain on the lumbar spine if the amputee tries to stand erect. Disabling back pain will result, which is likely to be intolerable to the amputee, and the prosthesis will be discarded.

In general, if there are no contraindications, the order of choice for an above-knee prosthesis is as follows:

1. total-contact quadrilateral suction socket
2. total-contact socket with auxiliary suspension
3. open-ended quadrilateral suction socket
4. open-ended socket with auxiliary suspension.

SOCKETS

QUADRILATERAL, TOTAL CONTACT

Indications

1. The optimum socket for most above-knee amputees.

2. It is necessary for the more sophisticated knee mechanisms such as the Henschke-Mauch S-N-S, which requires fine limb control.

Contraindications

1. Possibly an elderly amputee with a flabby limb with little strength.

2. Possibly a limb with painful neuromas, especially those caught in scars.

3. Draining osteomyelitis.

HARD

Indication

1. Soft, bulky residual limb where the femur can move with minimal resistance.

Contraindication

1. A firm residual limb.

SOFT END

Indications

1. A firm residual limb where there may be painful impingement of tissue between the femur and the socket.

2. When total contact during swing phase as well as stance phase is desired.

Contraindication

1. Soft, bulky residual limb where the femur can move with minimal resistance.

QUADRILATERAL, OPEN-ENDED

Indications

1. When there are painful bone spurs on the distal aspect of the residual limb.

2. When there is a problem with extreme perspiration.

Contraindications

1. If the limb will tolerate total contact.

2. If the problem of extreme perspiration can be solved by any other means.

SUSPENSION DEVICES

SUCTION ALONE

Indications

1. Residual limb long enough to maintain suction.

2. Stable body weight.

3. A pendulous abdomen owing to obesity or pregnancy.

4. Residual limb free from most skin disorders. Pressure boils (suppurative hidradenitis or folliculitis) usually disappear if they already exist secondary to an adductor roll.

5. Deep scar over end of limb or painful scars about the ilium. Deep scars over the distal end may smooth out and become more pliable with prosthetic use.

6. Willing to devote the time needed for adequate fitting and training.

7. Agility and strong limb muscles.

8. Adequate use of the upper extremities to don the prosthesis.

9. Cylindrical residual limb.

10. Well-shaped residual limb without excessive redundant tissue.

11. If a sophisticated knee mechanism is being used, since it will allow optimum functional control.

Contraindications

1. A residual limb of less than 7.6 cm (3 in), usually. It may be tried in cases of pregnancy when a conventional pelvic belt cannot be worn.

2. Rapid volumetric fluctuations of the residual limb.

3. Excessive subcutaneous fat of the residual limb.

4. Certain skin disorders, such as chronic dermatitis, fungus infection, eczematous rash of the residual limb, until they have cleared.

5. Deep linear scar near the socket brim which interferes with suction.

6. Psychological or emotional difficulties (impatient, discouraged, uncooperative, irresponsible).

7. Amputees who are debilitated and feeble, with weak muscles, poor coordination, and poor balance. Geriatric amputees may have difficulty donning a suction socket.

8. Amputee lives far from the prosthetic shop or for other reasons cannot be seen by prosthetist for frequent adjustments during the first few months.

9. Amputee who also has bilateral upper extremity amputations or other severe impairment of the upper extremities, since the hands are needed to don the prosthesis.

10. Conical or pointed residual limb.

11. Long, redundant, flabby mass of soft tissue beyond the end of the bone.

12. Open ulcers, draining sinuses, and osteomyelitis of the residual limb.

13. A large bony spur on the distal-lateral aspect of the bone with pain upon pressure (socket relief may not be enough).

14. In some cases of bilateral lower extremity amputation, especially if donning is a problem.

SUCTION WITH AUXILIARY SUSPENSION

Indications

1. If there is a tendency for the prosthesis to rotate, a Silesian bandage may be used.

2. If there is a tendency for the prosthesis to abduct, a pelvic belt may be used.

3. As a psychological aid for amputees who feel insecure without a belt around the waist. (Auxiliary suspension may not be needed after a transition period.)

Contraindications

1. If the prosthesis does not rotate with suction alone.

2. If the prosthesis does not abduct inadvertently with suction alone.

3. If the amputee feels secure with suction alone.

PELVIC BELT

Indications

1. Usually, short residual limb of less than 7.6 cm (3 in).

2. When mediolateral stability is needed. When the residual limb is weak or short.

3. If the amputee lives a long distance from the prosthetic center. (Suction sockets require frequent initial adjustments.)

4. No skin disorders around the hips at points of contact.

5. If the amputee is timid, feeble, or poorly coordinated, or does not have the strength to don a suction socket.

6. When additional shrinkage of the residual limb is anticipated.

7. If scars or an extremely tapered limb prohibit suction suspension.

Contraindications

1. Pregnancy, even with a short residual limb or an excessively obese amputee.

2. When there is good strength and motion about the hip.

3. Skin disorders, such as scars, warts, or moles, located at points of contact of the pelvic belt.

4. If the amputee has the strength and coordination to don a suction socket.

5. If limb size has stabilized sufficiently for the use of a suction socket.

6. If the shape of the limb and absence of scars permit the use of a suction socket.

7. If the amputee can tolerate skin contact with the socket wall and thus can use suction suspension.

8. If amputee becomes seriously dizzy when stooping, which is necessary for donning a suction socket.

9. Amputees who are allergic to socket finishes.

SILESIAN BANDAGE OR BELT

Indications

1. To control rotation or limit lateral displacement in the short or flabby residual limb.

2. In cases of weak musculature, may help by assisting adductor muscles in the swing phase, abductor muscles in the stance phase, and hip flexion at toe-off.

3. For amputees who feel insecure with suction alone and need the psychological security of a belt around the waist.

4. For amputees with short residual limbs who have difficulty with the socket coming off when they sit.

5. For amputees who work on roofs or scaffolds, where it would be dangerous if the prosthesis came off.

6. If a medial or lateral whip is present, a Silesian bandage may be added. If the bandage eliminates the whip, the flabby or weak residual limb is probably the cause and the Silesian bandage should be retained. If the whip is not corrected, then a prosthetic problem exists and alignment should be adjusted.

Contraindications

1. Mediolateral instability.

2. When musculature has good strength.

3. When the residual limb is not short.

SHOULDER SUSPENDER

Indications

1. Scarring on the area covered by a pelvic belt or Silesian bandage.

2. Excessive pistoning when using other methods of suspension.

Contraindications

1. If the skin around the pelvis is adequate or a suction socket can be worn.

2. If adequate suspension can be obtained from another method of suspension.

KNEE MECHANISMS

To function effectively, the knee mechanism depends on proper alignment of the prosthesis, a well-fitted socket, and a properly selected and fitted ankle/foot mechanism.

CONSIDERATIONS

ALIGNMENT

The most appropriate knee mechanism for any amputee is one that requires the least amount of alignment stability yet offers adequate security. The effort required to initiate swing phase is increased as more alignment stability is built into a prosthesis, thus affecting gait. The amount of alignment stability needed is inversely related to the length and strength of the residual limb. The amount of alignment stability needed is also determined by the type of knee mechanism used.

VOLUNTARY KNEE CONTROL

When the body weight is transmitted through a line posterior to the knee bolt, this is referred to as voluntary knee control. The knee bolt is usually aligned anterior to the trochanter-ankle (TA) vertical reference line (Fig. 19-1, *left*) for the long residual limb.

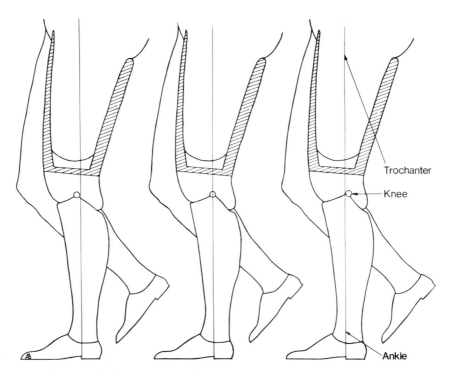

Trochanter

Knee

Ankle

FIGURE 19-1. Variations in the alignment of the knee bolt. *(Left)* Anterior to the TA line (voluntary knee control). *(Middle)* On the TA line (intermediate knee control). *(Right)* Posterior to the TA line (involuntary knee control).

Initial flexion in the socket is limited by the length of the limb. The shank and foot are inset. This alignment is for the active walker who has good use of the hip abductors and extensors and for special stance control units such as the Henschke-Mauch S-N-S, to take advantage of the high resistance to knee flexion and to facilitate the initiation of swing phase. Voluntary control of the knee with a minimum amount of alignment stability offers the smoothest and most effortless gait.

INTERMEDIATE KNEE CONTROL

For a residual limb of medium functional length, a vertical line passing through the knee bolt should pass through the center of the ankle bolt and fall just anterior to the heel of the shoe (Fig. 19-1, *center*; Fig. 19-2). The center of the heel is directly under the point of contact of the ischium.

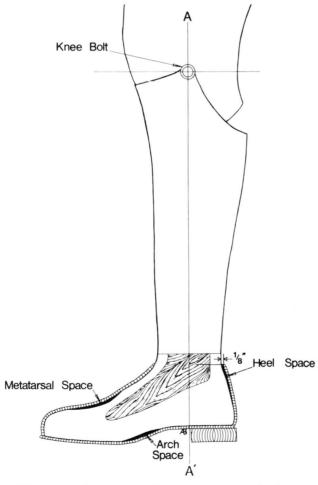

FIGURE 19-2. Alignment for intermediate knee control of an above-knee prosthesis. Metatarsal, arch, and heel spaces between the prosthetic foot and shoe are indicated.

INVOLUNTARY KNEE CONTROL

The knee bolt is usually placed posterior to the TA line for short residual limbs (Fig. 19-1, *right*). The amputee with short functional length has limited use of the hip abductors and extensors (which results in a slow, hesitant gait) and thus needs considerable alignment stability. The socket is slightly abducted, and the foot is somewhat outset. This is the usual alignment for the single-axis mechanical friction knee unit. If painful scars, neuromas, or skin problems exist on the posterior aspect of the limb, it may be difficult for the amputee to extend the hip with sufficient force to stabilize the knee. Increased alignment stability will lessen the hip extension force required for knee stability. Alignment of the knee bolt posterior to the TA line requires an excessive amount of energy to get the knee to break at toe-off and results in an unnatural gait. This excessive alignment stability should be avoided if possible.

EXTENSION AIDS

Internal extension aids may be adjustable, but they do not provide high forces in extension. These are indicated for amputees with medium or long residual limbs, amputees who do not work in confined areas, and when a cosmetic appearance is desired (external straps are not desirable).

External extension aids, although they are uncosmetic, nondurable, and may interfere with clothing, are indicated where high extension forces are needed (e.g., in cases of short residual limbs and for those whose activity pattern requires them to take short steps for lengthy periods).

ACTIVITY LEVEL

The active wearers usually need a sophisticated swing phase control. The more sedentary amputees who wear the prosthesis only for activities of daily living do not require a high degree of swing control. Stance phase control may be used by both active and sedentary amputees.

WEIGHT

Although hydraulic prostheses are usually heavier than other prostheses, they are not usually perceived as being heavier by the amputee. Most amputees feel that less effort is required to use a hydraulic limb and that it is less fatiguing. Although the hydraulic prosthesis may have more gross weight than another prosthesis, the center of the mass may be closer to the knee and thus require less force to move the mass. The additional weight of a hydraulic prosthesis should not be a contraindication for its use.

ENERGY EXPENDITURE

The amount of energy required to use various knee units depends on the resistance to be overcome rather than on whether it is a fluid or mechanical (sliding) friction unit. The idea that fluid units require more energy is probably based on the fact that fluid units can potentially operate at higher resistance settings than most sliding friction units. The choice of a knee unit, therefore, should be based on factors other than the amount of energy expenditure.

LIMB CONDITION

If the residual limb has painful scars, neuromas, or other skin problems on the posterior aspect, then it may be difficult for the amputee to extend the limb with sufficient force to stabilize the knee. Increased alignment stability may be necessary to reduce the amount of hip extension force needed. A stance control knee mechanism and a foot with minimal resistance to plantarflexion would address the problem even better.

COST

If function is compromised for cost, then the amputee may end up with a prosthesis that is eventually discarded. Costs should be compared only if two or more knee units of equal function are being considered.

COSMETIC APPEARANCE

Soft, resilient foam, which reduces weight and noise and has a more normal texture and shape, is used to cover the entire limb when the best cosmetic appearance is desired.

PRESCRIPTIONS

SHORT RESIDUAL LIMBS

Best: Constant or variable friction swing control with stance control.

Next best: A swing control only unit. Since this type of knee mechanism does not offer stance control, it can be used with an amputee with a short residual limb only if alignment stability is adequate. Increased alignment stability reduces the effort required by the amputee to stabilize the knee during early stance phase, but the initiation of swing phase becomes more difficult.

MEDIUM LENGTH RESIDUAL LIMBS

Either variable or variable, cadence responsive swing control knee mechanisms with stance control can be used with minimal alignment stability. Knee units with only variable or variable, cadence responsive swing control would require greater alignment stability. If there are no complications, constant friction knee mechanisms are not indicated, but rather those with more sophisticated swing controls.

LONG RESIDUAL LIMBS

Because patients with long residual limbs have greater muscular strength and are thus able to generate more force to stabilize the knee during stance phase, it would seem that they would have the least need for knee mechanisms offering stance phase control. However, they will still need stance phase control if they are engaged in activities such as walking on uneven terrains, climbing stairs, and walking on inclines. They also need sophisticated swing phase control because they are vigorous walkers. The choice would be variable or variable, cadence responsive swing control units with stance control, which would offer stance control when walking on uneven surfaces, minimal alignment stability, and versatile swing phase control.

UNRESTRICTED KNEE MECHANISMS

Indication
1. Amputees who walk very little and will usually use a manual lock when standing.

Contraindication
1. Amputees who desire a more normal gait appearance.

MANUAL LOCK

Indication
1. Amputees who require complete knee stability during walking because of special problems such as blindness, very short residual limbs, bilateral amputation, or being elderly or enfeebled.

Contraindication
1. If the amputee can achieve knee stability during walking by any other means.

SWING PHASE CONTROL

CONSTANT FRICTION

Indications
1. If cost is a primary factor, this type is relatively low in cost.

2. If the amputee lives far from the prosthetic shop, because it requires relatively little maintenance.

3. The bilateral amputee may prefer this type because of the sensory cue provided by the terminal-impact at full extension.

4. If the amputee has a heavy-duty occupation and is in need of low-maintenance components.

Contraindications
1. A very active walker who needs a knee that will respond to changes in walking speed.

2. Weak or short residual limbs or the elderly. (Without a locking mechanism, stability may be inadequate, stance control is poor.)

3. Very long above-knee or knee disarticulation amputations, because the prosthetic knee would be lower than the sound knee.

VARIABLE FRICTION

Indication
1. When a more natural gait is desired than that provided by the simple constant friction unit.

Contraindication
1. Usually not advised for the bilateral amputee.

VARIABLE, CADENCE RESPONSIVE

Indications
1. Active, vigorous amputees and those with long residual limbs, since these

Contraindications
1. Very long above-knee limbs or knee disarticulation amputations if the

units can operate at higher resistance settings than most mechanical friction units.

2. Amputees who desire a normal-looking gait at a wide variety of walking speeds.

3. Amputees who are located reasonably close to prosthetic and training facilities, since more sophisticated knee mechanisms usually require more maintenance.

4. Amputees who can maintain knee stability through muscular control.

5. If the prosthetist is qualified to install the mechanism and the therapist has the expertise to train the amputee.

prosthetic knee would be lower than the sound knee.

2. Short adults or children, because the shank would be too long and thus the knee center too high.

3. Amputees who have used mechanical friction knee mechanisms for a long period of time.

4. If the amputee has a heavy-duty occupation, at least for the work situation.

HYDRA-CADENCE UNIT

Indications

1. If the amputee will be sitting a great deal or traveling by public conveyance, since it offers dorsiflexion at the ankle and thus a more functional sitting posture.

2. Amputees who have jobs that require walking with short, rapid steps about a bench (need knee mechanism with substantial knee extension bias).

Contraindications

1. If the amputee has to wear boots (farmers, fishermen, or surveyors) or other restrictive footwear, since it would interfere with ankle action.

2. A very long above-knee limb or knee disarticulation amputation. This unit requires at least $3^2/5$ cm ($1^3/8$ in) above the knee center (Fig. 19-3) to the top of the plate. Additional space is needed between the plate and the bottom of the limb (distance C), depending upon the type of socket. A hard total-contact socket permits fitting of a longer limb than a soft-end total-contact or an open-ended socket.

SWING AND STANCE CONTROL

SWING: CONSTANT ADJUSTABLE FRICTION; STANCE: FRICTION UNDER WEIGHT-BEARING

Indications

1. Amputees who do not need to descend inclines frequently.

2. Amputees who require extensive

Contraindications

1. If the amputee needs to descend inclines frequently.

2. Amputees with average or better

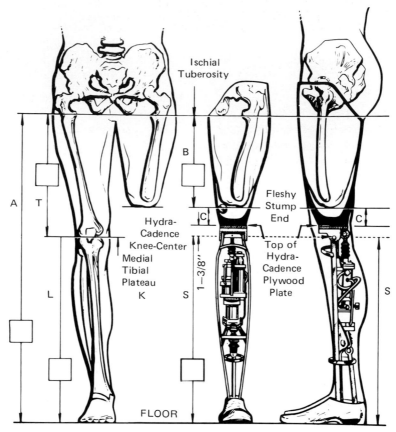

FIGURE 19-3. The Hydra-Cadence unit offers hydraulic resistance in swing phase at the knee, automatic ankle dorsiflexion at and beyond 20 degrees of knee flexion, and hydraulic resistance to plantarflexion. (From *Hydra-Cadence Guidebook.* Hydra-Cadence, Glendale, California, 1961, with permission.)

knee stability, such as the weak or elderly amputee, or a short residual limb.

3. Amputees with a long leg brace (KAFO) on the opposite side, since the concern is for knee stability rather than aesthetic swing characteristics.

4. If the amputee has a heavy-duty occupation and is in need of low-maintenance components.

musculature, coordination, or activity level.

SWING: VARIABLE FRICTION; STANCE: FRICTION
UNDER WEIGHT-BEARING OR POLYCENTRIC
(POSTERIOR DISPLACEMENT OF CENTER OF ROTATION)

FRICTION UNDER WEIGHT-BEARING

Indications

1. Amputees who do not need to descend inclines frequently.

2. Amputees who need extensive knee stability but also a more normal gait than that with a constant friction unit (especially for those on their feet a great deal).

3. Amputees with a KAFO on the opposite side, since the concern is for knee stability rather than sophisticated swing control.

Contraindications

1. If the amputee needs to descend inclines frequently.

2. Amputees with average or better musculature or coordination.

POLYCENTRIC

Indications

1. Extremely short above-knee limb.

2. Bilateral above-knee amputee.

3. Gives more auditory and proprioceptive feedback than most other units to the blind amputee while providing good knee stability.

4. The OHC four-bar-linkage for knee disarticulation or transcondylar residual limbs.

5. The OHC four-bar-linkage for bent-knee prosthesis.

Contraindication

1. If complete knee stability is needed.

SWING: VARIABLE, CADENCE RESPONSIVE; STANCE: FLUID CONTROL

Indications

1. Multiple amputations.

2. Amputees who are located reasonably close to prosthetic and training facilities, since more sophisticated knee mechanisms usually require more maintenance.

3. If the prosthetist is qualified to install

Contraindications

1. Very long above-knee limbs or knee disarticulation amputations, because the prosthetic knee would be longer than the sound knee.

2. Short adults or children, because the shank would be too long and thus the knee center too high.

the mechanism and the therapist has the expertise to train the amputee.

4. If the amputee will be walking over rough ground frequently, since it offers better knee control and toe clearance than other mechanisms.

3. If the amputee has a heavy-duty occupation, at least for the work situation.

BILATERAL AMPUTEES

PROSTHETIC FIT (MODIFICATIONS AND ALIGNMENT)

Although a precise and comfortable prosthetic fit is important for all amputees, it is particularly important for the bilateral amputee. Since a sound lower limb is not available, full weight must be borne on the prostheses at all times during standing. This will make the amputee more susceptible to excessive pressures and friction and the resulting skin problems during prosthetic wear. Immediate postoperative fitting is usually contraindicated for bilateral amputees since they cannot control the amount of weight on the residual limb. Weight-bearing does not begin until there is satisfactory wound healing—usually, 2 to 3 weeks after amputation. However, a rigid plaster dressing is indicated. Modifications of the standard prosthetic design are sometimes required for better comfort and stability. The feet are outset for a more stable walking base.

BILATERAL BELOW-KNEE AMPUTATIONS

The bilateral below-knee amputee is usually fitted prosthetically to restore full preamputation height. If the patient is in poor general condition or has poor balance, the decision may be made to shorten the over-all height. Stability is also enhanced by firm-heeled SACH feet, single-axis feet, or a thigh-lacer with sidebars.

BILATERAL ABOVE-KNEE AMPUTATIONS

Because they permit better sitting stability, thigh amputations are preferred over hip disarticulations.

STUBBY PROSTHESES

Stubby prostheses are generally prescribed only for patients with short bilateral above-knee amputations or bilateral hip disarticulations. They are occasionally used for above-knee/below-knee amputations and for long bilateral above-knee amputations.

Women usually find stubbies to be cosmetically unacceptable because of the extreme reduction in height. Ambulation in stubbies obligates exaggerated trunk rotation. Short canes or crutches are usually needed. The use of chairs and stair climbing are very difficult because of the shortness of the prostheses. Also, the limbs protrude markedly from the chair while the amputee is sitting, because of the lack of knee joints. Many elderly amputees prefer to remain in a wheelchair with or without cosmetic limbs while in the home and utilize cosmetic limbs when out of the home. Nevertheless, most elderly bilateral above-knee amputees should be provided with stubbies initially so that they can attempt early independence.

If the elderly bilateral above-knee amputee becomes proficient in walking with stubbies, then the question of whether to have full-length prostheses will be raised. Although the elderly amputee may be very stable when walking with stubbies, the lack of height will likely be a source of embarrassment. Factors to be weighed in the consideration of longer legs are the increased demand on the cardiovascular system and the decrease in balance and stability by virtue of raising the center of gravity. If good balance, endurance, and motivation are present, then standard limbs may be prescribed.

STANDARD PROSTHESES WITH ARTICULATED KNEES

Because there is no intact limb for balancing, the bilateral above-knee amputee requires a broader base for lateral stability; therefore, the feet are outset slightly more than usual. The center of gravity may be placed forward (shortened toe lever arm) to assist push-off (toe-off) and to add stability at the knee. Young amputees may be fitted with two single-axis, constant, sliding friction knee units with extension aids, two polycentric knee units, or a combination of one single-axis unit and one knee with a mechanical lock. Older amputees are usually fitted with two S-N-S units, two "safety" knee units, or one "safety" knee unit combined with an S-N-S unit, a single-axis constant friction unit, or a manual locking unit.

Slightly stiffer bumpers prevent backward tipping during standing and aid push-off in walking. The overall height may be lowered for better balance and coordination. Extension assists at the knees increase stability. Total-contact quadrilateral sockets are usually used.

Suction is often used for socket suspension, but it is generally augmented by Silesian bandages. Sometimes, pelvic band suspension is used in addition to or in place of suction suspension. Standard length above-knee prostheses increase the workload on the cardiovascular system and the hazard of falling when compared with stubby prostheses. Their main value to the bilateral amputee, especially the elderly amputee, is appearance.

BILATERAL HIP-DISARTICULATION AMPUTATIONS

A molded jacket or bucket socket will be necessary for the amputee to assume the erect position. In the case of amputation secondary to the skin complications of paraplegia, the amputee has the additional problems of distal sensory deficit and urogenital appliances. End weight-bearing thus needs to be avoided. An open-ended jacket that distributes weight over the chest wall, similar to that used for the hemicorporectomy amputee, may be necessary. The jacket is divided into two portions that are fastened with buckles or Velcro. The design should be such that the amputee can don and remove the jacket independently. Normal respiratory functions should not be compromised unduly by the prosthesis. Weight can be borne on the distal end of the socket if thick rubber reinforcement is applied externally to act as a shock absorber. Short hand crutches are used for a swing-through gait.

If the prosthesis is to have legs for ambulation, the molded socket of the Canadian-type prosthesis may need to be extended above the iliac crests to just below the lower costal margin. This design allows the amputee to use the trunk muscles to rotate or swivel to advance each leg individually. The amputee is thus able to use a four-point gait rather than a swing-through gait.

The amputee's total overall height with the prostheses is usually shortened to facilitate rising from a sitting position, standing balance, and walking. The hip joints may need a 90-degree anterior stop for stability during prolonged sitting; otherwise, the amputee may fall forward.

MODULAR SYSTEMS

Although interest in temporary limbs was revived and encouraged in the early 1960s (due in part to the relatively quick fabrication of plastic-laminate sockets), it was not until the introduction of immediate postoperative fittings that full impetus was given to the modular concept of quick-assembly, adjustable, interchangeable parts.

In recent years, tubular structures are being utilized in definitive prostheses (Fig. 19-4). In the definitive structure, a soft foam form (Prosmetic soft cover) is applied over

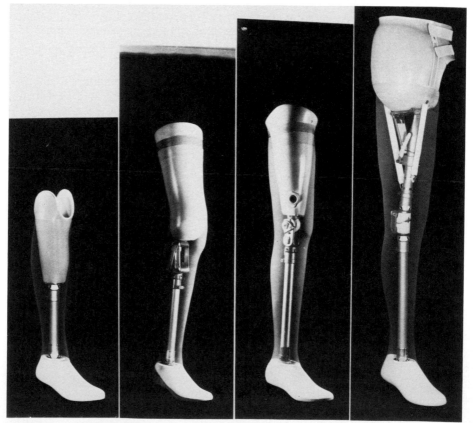

FIGURE 19-4. Modular prostheses with foam covers for (from left to right) below-knee, knee–disarticulation, above-knee, and hip-disarticulation amputees. (From *Otto Bock Modular Prostheses.* Otto Bock Orthopedic Industry, Minneapolis, with permission.)

the pylon and is sculpted to the shape of the sound leg. A stretch hose is used to cover the foam.

The endoskeletal concept is being merged with a modular concept in which components of standardized design and dimensions are readily interchangeable and adjustable. Through this system, various combinations of different components can be tried to find the optimum combination for a given patient.

The endoskeletal modular system offers simpler and faster maintenance. It also permits more frequent and easier adjustments of alignment as needed. It permits socket interchange without destroying the prosthesis. The flexible foam cover provides improved cosmetic appearance and can be removed for adjustments when necessary. Permanently adjustable devices are particularly beneficial to children because the growth process necessitates frequent adjustment.

ADVANTAGES

1. Cosmetic appearance. Natural outer contour. No distracting articulation separations.
2. Usually lighter in weight than the exoskeletal-type prosthesis. The tube structure offers a high strength-weight ratio.
3. Permits the use of a number of interchangeable modules for each segment of the system to permit any desired combination of function.
4. Foam covering gives a more natural feel to the touch and is easily removable to permit access to the internal structure.
5. Static and dynamic alignment is easier and can be done throughout the life of the prosthesis.
6. Can be assembled easier and quicker than the exoskeletal-type prosthesis through the use of mass-produced prefabricated modules. A functional prosthesis can be provided to the amputee in less time.
7. Various combinations of components can be tried with each amputee with minimal expenditure of time and effort.
8. The tube structure permits adjustment in length of various segments of the prosthesis.
9. The tube itself is an inexpensive structure.
10. Replacement of an individual module can be accomplished easily, which reduces subsequent costs.

DISADVANTAGE

1. The initial cost may be more than for an exoskeletal prosthesis.

BIBLIOGRAPHY

PROSTHETIC PRESCRIPTION

ALLEN, RW AND VERHOFF, JR: *Supracondylar suspension patellar-tendon-bearing prosthesis: Its evaluation in unselected cases.* South Med J 63:59–61, 1970.

BAKALIM, G: *Experiences with the PTB prosthesis*. Artificial Limbs 9:14–22, 1965.

BARCLAY, W: *Below-knee amputation prosthesis*. In MURDOCH, G (ED): *Prosthetic and Orthotic Practice*. Edward Arnold & Co, London, 1970, pp 69–78.

BECHTOL, CO: *The principles of prosthetic prescription*. In KLOPSTEG, PE AND WILSON, PD (EDS): *Human Limbs and their Substitutes*. Hafner Publishing, New York, 1954, pp 159–165.

BREAKEY, JW: *Criteria for use of supracondylar and supracondylar-suprapatellar suspension for below-knee prostheses*. Orthot Pros 27:14–18, 1973.

BREAKEY, JW: *Criteria for use of supracondylar and supracondylar-suprapatellar suspension for below-knee prostheses*. In *Selected Readings: A Review of Orthotics and Prosthetics*. American Orthotics and Prosthetics Association, Washington, DC, 1980, pp 163–168.

ERBACK, JR: *Hydraulic prostheses for above-knee amputees*. J Am Phys Ther Assoc 43:105–110, 1963.

FOORT, J: *The patellar-tendon-bearing prosthesis for below-knee amputees: A review of technique and criteria*. Artificial Limbs 9:4–13, 1965.

GILPIN, RE, DALE, GG, AND HARRIS, WR: *Canadian experience with the patellar-tendon-bearing below-knee prosthesis*. J Bone Joint Surg 44B:795–799, 1962.

GORDON, EJ AND ARDIZZONE, J: *Clinical experience with the S.A.C.H. foot prosthesis*. J Bone Joint Surg 42A:226–234, 1969.

HADDAN, CC AND THOMAS, A: *Status of the above-knee suction socket in the United States*. Artificial Limbs 1:29–39, 1954.

HAMPTON, FL: *Above-knee prostheses*. Orthop Clin North Am 3:359–372, 1972.

JONES, RF: *Amputee rehabilitation: Basic principles in prosthetic assessment and fitting*. Med J Aust 2:290–293, 1977.

KNAPP, ME: *Lower-extremity amputations and prosthetics. II. Prosthetics*. Postgrad Med J 44:259–264, 1968.

KNOTT, LW: *Basic principles in use of orthoses and prostheses*. Mod Treatm 5:900–905, 1968.

LAMBERT, CN: *Applicability of the patellar-tendon-bearing prosthesis to skeletally immature amputees*. Inter-Clinic Info Bull 3:7, 1964.

LEWIS, EA: *Fluid-controlled knee mechanisms: Clinical considerations*. Bull Prosthet Res 10–3:24–56, 1965.

MARSCHALL, K AND NITSCHKE, R: *Principles of the patellar tendon supra-condylar prosthesis*. Orth Pros Appl J 21:33–38, 1967.

MCCONVILLE, BE, KENNEDY, EH, AND SCHOUTEN, M: *An evaluation of the patellar-tendon-bearing prosthesis*. Int Surg 47:377–381, 1967.

MURDOCH, G: *Levels of amputation and limiting factors*. Ann R Coll Surg Engl 40:204–216, 1967.

MURPHY, EF: *The fitting of below-knee prostheses*. In KLOPSTEG, PE AND WILSON, PD (EDS): *Human Limbs and their Substitutes*. Hafner Publishing, New York, 1954, pp 693–735.

POETS, R: *The fitting of the above-knee stump*. Orthot Pros 28:28–32, 1974.

Program Guide: Selection and Application of Knee Mechanisms. Veterans Administration, Washington, DC, 1976.

RADCLIFFE, CW AND FOORT, J: *The Patellar-Tendon-Bearing Below-Knee Prosthesis*. Biomechanics Laboratory, University of California at San Francisco and Berkeley, 1961.

REDHEAD, RG: *Clinical requirements in the design of lower extremity prostheses*. Rehabil 97:21–24, 1976.

Selection and Application of Knee Mechanisms: Program Guide. Veterans Administration, Washington, DC, 1980.

Suggestions For Fitting and Alignment The SACH Foot. VA Prosthetics Center, 1970.

SYMINGTON, DC, LOWE, PJ, AND MACKAY, S: *Semi-flexible sockets for amputation below the knee.* Arch Phys Med Rehabil 56:399–404, 1975.

THOMPSON, RG: *The decline and fall of the PTB: With apologies to Edward Gibbons (The Decline and Fall of the Roman Empire).* Orth Pros Appl J 19:21–22, 1965.

THOMSON, HG AND BOCHMANN, D: *The skin-grafted below-knee stump: Can knee function be salvaged?* Can J Surg 13:37–40, 1970.

Varients of the PTB (patellar-tendon-bearing) below-knee prosthesis. Bull Prosthet Res 10–13:120–134, 1970.

WITTECK, FA: *Some experiences with patellar-tendon-bearing below-knee prostheses.* Artificial Limbs 6:74–85, 1962.

WOLCOTT, LE AND KOEPKE, GH: *Experience with patellar tendon-bearing below-knee prosthesis with total contact socket.* Arch Phys Med Rehabil 43:474–476, 1962.

BILATERAL AMPUTEES

ADAMS, IL: *Bilateral lower extremity dressing frame.* Am J Occup Ther 29:547–550, 1975.

BROWN, PW: *Rehabilitation of bilateral lower-extremity amputees.* J Bone Joint Surg 52A:687–700, 1970.

CHASE, RA AND WHITE, WL: *Bilateral amputation in rehabilitation of paraplegics.* Plast Reconstr Surg 24:445–455, 1959.

CICENIA, EF, ET AL: *Functional training of the bilateral above-knee amputee.* Int Rev Phys Med Rehabil 38:9–23, 1959.

CLARKE-WILLIAMS, MJ: *The elderly double amputee.* Geron Clin 11:183–192, 1969.

COSLA, HW, FORSTER, S, AND BENTON, JG: *Prosthesis fitted after bilateral hip disarticulation: Report of a case.* Arch Phys Med Rehabil 46:705–707, 1965.

DUNLAP, SW: *Bilateral amputation: Above-knee and hip disarticulation.* Phys Ther 49:500–502, 1969.

GEORGI, WH, ET AL: *Initial fitting of bilateral lower-extremity prostheses in the teen-ager.* Inter-Clinic Info Bull 9:1–5, 1969.

GHIULAMILA, RI, ET AL: *Prosthetic rehabilitation of a paraplegic with bilateral disarticulation and partial pelvectomy.* Arch Phys Med Rehabil 57:475–478, 1976.

GILLIS, L: *A new prosthesis for disarticulation at the hip.* J Bone Joint Surg 50B:389–391, 1968.

HAMILTON, EA, STRANGE, T, AND LUKER, C: *Modification of standard 8BL chair for the use of double amputees.* Rheumatol Rehabil 15:24–25, 1976.

HAMPTON, F: *Northwestern University suspension casting technique for hemipelvectomy and hip disarticulation.* Artificial Limbs 10:56–61, 1966.

HIGH, WJ: *Bilateral hip disarticulation.* Phys Ther 50:354–357, 1970.

HUBBARD, S AND MCLAURIN, CA: *The AK tie bar.* Artificial Limbs 16:54–59, 1972.

KERSTEIN, MD, ET AL: *Associated diagnoses which complicate rehabilitation of the patient with bilateral lower extremity amputations.* Surg Gynecol Obstet 140:875–876, 1975.

KERSTEIN, MD, ET AL: *Rehabilitation after bilateral lower extremity amputation.* Arch Phys Med Rehabil 56:309–311, 1975.

LOWENTHAL, M, POSNAIK, AO, AND TOBIS, JS: *Rehabilitation of the elderly double above-knee amputee.* Arch Phys Med Rehabil 39:290–295, 1958.

MACINNES, MSA: *Bilateral amputation of the legs: Patient care and rehabilitation.* Nurs Times 73:1033–1034, Jul 1977.

MAZET, R, JR: *The geriatric amputee.* Artificial Limbs 11:33–41, 1967.

MCCOLLOUGH, NC, III: *The bilateral lower extremity amputee.* Orthop Clin North Am 3:373–382, 1972.

MCCOLLOUGH, NC, III, JENNINGS, JJ, AND SARMIENTO, A: *Bilateral below-the-knee amputation in patients over fifty years of age: Results in thirty-one patients.* J Bone Joint Surg 54A:1217–1223, 1972.

MCDOUGALL, RV: *Case history: Bilateral above-knee amputee with "stubbies."* Phys Ther Rev 40:186–187, 1960.

MCLAURIN, CA: *The Canadian hip-disarticulation prosthesis.* In MURDOCH, G (ED): *Prosthetic and Orthotic Practice.* Edward Arnold & Co, London, 1970, pp 285–304.

PEIZER, E: *Socket flexion and gait of an above-knee bilateral amputee.* Artificial Limbs 7:43–49, 1963.

RIVERA, MC AND ANTIGUA, MY, JR: *Bilateral thigh amputation.* Phillipine J Surg 21:38–40, 1966.

SAKUMA, J, ET AL: *Rehabilitation of geriatric patients having bilateral lower extremity amputations.* Arch Phys Med Rehabil 55:101–111, 1974.

SPIRA, M AND HARDY, SB: *Our experiences with high thigh amputations in paraplegics.* Plast Reconstr Surg 31:344–352, 1963.

SPURGEON, MJ: *Chronic effects of bilateral leg amputations.* South Med J 70:1148, 1977.

VAN DE VEN, CMC: *A pilot survey of elderly bilateral lower-limb amputees.* Physiotherapy 59:316–320, 1973.

VAN DE VEN, C: *Bilateral amputees in North America.* Physiotherapy 60:316–317, 1974.

WARREN, MW: *The management of the elderly double amputee.* In *Old Age in the Modern World.* Livingstone, Edinburgh, 1955, pp 562–570.

WATKINS, AL: *Additional notes on rehabilitation of the bilateral lower extremity amputee.* Orth Pros Appl J 12:45–49, 1958.

WATKINS, AL AND LIAO, SJ: *Rehabilitation of persons with bilateral amputation of lower extremities.* JAMA 166:1584–1586, 1958.

WHITE, SA: *Treatment of a bi-lateral amputee using a pneumatic post-amputation mobility aid.* Physiotherapy 65:15, 1979.

MODULAR (ENDOSKELETAL)

BREAKEY, JW AND SMITH, CMT: *Below knee amputee program: Modular system for physiotherapists.* Physiotherapy Can 25:19–23, 1973.

CANTY, TJ: *Amputations and recent developments in artificial limbs.* US Armed Forces Med J 3:1147–1152, 1952.

CLARK, G: *The modular below-knee prosthesis.* Inter-Clinic Info Bull 8:11–12, 1969.

CONDIE, DN: *Amputee performance measurement.* Rehabilitation 92:5–7, 1975.

Cosmesis and Modular Limb Prostheses. A report of a conference sponsored by the Committee on Prosthetics Research and Development of the Division of Engineering, National Research Council, National Academy of Sciences, Washington, DC, 1971.

GARDNER, HF: *Endoskeletal structures for lower-extremity prostheses.* Bull Prosthet Res 10–13:113–119, 1970.

HAMPTON, FL: *Above knee prostheses.* Orthop Clin North Am 3:359–372, 1972.

JONES, RF AND BURNISTON, GG: *A conservative approach to lower-limb amputations: Review of 240 amputees with a trial of the rigid dressing.* Med J Aust 2:711–718, 1970.

KAY, HW AND NEWMAN, JD: *Report of a workshop on below-knee and above-knee prosthetics.* Orth Pros 27:9–25, 1973.

KROUSKOP, TA, NEWELL, PH, JR, AND LEAVITT, LA: *Cosmetic covers for lower limb prostheses.* Bull Prosthet Res 10–22:411–414, 1974.

LEAHEY, E, ET AL: *Clinical study of lower-extremity amputees: With emphasis on use of modular-unit prostheses.* NY State J Med 73:1186–1188, 1973.

LEAVITT, LA, ET AL: *Cosmetic cover for endoskeletal prosthetic systems: A new technique.* Arch Phys Med Rehabil 56:414–416, 1975.

LI, WK: *Ankle-knee synchronous in a new endoskeletal above-knee prosthetic mechanism: A preliminary report.* Arch Phys Med Rehabil 57:479–481, 1976.

MAUCH, HA: *Cosmetic covers for lower-limb prostheses.* Bull Prosthet Res 10–22:410, 1974.

MCDOUGALL, A AND EMMERSON, A: *The preformed socket and modular assembly for primary amputees.* J Bone Joint Surg 59B:77–79, 1977.

PELOSOF, HV, MUILENBERG, AL, AND LEAVITT, LA: *Endoskeletal prostheses: Use in a patient having ipsilateral fore- and hind-quarter amputations.* Arch Phys Med Rehabil 55:89–90, 1974.

RADCLIFFE, CW: *Cosmetic covers for lower-limb prostheses.* Bull Prosthet Res 10–22:415–416, 1974.

SAUTER, WF: *Cosmetic covers for modular prostheses.* Artificial Limbs 16:59–65, 1972.

SOKOLOW, J AND GRYNBAUM, BB: *Modular above-knee prostheses.* Arch Phys Med Rehabil 54:278–280, 1973.

SYMINGTON, DC, LOWE, PJ, AND MACKAY, S: *Semi-flexible sockets for amputation below the knee.* Arch Phys Med Rehabil 56:399–404, 1975.

WILSON, AB, JR: *Lower-limb modular prostheses: A status report.* Orth Pros 29:23–32, 1975.

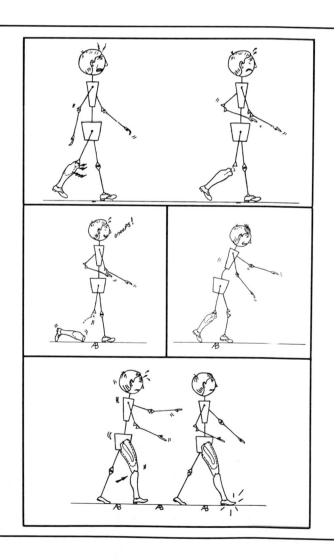

STATIC AND DYNAMIC ANALYSIS

STATIC ANALYSIS

Each individual has unique body proportions and a unique shape, which results in unique static and dynamic functions. It follows, therefore, that a prosthesis that was designed for all amputees of a particular level will not simulate the function of the lost limb for each particular amputee. Thus, a prosthesis needs to be custom-made to more closely replace the lost leg.

Fit is the relationship of the socket to the residual limb. Alignment is the relative position of various parts of the prosthesis with respect to each other, and the relationship of the whole prosthesis to the body. To a large extent, the alignment of a prosthesis will affect the gait pattern of the amputee. The amputee can walk with a narrow-based gait only if the prosthesis is constructed to give such a gait pattern. It should be remembered that socket fit and alignment are interdependent. Good alignment should always start with a good fit of the residual limb in the socket. Appropriate socket shape and orientation are essential for satisfactory gait. Variations in alignment depend upon such factors as the length of the residual limb, the strength of the residual limb, and the amputee's balance and coordination.

Adjustable alignment devices are used by the prosthetist to carry out the alignment procedure (Fig. 20-1). The device for amputations higher than the below-knee level has a pylon tube and a knee joint that connects the socket to the foot. The device is adjustable so that the position of the socket to the knee and foot may be altered in mediolateral and anteroposterior directions as well as angular and transverse rotational directions. The bench alignment—the initial alignment to a prescribed geometry—should be close to the final alignment. The adjustable alignment device is designed to offer adjustments ranging from an acceptable alignment to an optimum alignment. The dynamic alignment includes subsequent modifications after the amputee walks for a while. The alignment device is removed after static and dynamic alignments are completed.

Members of the prosthetic team need to pay attention to the finest details of fit and alignment. Optimum alignment provides stability and comfort, requires the least expenditure of energy, and results in a gait that more closely approximates normal

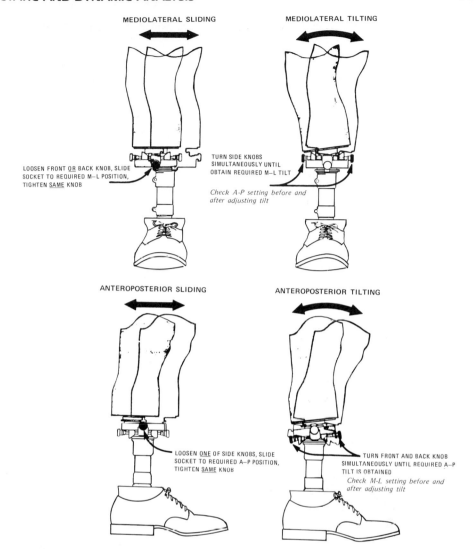

FIGURE 20-1. Adjustable alignment device for a PTB prosthesis. (From Fleer, B and Wilson, AB, Jr: *Construction of the patellar-tendon-bearing below-knee prosthesis.* **Artificial Limbs 6:46, 1962, with permission.)**

locomotion. The extent of prosthetic adjustment should be conservative and carefully planned.

SYME PROSTHESIS

FOOT

The Syme foot is set in slight dorsiflexion and in a valgus position relative to the shank. This alignment is necessary for the foot to be flat on the floor at mid-stance, since the long axis of the socket is set in slight flexion and adduction. The foot is also inset approximately 2 cm ($^3/_4$ in) medial to the center of the socket, with a normal stance base of 5 cm (2 in) between the heels (Fig. 20-2).

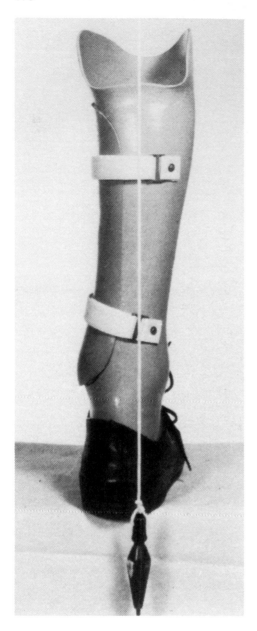

FIGURE 20-2. Medial placement of the foot relative to the socket. (From Hampton, FL: *Prosthetic principles in the lower extremity amputee.* Orthop Clin North Am 3:342, 1972, with permission.)

SOCKET

Alignment of the socket on the foot is similar to the alignment of the patellar-tendon-bearing (PTB) below-knee prosthesis. The knee is centered on a vertical line that passes midway between the front of the keel (metatarsal arch) on a SACH foot and the back of the heel (Fig. 20-3). The length of the Syme limb limits the amount of anterior placement of the socket relative to the foot. The knee flexion attitude is thus less than for a PTB prosthesis; however, it is desired when an effort is being made to enhance proximal weight-bearing.

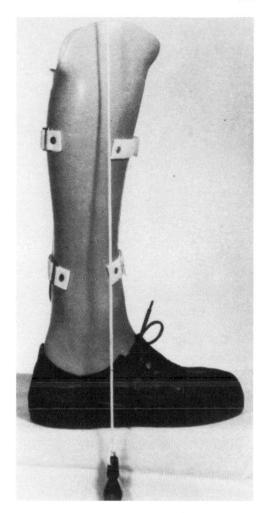

FIGURE 20-3. The Syme socket is set in an attitude of initial flexion. (From Hampton, FL: *Prosthetic principles in the lower extremity amputee.* Orthop Clin North Am 3:341, 1972, with permission.)

PTB PROSTHESIS

Alignment of the below-knee prosthesis involves the relationship between the position of the socket and the foot.

ANTERIOR-POSTERIOR VIEW

Proper Static Alignment	Malalignment Symptom	Cause (Problem)
Length of prosthesis equal to length on sound side. (Medial tibial plateau-to-floor and pelvis-to-floor equal on both sides.) The iliac crests and anterior superior iliac spines are used as pelvic landmarks.	The medial tibial plateau and anterior superior iliac spine are lower on the prosthetic side than the sound side when standing with the feet an equal distance apart and with equal weight on each foot.	The prosthesis is too short. The anterior tilt of the socket has been increased.

The medial tibial plateau and anterior superior iliac spine are higher on the prosthetic side.		The prosthesis is too long. Excessive upward pressure was placed on the cast during fabrication, causing elongation resulting in a socket that is too long. The limb is not seated well in the socket. Excessive socks. The socket has been tilted posteriorly.
Socket is set in 2 to 5 degrees adduction, like the sound tibial crest (Fig. 20-4).	Proximal-medial pressure.	Excessive adduction angle of socket.

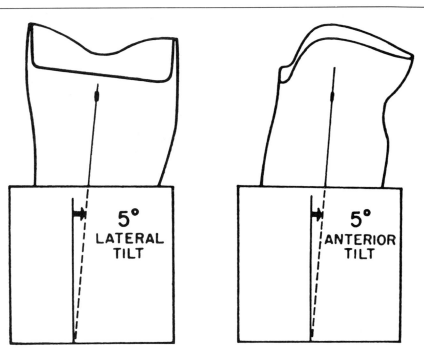

FIGURE 20-4. Pre-positioning of the socket in (A) 5 degrees of adduction and (B) 5 degrees of initial flexion. (From Fleer, B and Wilson, AB, Jr: *Construction of the patellar-tendon-bearing below-knee prosthesis.* Artificial Limbs 6:39, 1962, with permission.)

Medial-lateral placement of foot: A plumb line dropped from a mark 1.3 cm (½ in) medial to the center of the socket falls	Lateral motion of socket during stance, with pressure/pain in the proximal-medial and distal-lateral areas.	Plumb falls lateral to center of heel: foot is inset too far (socket is outset too far).

through the center of the heel (foot inset slightly relative to socket).

Generally, the shorter the residual limb, the more lateral the position of the foot.

Lateral bending of trunk toward prosthetic side during stance phase.

Pressure/pain in the proximal-lateral and distal-medial areas.

Weight-bearing on the medial tibial flare is less effective.

Plumb falls medial to center of heel: foot is outset.

LATERAL VIEW

Proper Static Alignment	Malalignment Symptom	Cause (Problem)
Socket suspension: Piston action should not exceed 1.3 to 1.9 cm ($^1/_2$ to $^3/_4$ in).	Excessive pistoning.	The negative cast of the limb is removed before the cast is hard, causing enlargement of the proximal third. The cast is rubbed or molded after it has started to harden, which causes the cast to enlarge.
Socket set in approximately 5 to 10 degrees of initial flexion (see Fig. 20-4). Amputee walks in a slightly flexed position throughout gait.	Pain at the distal tibia during weight-bearing. Knee is forced backward. (If the knee is brought forward, the heel does not contact the floor.)	Insufficient anterior tilt of socket; hence, distal weight-bearing is increased.
Socket and shank are aligned in 10 to 15 degrees of flexion with the perpendicular. (Affected by ankle dorsiflexion.)	Knee is forced forward.	Excessive anterior tilt of socket.
Anterior-posterior lever arms of foot: A plumb line dropped from a mark at the midpoint of the socket laterally falls 2.5 cm (1 in) anterior to the heel (Fig. 20-5).	Excessive anterior tilt of socket. End of limb is forced forward painfully against the socket as the amputee actively extends the knee at heel-strike to control the prosthesis.	The heel lever arm is too long (the plumb line falls more than 2.5 cm [1 in] anterior to the heel), and the toe lever arm is too short. The socket is too far forward.
A vertical reference line (B′B″) that passes through the midpoint of the socket at the level of the patellar tendon prox-	Knee is forced backward.	The heel lever arm is too short (the plumb line

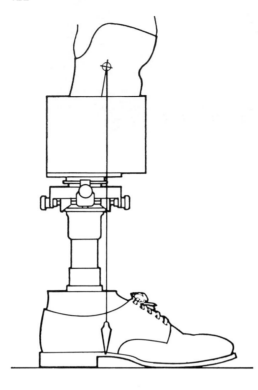

FIGURE 20-5. Ultimate anterior-posterior position of the socket with respect to the foot. (From Fleer, B and Wilson, AB, Jr: *Construction of the patellar-tendon-bearing below-knee prosthesis.* **Artificial Limbs 6:50, 1962, with permission.)**

imally should intersect the foot midway between the forward tip of the keel and the posterior aspect of the heel distally (Fig. 20-6).

falls less than 2.5 cm [1 in] anterior to the heel), and the toe lever arm is too long.

The socket is shifted too far back.

The heel cushion or plantarflexion bumper is too soft, thus not providing sufficient counterpressure.

SUPERIOR VIEW

Proper Static Alignment	Malalignment Symptom	Cause (Problem)
The medial-lateral midline of the socket (perpendicular to the posterior wall of the socket) is the same as the medial-lateral midline of the foot.	The medial-lateral midline of the socket is angled outwardly relative to the medial-lateral midline of the foot.	The foot is rotated inwardly relative to the socket (Fig. 20-7).
The foot should be in slight external rotation 5 to 7 degrees from the sagittal	The medial-lateral midline of the socket is angled inward relative to the	The foot is rotated too far outward relative to the socket.

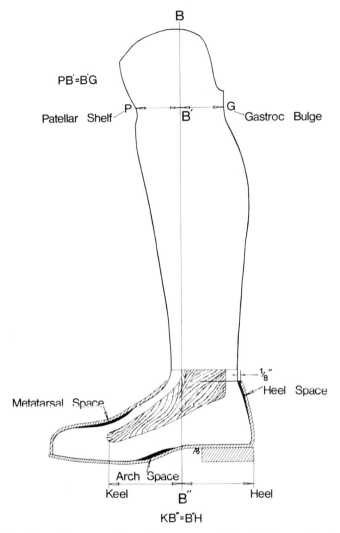

B

PB´=B´G

Patellar Shelf — P

B´

G — Gastroc Bulge

⅛″

Metatarsal Space

Heel Space

Arch Space

A´

Keel

B″

Heel

KB″=B´H

FIGURE 20-6. Anterior-posterior alignment of the PTB prosthesis. Metatarsal, arch, and heel spaces between the prosthetic foot and shoe are indicated.

plane.	medial-lateral midline of the foot.	
Anterior-posterior (sagittal) diameter of socket: Should equal ± 0.32 to 0.63 cm (¼ to ⅛ in) the distance from the patellar tendon anteriorly to the depression between the heads of the gastrocnemius posteriorly under pressure.	Constriction of limb causing edema and eventual deterioration of end of limb.	Too snug. Excessively tight fit in the popliteal area (bulge too large).
	Pressure at or on the distal end of the limb, causing pain.	Too loose.

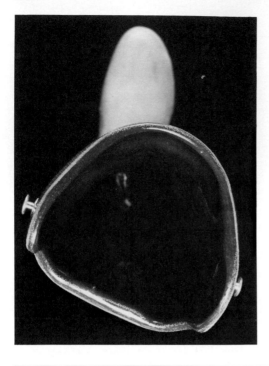

FIGURE 20-7. The foot is internally rotated relative to the socket.

Medial-lateral (coronal) diameter of socket: Must equal the greatest diameter between the outer aspects of the medial and lateral femoral condyles.	Pinching and pressure.	Too snug.
	Medial-lateral instability.	Too loose. During fabrication of the negative cast, the fingers exerted excessive pressure in the popliteal area, thus expanding the width of the cast.
The midline of the thigh should be perpendicular to the table during casting to ensure that the popliteal area is formed perpendicular to the line of progression.	Wrong orientation of the popliteal area in relation to the line of progression, or misalignment of the patellar tendon indentation.	External rotation of the femur during casting.
The patellar tendon shelf should be formed perpendicular to the line of progression and should not cause undue pressure. It should be located midway between the inferior aspect of the patella and the tibial tubercle.	Malalignment of the patellar tendon shelf.	Distortion of the patellar tendon during casting. Application of too much pressure with the thumb tips when molding the patellar shelf.

The limb should be held at a flexion angle of approximately 20 degrees during casting.	Gapping of the socket at the midpatellar level.	The knee was held in too much flexion during the fabrication wrap/casting procedure.

SITTING

Proper Static Alignment	Malalignment Symptom	Cause (Problem)
If the back of the socket extends up into the space between the hamstring tendons, medial and lateral grooves should be sufficient to relieve the tendons during knee flexion.	Forceful contact of the medial hamstrings with the socket when the knee is flexed (90 degrees), which produces skin abrasions.	The hamstring groove is inadequate.
The posterior brim of the socket should be a broad flared surface. The flare should begin approximately 2.5 cm (1 in) below the level of the patellar tendon protuberance.	Constriction of circulation in the popliteal area when standing or sitting.	The flare of the posterior edge of the socket is inadequate.
	The residual limb levers out of the socket when the knee is flexed.	The posterior wall is too high.
The prosthesis should allow at least 90 degrees of flexion (110 to 115 degrees of flexion needed for kneeling).	The limb slides off of the patellar bar, resulting in undue weight-bearing on the distal end.	The posterior wall is too low.

GENERAL CONSIDERATIONS

Proper Static Alignment	Malalignment Symptom	Cause (Problem)
There should be total contact of the socket over the entire surface of the residual limb, with primary pressure in the pressure-tolerant areas.	Abrasions, painful areas.	Excessive points of pressure.
	Distal coolness or edema.	Lack of distal contact. Excessive proximal pressure.

Suspension: The cuff should fit snugly over the suprapatellar area, with piston action no greater than 1.3 to 1.9 cm ($\frac{1}{2}$ to $\frac{3}{4}$ in). The suspension cuff should loosen when the amputee is sitting.

ABOVE-KNEE PROSTHESIS

Alignment of the above-knee prosthesis involves the relationship among the positions of the socket, knee, and foot.

ANTERIOR-POSTERIOR VIEW

Proper Static Alignment	Malalignment Symptom	Cause (Problem)
Medial-lateral alignment: A plumb line dropped from a point 2.5 cm (1 in) lateral to the inner posteromedial socket angle (the ischial seat) should pass through the center of the heel (Fig. 20-8). NOTE: If the residual limb is very short, the foot is outset more to relieve excessive pressure on the short femur.	A plumb line dropped from the ischial seat falls medial to the center of the heel. Compression of tissue on proximal-lateral and distal-medial aspects of the limb. There may be lateral bending of the trunk toward the prosthetic side.	Foot is outset (displaced away from midline); wide base for security at the expense of natural looking gait; may be indicated for short or weak residual limb.
	A plumb line dropped from the ischial seat falls lateral to the center of the heel. Increased pressure on the proximal-medial aspect of the limb. (This angular pressure is preferable to the opposite angular pressure caused by an outset foot.) Terminal femoral pressure.	Foot is inset (displaced toward midline); may be indicated for long, powerful residual limb.
Total length of the prosthesis: The pelvis should be level. Standing with equal weight on each leg, check the levels of the Iliac crests and the anterior superior iliac spines. Make sure the feet are an equal distance apart.	The iliac crest and anterior superior iliac spine are lower on the prosthetic side than on the sound side when standing with the feet an equal distance apart with equal weight on each foot.	The prosthesis is too short.
	The iliac crest and anterior superior iliac spine are higher on the prosthetic side than on the sound side when standing with the feet an equal distance apart with equal weight on each foot.	The prosthesis is too long. Limb is not seated well in the socket. Excessive socks.

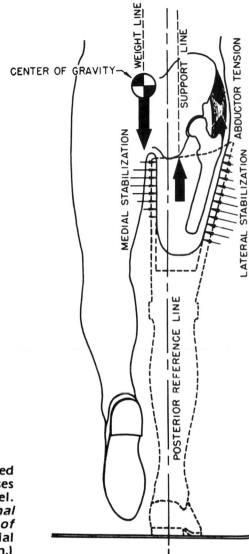

FIGURE 20-8. A plumb line dropped from the ischial tuberosity passes through the center of the heel. (From Radcliffe, CW: *Functional considerations in the fitting of above-knee prostheses.* Artificial Limbs 2:38, 1955, with permission.)

The medial brim should be 1.3 cm (½ in) below the inferior border of the pubic ramus with full weight-bearing on the prosthesis.	Pressure on the pubic ramus ("crotch pressure").	Medial brim is too high.
	Adductor roll present— bunching of soft tissue over the medial brim of socket.	Medial brim is too low. Medial-lateral diameter of socket is too small. The ischium is forced medially.
The ischial tuberosity should rest comfortably on the ischial seat. *To test:* Have the amputee	The tuberosity is anterior to the seat (limb has dropped into the socket). Discomfort in area of pu-	Anterior-posterior diameter of socket is too large. Weight loss since the fabrication measurements

bend forward at the waist while standing with equal weight on both legs and with the feet an equal distance apart. Place a finger on the ischial tuberosity. Ask the amputee to stand erect. The examiner's finger should be pinched between the ischial seat and the ischial tuberosity to the extent that it has to be withdrawn.

bic ramus. The amputee compensates by abducting the prosthesis or laterally bending toward the prosthetic side.

were taken.
Insufficient socks.

	The tuberosity is above the ischial seat. Sciatic nerve pressure causing pain or paresthesia in limb. Excessive pressure on the hamstring tendons originating from the ischial tuberosity will decrease the function of these muscles and thus reduce knee stability.	Anterior-posterior diameter of socket is too small. Limb edema or weight gain since the fabrication measurements were taken. Excessive socks.
	The adductor muscles are crowded, and there is a burning sensation in the skin around the ischial seat.	The ischial seat is too far medially. The fit is too tight over the gluteus maximus.
	There is excessive weight-bearing in the area of the ischial tuberosity, resulting in a burning sensation at the ischial seat.	The channel for the gluteus maximus is too large. The posterior brim is too low in the area of the gluteus maximus.
Anterior-posterior diameter: The correct diameter is the distance from the ischial tuberosity to the adductor longus tendon minus 1.3 cm (½ in), the horizontal length of the medial wall at the ischial level.	Paresthesia in femoral nerve distribution or discoloration of limb and edema owing to capillary congestion from constriction of vessels.	Scarpa's bulge is too thick—excessive pressure in Scarpa's triangle.
The lateral brim of the socket should maintain contact with the limb without gapping.	Lateral gapping of the socket.	Medial-lateral diameter of the socket is too large. In-slope of the posterior brim—amputee slides forward.
Posterior brim: The posterior brim should be parallel to the floor and sloped slightly forward.	Burning sensation at the ischial tuberosity. (This sensation is to be expected during the first few episodes of weight-bearing.)	The posterior seat is not sloped forward adequately.

	Pain or discomfort lateral to the ischial tuberosity.	
	Pain at the ischial tuberosity.	The posterior brim is not horizontal but slopes downward from medial to lateral. (The gluteus maximus does not share weight support; thus the ischial tuberosity is overloaded.)
	Pain or discomfort lateral to the ischial tuberosity.	The posterior brim slants upward from medial to lateral, causing undue pressure on the gluteus maximus.

LATERAL VIEW

Proper Static Alignment	Malalignment Symptom	Cause (Problem)
Anterior-posterior alignment: Trochanter-knee-ankle (TKA) line: T is a point on the lateral brim of the socket which closely corresponds to the greater trochanter of the femur. T is located on a transverse axis in the coronal plane drawn 2.5 cm (1 in) anterior to the inner posterior-medial angle of the socket.	Excessive alignment stability.	The socket is placed anterior to the knee axis.
	Inadequate alignment stability.	The socket is placed posterior to the knee axis.
K is the center of the knee bolt axis.	Knee stability during stance phase but difficulty in initiating swing phase.	K is posterior to the TA line (the center of gravity is anterior to K), resulting in inherent knee stability during stance: Involuntary Knee. Heel is too low for alignment.
	Knee instability standing (especially at heelstrike).	K is anterior to the TA line: Voluntary Knee. (Requires active hip extension to keep the knee locked.) Heel is too high for alignment.

A is the center of ankle rotation. Plumb line dropped from T should pass through A.	Tendency to fall backward.	A is anterior to the plumb line dropped from T (short heel lever arm: long toe lever arm).
For intermediate knee control, a vertical line (AA') passing through the knee bolt should pass through the center of the ankle bolt and fall just anterior to the heel of the shoe (Fig. 20-9).	Tendency to fall forward.	A is posterior to the plumb line dropped from T (long heel lever arm: short toe lever arm).
Initial socket flexion (ISF) equals the fixed flexion	Backache. Hyperlordosis (lumbar).	Insufficient initial flexion.

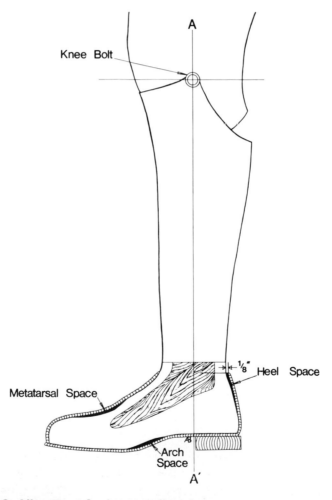

FIGURE 20-9. Alignment for intermediate knee control of an above-knee prosthesis. Metatarsal, arch, and heel spaces between the prosthetic foot and shoe are indicated.

contracture at the hip (FFC) minus 10 degrees (pelvic tilt) plus 15 degrees (hip extension necessary for proper push-off).

$$ISF = FFC - 10° + 15°$$

contracture at the hip (FFC) minus 10 degrees (pelvic tilt) plus 15 degrees (hip extension necessary for proper push-off). $ISF = FFC - 10° + 15°$	Knee instability if amputee stands erect without lumbar lordosis. Amputee bends forward at hips.	
For a total contact socket, the limb should be in uniform contact with the socket, with weight equally distributed on both legs. The limb can be palpated through the valve hole or roentgenograms can be made in two vertical planes or another method can be used to check fit.	Air pockets.	Contact with the socket wall is inadequate.
	Painful pressures, abrasions, edema, discoloration.	Contact with the socket wall is excessive.
If the amputee steps forward and bears weight on the prosthetic heel, the sole of the shoe should just barely touch the floor or should be within 1.3 cm (½ in) of the floor.	Foot is greater than 1.3 cm (½ in) from the floor.	Plantarflexion control is too strong. SACH heel is too stiff.
	Foot slap.	Plantarflexion control is too weak. SACH heel is too soft.
If the amputee stands with full weight on the prosthesis, it should be possible to just slide a piece of paper under the heel.	Paper slides under the heel too easily.	Too much plantarflexion alignment. Dorsiflexion bumper is too thick.
	Paper will not slide under the heel.	Too much dorsiflexion alignment. Dorsiflexion bumper is too thin.

SUPERIOR VIEW

Proper Static Alignment	Malalignment Symptom	Cause (Problem)
The channel for the adductor longus tendon should be adequate.	Pain over the adductor longus tendon. "Cutting" in this area. The amputee may externally rotate the leg.	The channel for the adductors is inadequate. Anterior-posterior diameter (medial wall) is too short.

The interior lateral wall should be set in adduction with a relief for the distal-lateral aspect of the femur and the greater trochanter.	Tenderness in the distal-lateral aspect of the limb during weight-bearing.	Insufficient relief in the distal-lateral socket for scar, skin graft, spur, neuromas, or the end of the femur.
	Adductor roll. Unable to maintain a level pelvis when weight-bearing on the prosthesis.	Femur is not adducted sufficiently in the socket.
	Pain at the proximal brim over the greater trochanter.	Insufficient relief for the greater trochanter.
The interior posterior wall should provide a conservative concavity for the hamstring tendons below the ischial seat.	Tightness in the socket below the ischial seat.	There is "undercutting" of the ischial seat without ample room for the functioning muscles.
The knee bolt is aligned in 5 degrees external rotation and is horizontal. (The femur rotates internally during swing phase, bringing the knee bolt to a position perpendicular to the line of progression so that the shank swings forward in a straight line.)	See Dynamic Analysis.	

SITTING

Proper Static Alignment	Malalignment Symptom	Cause (Problem)
The knee joints should be the same height.	The thigh component of the prosthesis is shorter than the sound side, and thus the knee may not flex to 90 degrees if the amputee is sitting back in the chair. The shank component of the prosthesis is longer than the	Prosthetic knee joint is too high.

	sound side, so the prosthetic thigh may be higher (farther from the floor).	
	The thigh component of the prosthesis is longer than the sound side and thus sticks out farther. The shank component of the prosthesis is shorter than the sound side, so the foot may not touch the floor.	Prosthetic knee joint is too low.
Height of the anterior brim: The anterior brim should be about 6.4 cm (2½ in) higher than the posterior or medial brim.	There is uncomfortable contact of the anterior brim with the anterior superior iliac spine when sitting. The amputee is unable to lean forward to tie shoes. Suction may be lost because the prosthesis is pushed off as the amputee leans forward.	Anterior brim is too high.
	There is a flesh roll over the anterior brim. If a pelvic belt is worn, there may be pinching of the flesh between the socket and the belt.	Anterior brim is too low.
Prosthetic shank and foot should be vertical when sitting. The back of the socket should be flat.	Shank and foot are rotated in or out when sitting.	Posterior wall of the socket is improperly shaped.
The ischial seat should be rounded and of proper thickness so that there is no discomfort when sitting.	Stretching of skin and discomfort (burning sensation) at the ischial tuberosity when sitting (may lose suction).	Ischial seat (posterior wall) is too thick. The limb is pushed anteriorly and the posterior brim loses contact with the soft tissue, permitting the entry of air. Gluteus relief is too large, causing rotation of the leg during sitting. Ischial seat is displaced medially.

GENERAL FEATURES

The socket interior should be smooth and comfortable. The knee should operate freely without binding. The entire limb should be the same shape and color as the normal leg.

CANADIAN-TYPE HIP-DISARTICULATION PROSTHESIS

ANTERIOR-POSTERIOR VIEW

Proper Static Alignment	Malalignment Symptom	Cause (Problem)
Medial-lateral alignment: A plumb line dropped from a point on the posterior wall in the sagittal plane where the ischium contacts the socket should fall in the center of the heel or no more than 2.5 cm (1 in) medial to it. The thigh piece should incline downward and medially (Fig. 20-10A).	A plumb line dropped from the point of contact of the ischium falls more than 2.5 cm (1 in) medial to the center of the heel.	Foot is outset too far.
	A plumb line dropped from the point of contact of the ischium falls lateral to the center of the heel.	Foot is inset.
Prosthetic length: With the amputee standing upright with equal weight on both the sound limb and the prosthesis, the pelvis should be level. (Check the height of the iliac crests or the straightness of the lumbar spine.) Some think that the prosthetic leg should be as much as 1 cm (²/₅ in) shorter than the normal leg for adequate clearance.	The iliac crest or anterior superior iliac spine is higher on the prosthetic side than on the sound side when standing with the feet an equal distance apart with equal weight on each foot.	Prosthesis is too long.
	The iliac crest or anterior superior iliac spine is lower on the prosthetic side when standing with the feet an equal distance apart with equal weight on each foot.	Prosthesis is too short.
Standing base: The distance between the medial borders of the heel should be between 5 and 7.6 cm (2 and 3 in).	Standing base is too wide.	Foot is outset too far.
	Standing base is too narrow.	Foot is inset too far.
Hip joint: The axis of the hip joint should be horizontal. It should be displaced laterally, with	Axis of hip joint is not horizontal.	Build-up on bottom of socket for attachment of hip joint is not properly aligned.

Canadian Hip Disarticulation Prosthesis

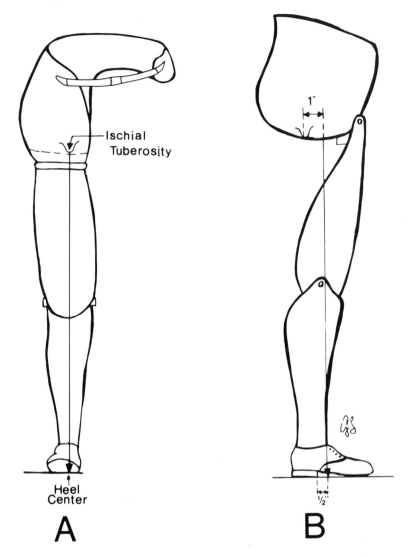

FIGURE 20-10. Static alignment of the Canadian-type hip-disarticulation prosthesis. *(A)* **Medial-lateral alignment.** *(B)* **Anterior-posterior alignment.**

two thirds of its length lateral to the midline of the socket.

Knee joint: The axis of the knee joint should be horizontal to the floor.	Axis of knee joint is not horizontal to floor.	Knee joint is not properly aligned.

LATERAL VIEW

Proper Static Alignment	Malalignment Symptom	Cause (Problem)
Anterior-posterior alignment: A plumb line dropped from a point 2.5 cm (1 in) anterior to the point where the ischium makes contact with the socket should fall at the breast of the heel or up to 1.3 cm (¹/₂ in) in front of it (see Fig. 20-10*B*).	Inadequate alignment stability.	The plumb line drops posterior to the breast of the shoe.
	Excessive alignment stability.	The plumb line drops more than 1.3 cm (¹/₂ in) in front of the breast of the shoe.
Hip joint: The hip joint should be located 4 cm (1¹/₂ in) above the bottom (lowest point) of the socket and as close to the socket as possible.	Prosthetic knee extends past normal knee during sitting.	Hip joint is too far forward.
Amputee's posture: Posture should be erect without excessive lordosis or kyphosis when the socket is against the bumper.	Excessive lumbar lordosis.	Hip joint bumper is too thick.
	Flat lumbar spine.	Hip joint bumper is too thin.
A line joining the hip joint to the back of the heel should pass about 1 cm (²/₅ in) anterior to the knee (in extension). This provides inherent knee stability. (The hip joint is forward to the weight-bearing line of the socket.)	Hip instability.	Hip joint is too far posterior.
	Knee instability.	Hip placed too far anterior, brings knee forward.
The thigh piece is diagonally downward and posterior. A straight line through the hip and knee joint should fall 2.5 cm (1 in) behind the heel of the shoe for the hip-disarticulation prosthesis and 4 cm (1¹/₂ in) behind the heel for the hemipelvectomy prosthesis.		

SUPERIOR VIEW

Proper Static Alignment	Malalignment Symptom	Cause (Problem)
The axis of the hip joint should be externally rotated 5 degrees to the line of progression.	Toe-out is inadequate.	Axis of hip joint is at neutral or is inwardly rotated.
	Toe-out is excessive.	Axis of hip joint is outwardly rotated more than 5 degrees.
The axis of the knee bolt should be outwardly rotated 3 degrees to the line of progression.	Toe-out is inadequate.	Axis of knee bolt is at neutral or is inwardly rotated.
	Toe-out is excessive.	Axis of knee bolt is outwardly rotated more than 3 degrees.

SITTING

Proper Static Alignment	Malalignment Symptom	Cause (Problem)
The pelvis should be level.	Pelvis is higher on the prosthetic side.	Excessive build-up on bottom of socket.
	Pelvis is lower on the prosthetic side.	Inadequate build-up on bottom of socket.
There should be no discomfort or restriction. All edges should be smooth and flared.	Pain at the thigh on the sound leg (the patient is asked to move the normal leg in every direction).	The medial side of the socket is too wide. It should be cut away to relieve the rubbing, leaving the ischial seat intact.
	Pain at the rib cage or lumbar area.	The socket is too high.
	Motion at the hip is impeded.	The hip joint is set too far anterodistally.
Length of the prosthetic thigh should be the same as on the sound side.	Prosthetic thigh is longer than the normal leg.	The hip joint is set too far anteroproximally. The thigh section is too long; knee axis is located too far distally.
	Prosthetic thigh is shorter than the normal leg.	The hip joint is set too far posterodistally. The

		thigh section is too short; the knee axis is located too proximal.
The shin piece should be vertical.	Shin is not vertical.	Knee bolt is not horizontal. Foot is attached in varus or valgus attitude.
Toe-out should be equivalent to the normal side.	Toe-out is inadequate.	Knee bolt is not sufficiently outwardly rotated.
	Toe-out is excessive.	Knee bolt is excessively outwardly rotated.

GENERAL CONSIDERATIONS

Proper Static Alignment	Malalignment Symptom	Cause (Problem)
Suspension: Piston action of the socket should not exceed 0.6 cm (¼ in). This will be greater (1.3 to 2 cm [½ to ¾ in]) with the hemipelvectomy amputee.	Excessive pistoning causing chafing and painful pressures.	The body has not been sufficiently stabilized in the socket. The amputee has lost weight.
Comfort: Check for socket comfort. There should be no pain when full weight is borne in the socket or when sitting.	Ramus pressure.	The ischial seat and other weight-bearing areas are too low and need to be built up.

Cosmetic appearance: The prosthesis should duplicate the sound limb in color and contour.

METHODS OF EVALUATING RESIDUAL LIMB/SOCKET FIT

A properly fitting prosthesis is necessary for maximum comfort and function. A socket that does not fit can result in edema in the residual limb, painful ambulation, skin breakdown, and gait deviations. Many amputees have diminished sensation in the residual limb because of skin grafts or neuropathy, or they have cerebral insufficiency that compromises reliance on subjective complaints. Skin breakdown may precede complaints of discomfort. In such cases, objective evaluation of socket fit is especially important.

Many methods of varying sophistication are utilized to evaluate the critical relationship between the residual limb and the socket. The information gained contributes to the overall knowledge of prosthetics, and the methods used aid in teaching proper socket fabrication.

CHALK, TALCUM, CLAY, LIPSTICK

Chalk, talcum, clay, or lipstick are placed within prosthetic sockets to determine the adequacy of prosthetic fit and the achievement of total contact. Because these methods are adequate for showing contact status at the distal end of the residual limb but not around the periphery, they have met with limited success in the accurate diagnosis of fitting problems.

ELECTRONIC PRESSURE TRANSDUCER

Attempts have been made to use pressure transducers to determine the distribution of forces over the amputation limb. The results have generally been unreliable. The measurement of pressure over a small area, as is done by many pressure transducers, is not as relevant to the assessment of socket-limb relationships as measurement over a large segment of the socket. Most pressure transducers are expensive and fragile, breaking frequently.

RADIOGRAPHIC TECHNIQUE

Roentgenograms of the residual limb in the socket under weight-bearing conditions, which are taken after static and dynamic alignment have been completed, can be used to determine total contact, fit, and alignment. Anterior-posterior and lateral views are needed. Sometimes a third view is taken while the amputee is sitting.

A clear demarcation between the skin and the inner surface of the socket is not usually seen with conventional films. If an x-ray contrast material, such as a saturated solution of sodium iodide in absolute or isopropyl alcohol, is applied topically to the skin of the residual limb, then an adequate visualization of the interface can be made. The contrast medium or lead foil on pressure-sensitive tape can also be applied to the inner surface of the socket or socket insert as a radiopaque marker. However, this is not usually necessary because the insert, if it is leather or hard rubber, and the plastic or wood of the socket are adequately radiopaque for clear visualization of the inner surface of the prosthesis without contrast material.

The utilization of radiologic evaluation of PTB fit and alignment was first reported by R.E. King in 1963. Areas of compression, such as over the patellar tendon, show increased density of the contrast material. Gapping occurs most often between the distal aspect of the limb and the socket.

From an anterior-posterior view, the fit around the femoral condyles and the location of the mediotibial flare on the mediotibial shelf are checked. The distal end of the residual limb is viewed for total contact. Adequacy of relief is checked over the head of the fibula and the distal end of the cut fibula.

From a lateral view, it can be determined if the patellar shelf of the PTB prosthesis makes contact with the patellar tendon midway between the distal patella and the tibial tubercle. The height and flare of the posterior brim in relation to the patellar tendon shelf are assessed. To provide optimum mechanical support, the popliteal bulge may be slightly higher than the patellar tendon shelf, but it is never lower. Relief over the tibial tubercle should be adequate. Total contact is checked, including the distal end, as well as the flexion angle of the socket. Black areas, which denote incomplete contact, require immediate attention.

Pistoning is evaluated by comparing weight-bearing to non–weight-bearing

views. Abrasions on the limb are associated with significant air gaps between the prosthesis and the skin. Roentgenograms may also show bony pathology in the residual
limb, and in some instances, they will even outline arteriosclerotic vessels.

SOCK THAT CONTAINS PRESSURE-SENSITIVE MICROCAPSULES

Paul Brand and colleagues at the United States Public Health Service Hospital, Carville,
Louisiana, developed a pressure-sensitive fabric in which pressure-sensitive microcapsules are embedded in a cloth-backed polyurethane-foam sheet. The socks come in
various sizes, are inexpensive, and are disposable after use.

When external pressure is applied, the microcapsules rupture, releasing a dye
that stains the overlying fabric. In this particular sock, the color remains yellow over
areas of no pressure, changes to green over areas of moderate pressure, and changes to
blue over areas of high pressure. The colors can be better visualized by turning the sock
inside out.

This evaluation method is quick and easy and can be done in the clinic area,
unlike radiographic methods. It produces a three-dimensional picture that can be easily
related to the socket surface, unlike radiographic or pressure transducer methods. It
also differs from pressure transducers in that areas of intense blue may represent areas
of high shear or friction rather than high perpendicular pressure. For example, an area
of deep blue may be seen where the direct pressure measurement is less than 5 psi and
yet an open lesion exists. Neither the pressure transducer nor the pressure-sensitive
sock can be used to determine the amount of pistoning or the presence of bony abnormalities.

TRANSPARENT SOCKETS

The relationship of the residual limb to the socket is masked by the opaqueness of the
socket material. Transparent sockets are used to assess relative motion between the
limb and the socket, as well as to study stress patterns. Pressure points can be readily
observed by soft-tissue blanching. Transparent sockets are used mostly as a research
tool for studying socket design, fitting, and alignment, thus improving fitting practice.

Early attempts at using Plexiglas and Lucite were abandoned because difficulty
was encountered in controlling contours and they required extreme care and an inordi-
nate amount of time because the socket was formed in two parts that were bonded
together. Sockets that are vacuum-formed from transparent polycarbonate material
have proven to be satisfactory. They can be sawed, trimmed, ground, sanded, cut, or
drilled with ordinary tools and bonded with an acrylic cement. A 1 sq ft piece of
polycarbonate is sufficient for most sockets. There is a problem with breakage at the
point of transition where the flexible socket is cemented to the rigid block. Excellent
results have also been claimed with the use of clear polyester casting resin for both
above-knee and below-knee sockets. The role of the transparent socket is still mostly
that of a check or study socket.

THERMOGRAPHY

In thermography, the skin temperature is measured by sensing infrared energy emitted
by the body's surface. Thermography provides a means of mapping warmer and cooler
areas of skin by displaying a white-to-gray-to-black image via cathode-ray tube. The

temperature picture is called a thermogram. Warmer areas can be set to register as either white or black, with cool areas being the opposite. For example, at a base temperature of 90°F, a temperature of 95°F and above may register as absolute white, 85°F and below as absolute black, and the intermediate temperatures as gray.

Warmer areas indicate localized pressure irritation or infection. Thermography can possibly be used to predict future problem areas. Comparative thermographs may show the effect of the socket on the limb over a period of time. Thermography is not considered absolute and should be used along with visual evidence and the subjective report of the amputee. This procedure can be performed quickly and without danger or discomfort to the amputee.

GENERAL INSTRUCTIONS TO AMPUTEES REGARDING A PROSTHESIS

1. The residual limb may undergo changes such as shrinkage, minor skin problems, or some discomfort.
2. Check the residual limb frequently for red spots, abrasions, or skin breakdown.
3. Change the socks daily and use clean socks.
4. Wrap the residual limb when not wearing the prosthesis.
5. Heel heights should not be changed because this will change the alignment.

DYNAMIC ANALYSIS

Dynamic analysis is the evaluation of the amputee and the prosthesis during functional use. A team effort by the physician, prosthetist, and therapist is necessary to evaluate and correct the many possible dynamic problems since they may be due to improper surgery, improper prosthetic construction, or improper gait training, or to amputee factors such as contractures, insecurity, pain, or weakness. Dynamic analysis is performed when the amputee is fairly skilled in the use of the prosthesis.

The following rules are important for a thorough analysis:

1. Analyze gait while the amputee is walking on a level surface.
2. View the amputee laterally, anteriorly, and posteriorly.
3. Pinpoint the exact phase in gait where the deviations occur.
4. Note specific deviations.
5. Analyze gait on uneven terrains and while ascending and descending stairs and inclines.
6. After ambulation, check the residual limb for pain, tenderness, or skin abrasions.

The amputee's gait should be formally evaluated several times during the training process as well as at its termination. The therapist, of course, will analyze various aspects of gait during every training session. The final evaluation will indicate how well the amputee has learned to make use of the prosthesis in all ambulatory activities encountered in daily living.

It should be remembered that a poorly fitted prosthesis may be reasonably comfortable if the amputee uses gait deviations to compensate for errors in fit and alignment. If the same amputee changes to a more normal gait, the prosthesis may be very uncomfortable.

PTB PROSTHESIS

STANCE PHASE

HEEL-STRIKE

Lateral View

Normal	Symptom (Gait Deviation)	Possible Cause (Potential Problem)
The ball of the foot not more than 4 cm (1½ in) from the floor.	Ball of foot dorsiflexed >4 cm (1½ in) from floor. (Fig. 20-11, *left*)	Stride length too long on prosthetic side. Too much dorsiflexion. Excessive socket flexion.
Knee flexed at least 10 to 15 degrees.	Full extension of the knee.	Inadequate cuff suspension. Inadequate socket flexion. Heel lever arm too short.
	Excessive knee flexion.	Knee extensors weak. Knee flexion contracture

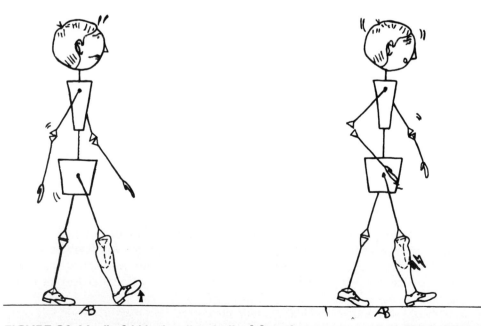

FIGURE 20-11. *(Left)* **Heel-strike: ball of foot is too high off of floor.** *(Right)* **Heel-contact to foot-flat: hyperextension force on knee with anterior distal pressure.**

not compensated for in the prosthesis.
Excessive flexion built into the socket.

Anterior-Posterior View

Normal	Symptom (Gait Deviation)	Possible Cause (Potential Problem)
Foot remains in plane of progression without rotating or exerting a torque on the limb.	External rotation of the prosthesis with resulting torque on the residual limb.	Plantarflexion bumper is too stiff. SACH heel is too hard. Socket is too loose. Too much toe-out built into the prosthesis. Poor muscle control of the prosthesis by the residual limb.

HEEL-CONTACT TO FOOT-FLAT

Lateral View

Normal	Symptom (Gait Deviation)	Possible Cause (Potential Problem)
Knee flexes quickly and smoothly (15 to 20 degrees average range) or same as normal side.	Excessive knee extension. Anterior-distal tibial pressure. Hyperextension force on knee at heel-strike. (See Fig. 20-11, *right*)	Weakness of quadriceps (lean head and shoulders forward). Excessive use of quadriceps. (Bad gait habit.) Too little flexion built into the socket. SACH heel is too soft. Plantarflexion bumper is too soft or is worn. Foot is set too far anterior in relation to socket. (Socket is too far posterior.) Heel lever arm is too short. Suspension strap is too tight.
	Knee is forced into excessive flexion at heel-strike (flexes abruptly, ''jack-knifes'').	Historic foot: plantarflexion bumper too stiff. SACH heel not compressing.

The limb may be forced forward painfully against the socket as the amputee attempts to control the prosthesis by active extension of the knee. (Fig. 20-12, *left*)

a. Heel too firm.
b. SACH foot fits too tight in shoe.

Insufficient relief along anterior-distal tibia.

Shoe heel changed by amputee from low to high.

Too much flexion built into the socket.

Weak quadriceps.

Foot in too much dorsiflexion.

Foot is set too far posterior in relation to socket. (Socket is too far anterior.)

Heel lever arm is too long.

The molded convexity over the patella on the supracondylar/suprapatellar prosthesis is excessive, restricting extension.

Supracondylar cuff attaches too far posterior on the prosthesis. (Sus-

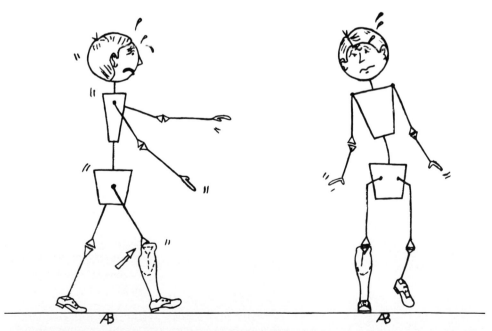

FIGURE 20-12. *(Left)* **Heel-contact to foot-flat: the knee "jackknifes."** *(Right)* **Mid-stance: excessive lateral bending toward the prosthetic side.**

		pension tabs tighten and prevent adequate knee extension.) Knee flexion contracture (without prosthetic compensation).
Compression of SACH heel 1.3 to 1.9 cm (¹/₂ to ³/₄ in) or plantarflexion bumper allows smooth progression to foot-flat.	Toe stays off floor after heel-strike.	Heel wedge is too stiff. Plantarflexion bumper is too stiff. Heel lever arm is too long. (Foot is too far posterior.) Too much dorsiflexion. Inadequate knee flexion built into the socket.
	Foot-slap.	Plantarflexion bumper or SACH heel is too soft. Heel lever arm is too short.

MID-STANCE

Anterior-Posterior View

Normal	Symptom (Gait Deviation)	Possible Cause (Potential Problem)
Lateral bending of trunk not more than 2.5 cm (1 in).	Lateral bending of trunk exceeds 2.5 cm (1 in). Head sway more than 2.5 cm (1 in) toward the prosthetic side. (See Fig. 20-12, right)	Prosthetic foot is outset too far. Prosthesis is too short. Weak gluteus medius (compensated Trendelenburg gait) or arthropathy of the hip. Medial-lateral diameter of socket is too great.
	Inadequate weight shift toward the prosthetic side.	Pain in the residual limb. a. Improper donning. b. Improper socket fit. Insecurity in weight-bearing on the prosthesis. a. Muscular weakness in the amputated limb. b. Improper or inadequate gait training. c. Use of a cane or crutch on the sound side.

		d. Unstable prosthetic alignment.
Foot is flat on the floor.	Inversion or eversion of foot (walks on medial or lateral border of foot). (Fig. 20-13, *left*)	Improper abduction or adduction of socket. Excessive medial-lateral diameter of socket. Malalignment of foot (inverted or everted).
Lateral View. Foot is flat on the floor.	Toe is off of the floor or knee is flexed too much. (See Fig. 20-13, *right*)	Foot is too dorsiflexed. Insufficient initial flexion built into the socket.

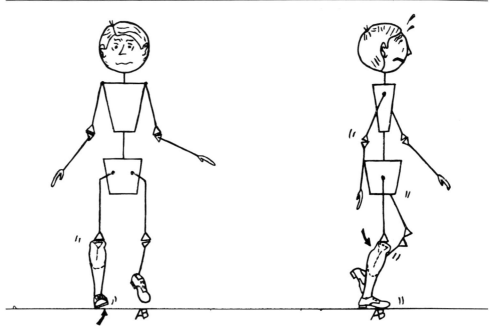

FIGURE 20-13. *(Left)* **Mid-stance: Inversion of the foot.** *(Right)* **Mid-stance: knee is flexed excessively.**

Socket is displaced 0.6 to 1.3 cm (1/4 to 1/2 in) laterally. In general, the longer the limb, the more medial the foot placement.	Valgus moment at knee during stance phase. Excessive pressure proximal-lateral surface of knee and distal-medial area of residual limb. (Fig. 20-14, *left*)	Prosthetic foot is outset too far. (No lateral displacement of socket or some medial displacement.) Pain in peroneal nerve area. (Patient tries to get away from it.) Short amputation limb. (Amputee has to get far over it for balance.) Distal fibular pressure, causing pain.

Knee joint pathology (ligamentous laxity).

	Varus moment at knee during stance phase. Pain on distal-lateral stump. (Lateral displacement exceeds 1.3 cm [1/2 in].) (See Fig. 20-14, *right*)	Short residual limb (short lever arm). Prosthetic foot is inset too far. (Lateral displacement of socket exceeds 1.3 cm [1/2 in].) Excessive medial-lateral diameter (loose socket). Ligamentous laxity.

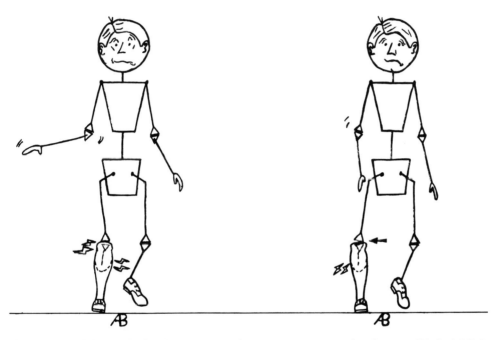

FIGURE 20-14. *(Left)* **Mid-stance: valgus moment at the knee.** *(Right)* **Mid-stance: varus moment at the knee.**

Gait base not more than 5 cm (2 in) wide.	Abducted gait. (Gait base exceeds 5 cm [2 in].) (Fig. 20-15, *left*)	Foot is outset too far. Prosthesis is too long. Limb is not seated well in the socket. Excessive socks. Hip pathology or abduction contracture. Insecurity—intentional for wider base of support.
Equal stance duration on each side.	Short stance on prosthetic side.	Inadequate shift of weight to prosthetic side (see

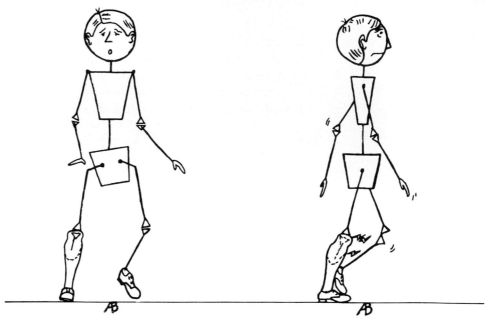

FIGURE 20-15. *(Left)* Mid-stance: abduction of the prosthesis. *(Right)* Mid-stance to toe-off: anterior knee and shin pressure.

		above reasons). Abducted gait.
Equal arm swing.	Arm on prosthetic side held close to body.	Insecurity in weight-bearing on the prosthesis (see above reasons). Pain in the residual limb upon weight-bearing (see above reasons). Unequal step length. Uneven timing. Bad gait habit.

MID-STANCE TO TOE-OFF

Lateral View

Normal	Symptom (Gait Deviation)	Possible Cause (Potential Problem)
Weight is shifted to sound side without perceptible rise of head and torso.	"Hill climbing" sensation toward the end of stance phase—pelvic rise—inability to go over the toe. Anterior knee and shin pressure. (See Fig. 20-15, *right*)	Forefoot is too stiff. Toe lever arm is too long. (Foot is too far anterior.) Too much plantarflexion (insufficient dorsiflexion). Insufficient initial socket flexion.

		Bad gait habit. (Amputee does not try to keep knee bent.) Keel of SACH foot is too long. Change in heel height (high to low).
	Heel is off the floor early. High pressure on patella through most of stance phase.	Foot is too plantarflexed. Excessive knee flexion contracture or hip flexion contracture.
Weight is shifted to sound side without perceptible drop of head or torso.	Drop off: Hips are level but the prosthesis seems short (shortening of prosthetic stance phase and early knee flexion).	Too much initial flexion in socket. Toe lever arm is too short. a. Foot is too far posterior. (Socket is too far anterior in relation to foot.) b. Keel of SACH foot is too short. c. Distance between ankle joint and toe break is too short. Foot is too dorsiflexed. Dorsiflexion bumper has insufficient stiffness. Hip flexion contracture on prosthetic side. Stride is too long on sound side. Hip or knee extensor weakness.
Knee flexion increases smoothly on prosthetic side as center of gravity passes over the prosthesis.	Knee flexes jerkily.	Excessive anterior tilt of socket. Weak knee musculature. Bad gait habit (possibly change from historic to PTB prosthesis). Toe lever arm is too short.
	Knee extends (pressure on front of socket). Inadequate knee flexion. (Fig. 20-16, *left*)	Insufficient anterior tilt of socket (initial socket flexion). Toe lever arm is too long. Toe break is too stiff (results in long toe lever arm). Heel height change (high to low).

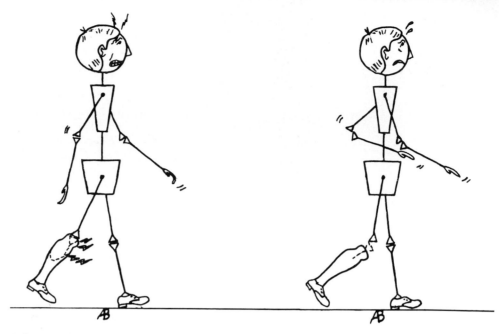

FIGURE 20-16. *(Left)* **Mid-stance to toe-off: knee extends; pressure on front of socket.** *(Right)* **Toe-off: early piston action.**

Normal	Symptom (Gait Deviation)	Possible Cause (Potential Problem)
		Shoe vamp is too tight. Forefoot is too stiff. Intentional due to fear of knee collapse (weak knee extensors).
Socket remains securely on residual limb.	Early piston action. (See Fig. 20-16, *right*)	Inadequate suspension device.

SWING PHASE

LATERAL VIEW

Normal	Symptom (Gait Deviation)	Possible Cause (Potential Problem)
Socket remains securely on the limb.	Piston action. (Fig. 20-17)	Faulty suspension device. Improper donning. Improper socket fit. a. Inadequate socks. b. Loss of weight. c. Muscle atrophy.
Ball of foot is not over 2.5 cm (1 in) from the floor.	Ball of foot >2.5 cm (1 in) from the floor.	Stride length is too long (gait training problem).

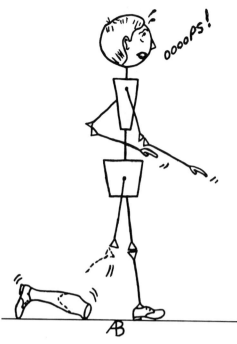

FIGURE 20-17. Swing phase: loss of suspension.

		Excessive anterior tilt of socket. Excessive dorsiflexion of foot.
Ample toe clearance.	Drags toe on floor—toe stubbing. (Fig. 20-18) OR Vaulting—rising on the toe of the sound foot to permit the prosthesis to swing through.	Weak hip or knee flexors. Prosthesis is too long. Inadequate initial knee flexion in socket. Foot is set in plantarflexion or inadequate dorsiflexion. Limb not seated in socket. a. Improper donning. b. Excessive socks. c. Edema of the residual limb.
Equal stride length.	Unequal stride length. a. Longer on prosthetic side.	Pain from a malfitting socket (stance phase is shorter on prosthetic side). Prosthesis is too long. Insecurity during stance phase (shorter stance phase) on prosthesis. Hip flexion contracture on amputated side. Knee flexion contracture on sound side.

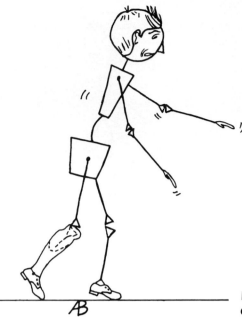

AB

FIGURE 20-18. Swing phase: toe stubs on floor.

b. Shorter on the prosthetic side.	Excessive initial socket flexion. Prosthesis is too short. Hip flexion contracture on sound side. Inadequate strength to advance prosthetic leg. Knee flexion contracture on prosthetic side (exceeds flexion built into the socket).

POSTERIOR VIEW

Normal	Symptom (Gait Deviation)	Possible Cause (Potential Problem)
Shank and foot swing through on line of progression.	Whip—axial rotation of prosthesis in swing phase.	Rotation of limb within socket. a. Socket is too large. b. Shrinkage of residual limb. c. Inadequate socks. Prosthesis donned incorrectly. Improper placement of cuff suspension studs. Bad gait habit.

a. Medial whip (medial deviation of heel during swing phase). (Fig. 20-19, *left*)	Medial stud is anterior to the lateral stud (external rotation of socket).
b. Lateral whip (lateral deviation of the heel during swing phase). (See Fig. 20-19, *right*)	Lateral stud is anterior to the medial stud (internal rotation of socket).

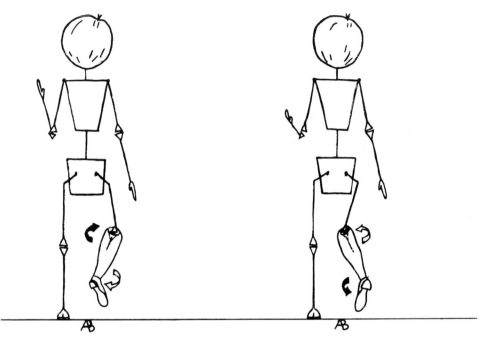

FIGURE 20-19. *(Left)* **Swing phase: medial whip.** *(Right)* **Swing phase: lateral whip.**

ANTERIOR-POSTERIOR VIEW

Normal	Symptom (Gait Deviation)	Possible Cause (Potential Problem)
The shank and foot swing through on the line of progression.	Circumduction—a semicircular swing of the prosthesis to the side. (Fig. 20-20)	Prosthesis is too long. Limb is not seated in the socket. a. Improper donning. b. Excessive socks. c. Edema of residual limb. Knee flexion is limited or painful.

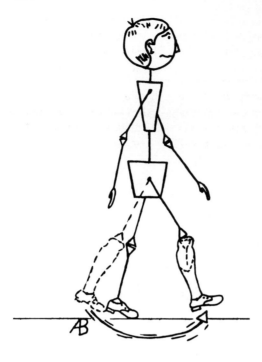

FIGURE 20-20. Swing phase: circum-duction of the prosthesis.

		Inadequate suspension. Substitution for inadequate hip or knee flexion.
The pelvis should be level.	Pelvic rise.	Prosthesis is too long. Foot is in too much plantarflexion. Keel of SACH foot is too long. Substitute for inadequate hip or knee flexion. Foot designed for a high heel and using a low heel. Inadequate suspension.

INSPECTION OF RESIDUAL LIMB

Normal	Symptom (Gait Deviation)	Possible Cause (Potential Problem)
There should be no skin abrasions.	Abrasions over: a. Head of fibula. b. Tibial tubercle. c. Anterodistal tibia.	Foot is outset too far. Pistoning. a. Limb shrinkage. b. Inadequate suspension device. c. Inadequate sock thickness.

	d. Socket diameter is too great. Inadequate relief areas. Improper donning.
Abrasions over the hamstring tendons. (Limb comes out of the socket with knee flexion—sitting.)	Inadequate relief area for the hamstring tendons. Limb is too deep in the socket. a. Limb shrinkage. b. Inadequate socks.

ABOVE-KNEE PROSTHESIS

STANCE PHASE

HEEL-CONTACT TO FOOT-FLAT

Lateral View

Normal	Symptom (Gait Deviation)	Possible Cause (Potential Problem)
Knee is stable in extension.	Knee is forced into flexion (instability of prosthetic knee). (Fig. 20-21, *left*)	SACH heel not compressing adequately. a. Heel is too firm. b. SACH foot fits too tight in shoe. Plantarflexion bumper is too stiff. Foot is in too much dorsiflexion. Heel lever arm is too long. (Socket is too far anterior.) Knee axis is too far anterior to hip and ankle joints. Severe hip flexion contracture. Insufficient initial flexion built into the socket. Weak hip extensors (when using mechanical friction knee unit), especially if knee axis is anterior to the TA line. Shoe heel changed by amputee from low to high. Anterior-posterior diameter of socket is too

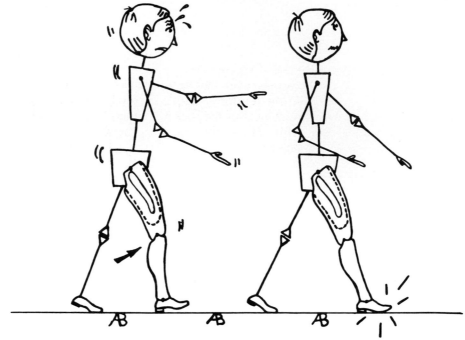

FIGURE 20-21. *(Left)* **Heel-contact: knee is forced into flexion.** *(Right)* **Heel-contact to foot-flat: foot slap.**

		small—excessive pressure on the hamstring tendons at the ischial tuberosity, reducing the functioning of these muscles.
Forefoot descends gradually. Smooth and controlled plantarflexion.	Foot slap. (See Fig. 20-21, *right*)	SACH foot—heel is too soft. Heel lever arm is too short. Plantarflexion bumper is too soft or worn out.
Heel into contact with floor gently.	Forceful impact of heel with floor. (Fig. 20-22, *left*)	Insufficient gait training. Lack of confidence. (Amputee forcefully brings heel into contact with floor to ensure knee stability.)

Anterior-Posterior View

Normal	Symptom (Gait Deviation)	Possible Cause (Potential Problem)
Foot remains in plane of progression without rotating or exerting a torque on the limb.	External rotation of prosthesis with resulting twisting torque on residual limb. (See Fig. 20-22, *right*)	Plantarflexion bumper is too stiff. SACH heel is too hard. Anterior-medial rim pressure on pelvis. Too much toe-out built into the prosthesis. Socket is too loose. Poor muscle control of the prosthesis by residual limb (such as a new suction socket wearer). Amputee may extend limb too vigorously.

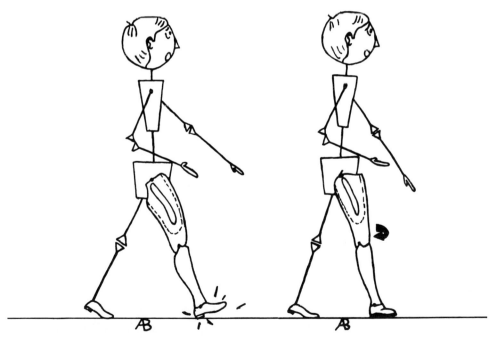

FIGURE 20-22. *(Left)* **Heel-contact: forceful impact of heel with floor.** *(Right)* **Heel-contact to foot-flat: external rotation of prosthesis.**

MID-STANCE

Anterior-Posterior View

Normal	Symptom (Gait Deviation)	Possible Cause (Potential Problem)
The pelvis drops only 5 degrees on the non–weight-bearing side during normal locomotion. The pelvis is stabilized by the action of the gluteus medius.	Excessive drop of the pelvis on the sound side, which results in crotch pressure and pain as the pubic ramus comes into hard contact with the medial brim. (Medial-lateral instability.) The amputee usually compensates by abducting the prosthesis or laterally bending toward the prosthetic side to avoid the pain.	Inadequate adduction of the femur in the socket. Weak hip abductors (uncompensated Trendelenburg gait). Inadequate support to the lateral side.
Lateral bending of the trunk (2.5 cm [1 in] at the head). (Those with short amputation limbs will bend more.) Medial-lateral stability.	Lateral bending of the trunk toward the prosthetic side. (Excessive bending laterally from the midline.) This is usually present when the amputee walks with an abducted gait. (Fig. 20-23, *left*)	Lateral wall of the socket is abducted too much (does not provide adequate support to the femur; inadequate adduction angle to the socket). Medial wall of socket causing painful pressure on the pubic ramus. a. Medial wall is too high. b. Anterior-posterior diameter is too great. Weakness of hip abductors (compensated Trendelenburg gait) on prosthetic side. Contracture of hip abductors. Foot is outset too far. Prosthesis is too short. Lateral side of limb is painful (improper contouring of lateral wall). Medial-lateral diameter of socket is too great. A short amputation limb

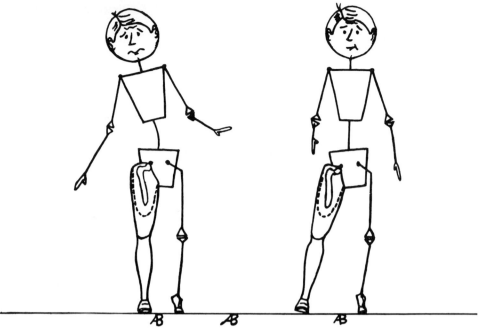

FIGURE 20-23. *(Left)* **Mid-stance: excessive lateral bending toward the prosthetic side.** *(Right)* **Mid-stance: abduction of the prosthesis.**

		(inadequate support to the femur).
Width of gait base should not exceed 5 cm (2 in) between the medial borders of the heel as the swing foot passes the stance foot. Narrow-base gait.	Abducted gait (a very wide base with the prosthesis held away from the midline at all times). This results in a side-to-side swaying. (See Fig. 20-23, *right*)	Prosthesis is aligned in too much abduction. a. Shank is aligned in valgus position with respect to thigh. b. Mechanical hip joint of pelvic band is set so that the socket is in abduction. c. Too much abduction built into the socket. Medial wall is causing painful pressure on the pubic ramus. a. Medial wall is too high. b. Anterior-posterior diameter of socket is too great; ischial tuberosity is not on the shelf but is forward in the socket.

c. Hip flexion contracture causing excessive anterior pelvic rotation results in medial brim pressure.

Prosthesis is too long.

Poor balance; therefore, widened base of support.

Contracture of abductor muscles.

Painful pressure on lateral distal femur in socket (improper contouring of lateral wall).

Bad gait habit.

Weak hip extensors (abduct prosthesis to avoid flexing the knee, which requires hip extension at heel-strike for stability).

The ischial tuberosity should be centered over the heel, and the pelvis should be level.	Lateral gapping of the socket. (Fig. 20-24)	Medial-lateral diameter of the socket is excessive. Foot is inset too far. Inward slope of the posterior brim causing the residual limb to slide inward, resulting in adductor pressure.

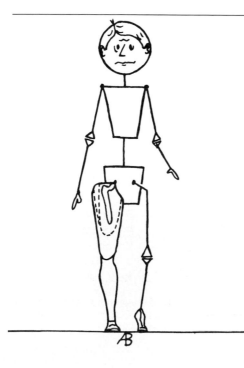

FIGURE 20-24. Mid-stance: lateral gapping of the socket.

MID-STANCE TO TOE-OFF

Lateral View

Normal	Symptom (Gait Deviation)	Possible Cause (Potential Problem)
Smooth heel-rise without excessive rise of center of gravity.	Premature heel-rise with sudden knee bend. (Fig. 20-25A)	Foot set in plantarflexion. Hip flexion contracture not adequately compensated for by initial flexion built into the socket.
	Late heel-rise. (See Fig. 20-25B)	Foot set in dorsiflexion. Dorsiflexion bumper is too soft or worn.
Torso does not rise or fall more than 4 cm (1½ in).	Pelvic rise—"hill climbing"—as the amputee rolls over the ball of the prosthetic foot. (See Fig. 20-25C)	Toe lever arm is too long. (Distance between ankle and toe break is too great.) a. Toe break is too far forward. b. Keel of SACH foot is too long. SACH foot is too tight in the shoe (stiff shoe vamp). Change in heel height (high to low).

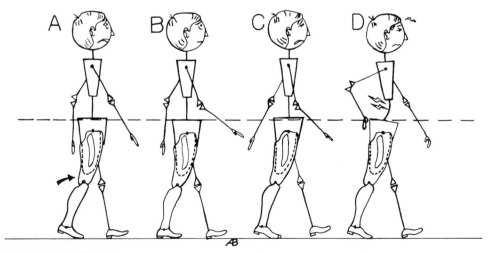

FIGURE 20-25. Mid-stance to toe-off: *(A)* premature heel-rise with sudden knee bend, *(B)* late heel-rise, *(C)* pelvic rise ("hill climbing"), and *(D)* excessive lumbar lordosis.

		Too much plantarflexion (insufficient dorsiflexion).
The hip extends without excessive lumbar lordosis.	Excessive lumbar lordosis. (See Fig. 20-25D)	Flexion contracture of the hip or joint pathology limiting extension not compensated for by initial flexion built into the socket. Posterior wall of socket improperly shaped. (Amputee is trying to avoid weight-bearing on the ischium.) Weak abdominal muscles. Weak hip extensors.
As the residual limb extends at push-off, the ischial tuberosity remains on the ischial seat.	The hamstring muscles force the ischial tuberosity off of the ischial seat, causing pressure on the hamstring muscles.	Overdeveloped hamstring musculature. Contour of socket wall is inadequate for muscle bulk. Inadequate initial socket flexion.

Center of gravity follows a smooth, uninterrupted fall.
No knee flexion.
	Drop off—excessive pelvic drop just prior to swing phase as the body moves over the prosthesis. (Fig. 20-26)	Toe lever arm is too short.
		  a. Distance between ankle joint and toe break is too short.
		  b. Keel of SACH foot is too short.
		  c. Socket is too far anterior in relation to the foot.
		Weak or worn dorsiflexion bumper.
		Foot is too dorsiflexed.
		Sponge rubber toe is too soft.
		Stride is too long on the sound side.

Knee should feel secure during the transition from stance to swing phase.	Knee feels insecure.	Excessive ankle dorsiflexion. Soft dorsiflexion bumper. Toe break is not at right angles to the line of progression, resulting in a rapid shift of the center of pressure during push-off.

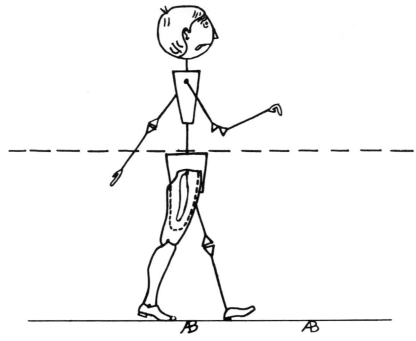

FIGURE 20-26. Mid-stance to toe-off: excessive pelvic drop.

Effortless flexion of the hip.	Delay in the initiation of swing phase (knee flexion).	Prosthetic knee axis is posterior to the TA line (too much alignment stability). Hydraulic knee mechanism fluid is too viscous. Knee mechanical friction is too great. Toe lever arm is too long.

SWING PHASE

ACCELERATION

Posterior View

Normal	Symptom (Gait Deviation)	Possible Cause (Potential Problem)
The prosthetic leg swings forward in the line of progression. The knee axis is set in 5 degrees of external rotation to compensate for the tendency	Whips are best observed when the patient walks away from the observer. Medial whip: inward movement of heel, outward movement of knee	Bad gait habit. Axis of knee joint is rotated too far externally. Varus knee.

of the femur to rotate medially as the hip is flexed.

on initial flexion at the beginning of swing phase.
(Fig. 20-27, *left*)

Prosthesis may be donned with the socket externally rotated.

Socket is too tight or insufficient socket contour to accommodate muscle contraction. The contracting muscle bellies cause the prosthesis to rotate on its long axis.

Toe break is not set at a right angle to the line of progression.

Silesian bandage is too tight.

Residual limb is weak. The musculature rotates around the femur.

Lateral whip: outward movement of the heel, inward movement of the knee on initial flexion at the beginning of swing phase.
(See Fig. 20-27, *right*)

Axis of knee joint is rotated too far internally.

Valgus knee.

Prosthesis may be donned with the socket internally rotated.

Socket is too tight or insufficient socket contour to accommodate muscle contraction. The contracting muscle bellies

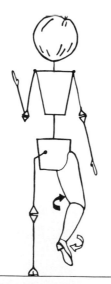
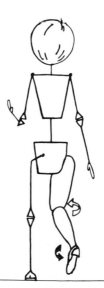

FIGURE 20-27. *(Left)* Swing phase: medial whip. *(Right)* Swing phase: lateral whip.

cause the prosthesis to rotate on its long axis.

Toe break is not set at a right angle to the line of progression.

Residual limb is weak. The musculature rotates around the femur.

Lateral View

Normal	Symptom (Gait Deviation)	Possible Cause (Potential Problem)
Smooth heel-rise equal to sound side.	Excessive heel-rise. (Excessive knee flexion at the beginning of swing phase.) It is often associated with terminal-impact. (Fig. 20-28, *left*)	Insufficient knee friction. (Insufficient knee flexion resistance.) Inadequate extension aid. Amputee flexes the hip too vigorously at the initiation of swing phase.
	Insufficient heel-rise.	Excessive friction on the prosthetic knee or manual knee lock. Extension aid is too tight. Insecurity. Amputee walks with little or no knee flexion.

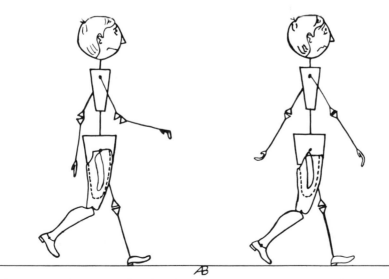

FIGURE 20-28. *(Left)* **Swing phase: excessive heel-rise.** *(Right)* **Swing phase: excessive piston action.**

| No piston action. (Socket remains secure on residual limb.) | Excessive piston action. (See Fig. 20-28, *right*) | Socket is too large. Loose suspension. Improper donning. Excessive shrinkage. Inadequate socks. |

SWING-THROUGH

Anterior-Posterior View

Normal	Symptom (Gait Deviation)	Possible Cause (Potential Problem)
Smooth pelvic rise on the sound side.	Vaulting—rising on the toe of the sound foot to permit the prosthesis to swing through (with little or no knee flexion) without stubbing the prosthetic toe. Pelvic hike on the prosthetic side. OR The toe stubs.	Prosthesis is too long. a. Excessive length. b. Inadequate donning (not seated in socket). Excessive pistoning. a. Socket is too large. b. Inadequate suspension device. Limited prosthetic knee flexion. a. Excessive knee friction. b. Excessive alignment stability. c. Excessive extension aid. d. Knee locked. e. Gait pattern—amputee does not initiate knee flexion because of poor balance or fear of falling, or amputee vaults because of fear of stubbing the toe. Amputee is walking at a faster speed without a mechanical adjustment of the knee friction. (If the amputee did not vault, the knee would not have time to reach full extension before heel-strike.) Excessive plantarflexion. The toe lever arm is too long.

		Substitute for inadequate hip flexion.

The prosthesis swings through on the line of progression.	Circumduction (a swinging of the entire prosthesis laterally in a wide arc—returning to the line of progression).	Prosthesis is too long.
		a. Excessive length.
		b. Inadequate donning (not seated in socket).
		Limited prosthetic knee flexion. (Difficulty in bending the knee during swing-through.)
		  a. Excessive knee friction or hydraulic resistance.
		  b. Excessive alignment stability.
		  c. Lack of confidence by the amputee because of muscle weakness, lack of balance, or fear of stubbing the toe.
		  d. Excessive extension aid.
		  e. Knee locked.
		Gluteus medius weakness on the unamputated side.
		Abduction contracture on the prosthetic side.
		Medial wall of the socket is too thick proximally.
		Bad gait habit.
		Inadequate socket suspension.
		Substitute for inadequate hip flexion.
		Foot is set in plantarflexion.

DECELERATION

Lateral View

Normal	Symptom (Gait Deviation)	Possible Cause (Potential Problem)
Knee extension is smooth and noiseless to neutral.	Terminal-impact. (A rapid forward movement of the shin piece, which reaches maximum extension with excessive	Insufficient knee friction. Extension aid is too strong. Rapid, forceful extension of the limb by the amputee. (This cue tells the

	force just before heel-strike.)	amputee that the knee is extended and thus stable.)
Equal stride length to the sound side.	Unequal step length. a. Longer on the prosthetic side. Shorter step with the sound leg.	Pain from a malfitting socket. (Stance phase is shorter.) Hip flexion contracture is not accommodated by initial socket flexion. Prosthesis is constructed too long. Excessive pistoning. Excessive socks. Insecurity during stance phase. (Stance phase is shorter.)
	b. Shorter on the prosthetic side.	Prosthesis is too short. The heel lever arm is too short.
Knee extension is to neutral.	Hyperextension of the knee.	The knee axis is excessively posterior to the TA line, resulting in a worn extension bumper. Insufficient flexion of the posterior wall.
Arm swing is equal bilaterally.	Uneven arm swing. (Arm on the prosthetic side is held close to the body.)	Unequal step length. Poor balance. Uneven timing. Fear and insecurity. Painful limb. Bad gait habit.
Steps should be of even duration.	Uneven timing. (Steps of uneven duration, usually shorter on prosthetic side.)	Pain from malfitting socket. Knee bolt is higher or lower than the sound knee axis. Prolonged prosthetic swing-through. a. Weak extension aid causing excessive heel-rise. b. Insufficient knee friction or hydraulic resistance causing excessive heel-rise. c. Excessive knee friction or hydraulic re-

sistance (takes longer step to allow time for shank to swing forward).

Poor balance, fear, or insecurity.

Bad gait habit.

CANADIAN-TYPE HIP-DISARTICULATION PROSTHESIS

STANCE PHASE

HEEL-CONTACT TO FOOT-FLAT

Lateral View

Normal	Symptom (Gait Deviation)	Possible Cause (Potential Problem)
Heel-Strike Hip joint is flexed and free of the hip extension bumper. Knee is fully extended. Line of support passes through the posterior tip of the heel and center of the hip joint.	Hip extension bumper comes into contact before the foot is flat. Knee buckles.	Hip extension bumper is too thick. SACH heel is too firm. Plantarflexion bumper is too firm.
Foot-Flat Foot goes flat to the floor by action of the ankle joint or compression of the SACH heel. The heel should be very soft, providing added stability at the knee. The hip bumper has not made contact.		

MID-STANCE

Lateral View

Normal	Symptom (Gait Deviation)	Possible Cause (Potential Problem)
Contact is made with the hip bumper. The hip	Drop in socket just before the hip bumper makes	Hip joint is mounted too far forward.

| joint becomes stable, making it safe to lift the opposite leg. Prosthetic motion now occurs at the ankle (foot). | contact. Hyperextension of the prosthetic hip. | Excessive compression of the hip bumper. Worn rubber hip extension stop. |

Anterior-Posterior View

Normal	Symptom (Gait Deviation)	Possible Cause (Potential Problem)
Lateral bending of the trunk is not excessive. Medial-lateral stability.	Excessive lateral bending toward the prosthetic side.	Walking base is too wide. (Foot is outset too far.) Inadequate medial-lateral stability.

MID-STANCE TO TOE-OFF

Lateral View

Normal	Symptom (Gait Deviation)	Possible Cause (Potential Problem)
Ankle (foot) provides a smooth, rolling action from heel to toe. Body weight produces a downward force in the socket behind the hip joint. Knee flexion is initiated before toe-off by a posterior pelvic tilt (effort to keep the pelvis vertical) in combination with the weight passing posterior to the knee axis. The amputee does not lift the pelvis to swing the prosthetic leg forward but rather sits hard on the prosthesis to initiate knee flexion.	Difficulty in flexing the knee.	Torso is not kept vertical. The patient is leaning forward on crutches or parallel bars. Amputee lifts the pelvis to swing the leg forward rather than sitting hard in the socket to initiate knee flexion.

SWING PHASE

LATERAL VIEW

Normal	Symptom (Gait Deviation)	Possible Cause (Potential Problem)
Early The hip joint is in contact with the bumper, and the check-strap is assisting knee extension. The prosthetic leg swings forward in the line of progression. The knee axis is set in 5 degrees of external rotation.	Medial whip	Knee externally rotated more than 5 degrees.
	Lateral whip	Knee externally rotated less than 5 degrees or medially rotated.
The prosthetic foot lifts clear of the floor, but not excessively. The prosthesis swings forward like a pendulum.	Since there is no means to actively flex the hip, vaulting or hip hiking on the prosthetic side (pelvic list), causing the limb to abduct, may be the only way to get toe clearance. OR The toe drags.	Prosthesis is too long. Inadequate suspension (pistoning). Foot in plantarflexion. Knee flexion is inadequate. a. Kick-strap tension is too great. b. Knee friction is too great.
	Excessive heel-rise.	Stride length control strap is too loose. Knee friction is inadequate.
Firm fit between the stump and socket allows control and minimal motion.	Pistoning.	Socket is too loose. a. Socket is too large. b. Inadequate contour over iliac crest(s).
Late After the knee extends completely, hip flexion is limited by the check-strap. The distance between toe-off and heel-strike should be the same for the two legs.	Stride length is longer on the prosthetic side.	Check-strap is too loose. Hip extension bumper is too thick. (Shortens step on sound side.)
	Stride is shorter on the prosthetic side.	Check-strap is too tight. Hip extension bumper is too thin. (Lengthens step on sound side.)

| Knee extension is smooth and noiseless to neutral. | Terminal-impact. | Kick-strap is too tense. Inadequate friction in knee. |

BIBLIOGRAPHY

STATIC ANALYSIS

ANDERSON, MH, BRAY, JJ, AND HENNESSY, CA: *Prosthetic Principles: Above Knee Amputations.* Charles C Thomas, Springfield, Ill, 1960.

APPOLDT, FA, BENNETT, L, AND CONTINI, R: *Socket pressure as a function of pressure transducer protrusion.* Bull Prosthet Res 10–11:236–249, 1969.

APPOLDT, FA, BENNETT, L, AND CONTINI, R: *Tangential pressure measurements in above-knee suction sockets.* Bull Prosthet Res 10–13:70–86, 1970.

Below-Knee and Above-Knee Prostheses. A Report of a Workshop Sponsored by the Committee on Prosthetics Research and Development, Division of Medical Sciences, National Research Council, National Academy of Sciences, 1973.

BERGTHOLDT, HT, AND BRAND, PW: *Thermography: An aid in the management of insensitive feet and stumps.* Arch Phys Med Rehabil 56:205–209, 1975.

BERME, N, PURDEY, CR, AND SOLOMONIDIS, SE: *Measurement of prosthetic alignment.* Prosthet Orthot Int 2:73–75, 1978.

BYER, JL: *X-rays: A "fitting tool" for the prosthetist.* Orth Pros 28:55–57, 1974.

CANZONERI, J, 3RD, LEAVITT, LA, AND PETERSON, CR: *Prosthetic ambulation: Automatic analysis of gait and stump socket pressure dynamics.* Automedia 1:13–18, 1973.

ERIKSON, U AND JAMES, U: *Roentgenological study of certain stump-socket relationships in above-knee amputees with special regard to tissue proportions, socket fit and attachment stability.* Ups J Med Sci 78:203–214, 1973.

FAULKNER, V AND PRITHAM, C: *A preliminary report on the use of thermography as a diagnostic aid in prosthetics.* Orth Pros 20:26–69, 1973.

FOORT, J: *Construction and fitting of the Canadian-type hip-disarticulation prosthesis.* Artificial Limbs 4:39–51, 1957.

GARDNER, HF AND CLIPPINGER, FW, JR: *A method for location of prosthetic and orthotic knee joints.* Artificial Limbs 13:31–35, 1969.

GOLLER, H, LEWIS, DW, AND McLAUGHLIN, RE: *Thermographic studies of human skin subjected to localized pressure.* Am J Roentgenol Radium Ther Nucl Med 113:749–754, 1971.

GRILLE, T, LIPSKIN, R, AND HANAK, R: *The NYU transparent socket fabrication procedure.* Artificial Limbs 13:13–30, 1969.

HAMONTREE, S AND SNELSON, R: *The use of check sockets in lower-limb prosthetics.* Orth Pros 27:30–33, 1973.

HAMONTREE, S AND SNELSON, R: *The use of check sockets in lower-limb prosthetics.* In *Selected Readings: A Review of Orthotics and Prosthetics.* American Orthotics and Prosthetics Association, Washington, DC, 1980, pp 83–86.

HAMPTON, FL: *Above-knee prostheses.* Orthop Clin North Am 3:359–372, 1972.

HAMPTON, FL: *Prosthetic principles in the lower extremity amputee.* Orthop Clin North Am 3:339–347, 1972.

IULIUCCI, L AND DeGAETANO, R: *VAPC Technique for Fabricating a Plastic Syme Prosthesis with*

Medial Opening: Fabrication Manual. Veterans Administration Prosthetics Center, New York, 1969.

KAY, HW, AND NEWMAN, JD: *Report of a workshop on below-knee and above-knee prosthetics.* Orth Pros 27:9–25, 1973.

LEAVITT, LA, ET AL: *Quantitative method to measure the relationship between prosthetic gait and the forces produced at the stump-socket interface.* Am J Phys Med 49:192–203, 1970.

LECONTE, RG: *New war methods in amputations, stumps and prosthesis of the lower limbs.* US Nav M Bull 13:244–254, 1919.

MARGETIS, PM, ET AL: *A fluid resin technique for the fabrication of check sockets.* Orth Pros 22:8–27, 1968.

MCCOLLOUGH, NC AND GILMER, RE, JR: *A method of determining total contact in prostheses.* Inter-Clinic Info Bull 6:9–13, 1967.

MCLAURIN, CA: *The Canadian hip-disarticulation prosthesis.* In MURDOCH, G (ED): *Prosthetic and Orthotic Practice.* Edward Arnold & Co, London, 1970, pp 285–304.

MCQUIRK, AW: *The Canadian hip disarticulation prosthesis and modifications required for the hemipelvectomy.* In MURDOCH, G (ED): *Prosthetic and Orthotic Practice.* Edward Arnold & Co, London, 1970, pp 305–311.

MEIER, RH, 3RD, MEEKS, ED, JR, AND HERMAN, RM: *Stump-socket fit of below-knee prostheses: Comparison of three methods of measurement.* Arch Phys Med Rehabil 54:553–558, 1973.

MOONEY, V AND SNELSON, R: *Fabrication and application of transparent polycarbonate sockets.* Orth Pros 26:1–13, 1972.

MOONEY, V AND SNELSON, R: *Feasibility Study of the Use of Transparent Sockets and Modular Prostheses in Clinical Practice: Final Report.* Department of Health, Education and Welfare, Social and Rehabilitation Service, Washington, DC, 1973.

RADCLIFFE, CW: *Alignment of the above-knee artificial leg.* In KLOPSTEG, PE AND WILSON, PD: *Human Limbs and their Substitutes.* Hafner Publishing, New York, 1954, pp 676–692.

RADCLIFFE, CW: *Functional considerations in the fitting of above-knee prostheses.* Artificial Limbs 2:35–60, 1955.

RADCLIFFE, CW: *The biomechanics of the Canadian-type hip-disarticulation prosthesis.* Artificial Limbs 4:29–38, 1957.

RADCLIFFE, CW: *Biomechanics of above-knee prostheses.* In MURDOCH, G (ED): *Prosthetic and Orthotic Practice.* Edward Arnold & Co, London, 1970, pp 191–198.

RADCLIFFE, CW: *Functional considerations in the fitting of above-knee prostheses.* In *Selected Articles from Artificial Limbs: January 1954–Spring 1966.* Robert E. Krieger Publishing, Huntington, New York, 1970, pp 5–30.

RADCLIFFE, CW AND FOORT, J: *The Patellar-Tendon-Bearing Below-Knee Prosthesis.* Biomechanics Laboratory, University of California at San Francisco and Berkeley, 1961.

RADCLIFFE, CW, JOHNSON, NC, AND FOORT, J: *Some experience with prosthetic problems of above-knee amputees.* Artificial Limbs 4:41–75, 1957.

RAJESWARAMMA, V, ET AL: *Pressure-sensitive stump sock.* Arch Phys Med Rehabil 54:142–144, 1973.

REGER, SI, ET AL: *Applications of transparent sockets.* Orth Pros 30:35–39, 1976.

SEEBER, JJ, MAGILNER, A, AND REYES, T: *Radiologic technique to evaluate patellar-tendon-bearing prosthesis.* Arch Phys Med Rehabil 53:65–69, 1972.

SHEPLAN, L, LIEBERMAN, B, AND SARMIENTO, A: *Patellar tendon bearing prostheses: Value of routine x-ray studies.* South Med J 62:1223–1226, 1969.

SNELSON, R: *Fabrication of vacuum-formed sockets for limb prostheses.* Orth Pros 27:3–13, 1973.

SNELSON, R: *Fabrication of vacuum-formed sockets for limb prostheses.* In *Selected Readings: A*

Review of Orthotics and Prosthetics. American Orthotics and Prosthetics Association, Washington, DC, 1980, pp 72–82.

STROHM, BR AND OGG, L: *Patellar tendon bearing-cuff suspension below-knee prosthesis: An evaluation procedure.* Phys Ther Rev 41:339–347, 1961.

Suggestions for Fitting and Aligning the SACH Foot. VA Prosthetics Center, 1970.

TAFT, CB: *Radiographic evaluation of stump-socket fit.* Artificial Limbs 13:36–40, 1969.

TOSBERG, WA: *Prosthetic management of the proximal A-K amputations.* In *Prosthetics International, Proceedings of the Second International Prosthetics Course, Committee on Prostheses, Braces and Technical Aids, International Society for the Welfare of Cripples.* Copenhagen, 1960, pp 111–112.

TOSBERG, WA: *Relationship of socket shape to anatomy and biomechanics.* In *Prosthetics International, Proceedings of the Second International Prosthetics Course, Commiteee on Prostheses, Braces and Technical Aids, International Society for the Welfare of Cripples.* Copenhagen, 1960, pp 109–110.

WILSON, AB, JR: *The connection.* Acta Orthop Scand 44:583–588, 1973.

WILSON, LA AND LYQUIST, E: *Plaster bandage wrap cast: Procedure for the below-knee stump.* Prosthet Int 3:3–7, 1968.

DYNAMIC ANALYSIS

ANDERSON, MH, BRAY, JJ, AND HENNESSY, CA: *Prosthetic Principles: Above Knee Amputations.* Charles C Thomas, Springfield, Ill, 1960.

BARCLAY, W: *Below-knee amputation-prosthesis.* In MURDOCH, G (ED): *Prosthetic and Orthotic Practice.* Edward Arnold & Co, London, 1970, pp 69–78.

BREAKEY, J: *Gait of unilateral below-knee amputees.* In *Selected Readings: A Review of Orthotics and Prosthetics.* American Orthotics and Prosthetics Association, Washington, DC, 1980, pp 154–162.

CHODERA, JD: *Analysis of gait from footprints.* Physiotherapy 60:179–181, 1974.

FLEER, B AND WILSON, AB, JR: *Construction of the patellar-tendon-bearing below-knee prosthesis.* Artificial Limbs 6:25–73, 1962.

FOORT, J: *Construction and fitting of the Canadian-type hip-disarticulation prosthesis.* Artificial Limbs 4:39–51, 1957.

FOORT, J: *The patellar-tendon-bearing prosthesis for below-knee amputees: A review of technique and criteria.* Artificial Limbs 9:4–13, 1965.

HAMPTON, FL: *Above-knee prostheses.* Orthop Clin North Am 3:359–372, 1972.

HAMPTON, FL: *Prosthetic principles in the lower extremity amputee.* Orthop Clin North Am 3:339–347, 1972.

LEAVITT, LA, ET AL: *Quantitative method to measure the relationship between prosthetic gait and forces produced at the stump-socket interface.* Am J Phys Med 49:192–203, 1970.

LEAVITT, LA AND ZUNIGA, EN: *Gait analysis in a series of normal subjects as related to above-the-knee amputees.* Isr J Med Sci 9:592–598, 1973.

LEAVITT, LA, ET AL: *Gait analysis and tissue-socket interface pressures in above-knee amputees.* South Med J 65:1197–1207, 1972.

McLAURIN, CA: *The Canadian hip-disarticulation prosthesis.* In MURDOCH, G (ED): *Prosthetic and Orthotic Practice.* Edward Arnold & Co, London, 1970, pp 286–304.

MITAL, MA AND PIERCE, DS: *Amputees and Their Prostheses.* Little, Brown & Co, 1971, pp 150–154; 158–164.

MURPHY, EF: *Swing phase of walking with above-knee prostheses.* Bull Prosthet Res 10–1:5–39, 1964.

RADCLIFFE, CW: *Alignment of the above-knee artificial leg.* In KLOPSTEG, PE AND WILSON, PD: *Human Limbs and their Substitutes.* Hafner Publishing, New York, 1954, pp 676–692.

RADCLIFFE, CW: *Functional considerations in the fitting of above-knee prostheses.* Artificial Limbs 2:35–60, 1955.

RADCLIFFE, CW: *The biomechanics of the Canadian-type hip-disarticulation prosthesis.* Artificial Limbs 4:29–38, 1957.

RADCLIFFE, CW: *Functional considerations in the fitting of above-knee prostheses.* In *Selected Articles from Artificial Limbs:* January 1954–Spring 1966. Robert E. Krieger Publishing, Huntington, New York, 1970, pp 5–30.

RADCLIFFE, CW AND FOORT, J: *The Patellar-Tendon-Bearing Below-Knee Prosthesis.* Biomechanics Laboratory, University of California at San Francisco and Berkley, 1961.

RUBIN, G: *Some problems of the above-knee amputee.* Bull Hosp Joint Dis 31:53–68, 1970.

SHAMBES, GM AND WATERLAND, JC: *Stance characteristics of a quadrilateral amputee.* Bull Prosthet Res 10–13:173–183, 1970.

SHAMBES, GM AND WATERLAND, JC: *Stance characteristics of a quadrilateral amputee: addendum.* Bull Prosthet Res 10–15:102–106, 1971.

STROHM, BR AND OGG, L: *Patella tendon bearing-cuff suspension below-knee prosthesis: An evaluation procedure.* Phys Ther Rev 41:339–347, 1961.

SYMINGTON, DC, LOWE, PJ, AND OLNEY, SJ: *The pedynograph: A clinical tool for force measurement and gait analysis in lower extremity amputees.* Arch Phys Med Rehabil 60:56–61, 1979.

WALLACH, J AND SAIBEL, E: *Control mechanism performance criteria for an above-knee leg prosthesis.* J Biomech 3:87–97, 1970.

ZARRUGH, MY AND RADCLIFFE, CW: *Simulation of swing phase dynamics in above-knee prostheses.* J Biomech 9:283–292, 1976.

ZUNIGA, EN, ET AL: *Gait patterns in above-knee amputees.* Arch Phys Med Rehabil 53:373–382, 1972.

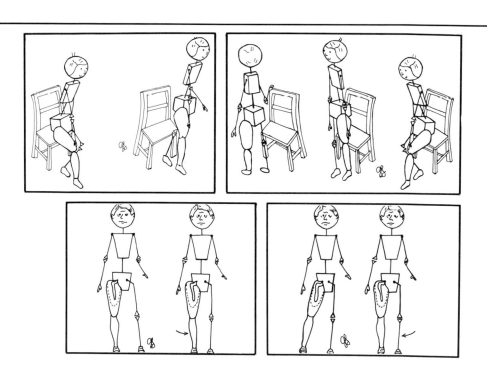

CHAPTER 21

PROSTHETIC MANAGEMENT

BELLA J. MAY, Ed.D., R.P.T.

Training the lower extremity amputee is similar to the teaching of any psychomotor skill; it is sequenced to allow the individual to learn first the parts, then the whole, and then to adapt the skill to changing situations. Time spent in the initial training of an amputee is critical to the eventual level of skill obtained. Bad habits developed early are stubbornly resistant to later attempts at elimination. Bad habits need not develop if adequate time and attention are given to the process of gait training.

FUNCTIONAL CONSIDERATIONS

AGE

Age, in and of itself, is not a deterrent to the achievement of functional independence. However, many elderly amputees have other problems that may delay the rehabilitation process and influence the final level of rehabilitation. Kerstein and associates, in a study of 194 male amputees who ranged in age from 20 to 84, found that older patients had a greater incidence of multiple medical problems, were more frequently amputated at above-knee levels, and were more likely to be bilateral amputees. All of these factors could delay the rehabilitation process. The most frequent causes of delayed rehabilitation were localized stump problems and delayed healing. These occurred more frequently in the older population.

Kegel and associates reviewed the questionnaire responses of 156 amputees who ranged in age from 3 to 89 years. Her findings were similar to those of Kerstein and associates in that functional rehabilitation level was related more to level of amputation and medical complications than to age in itself. Since older patients have more medical problems and many become bilateral amputees, their expected level of function is not as high as that of the younger unilateral amputee.

In general, then, functional expectations are determined by factors other than the age of the amputee. Medical complications that delay or prevent the rehabilitation process will affect functional expectations. These include uncontrolled diabetes, cardiopulmonary disease, severe peripheral vascular disease, cerebral vascular accidents, previous amputation, and neuropsychiatric disease. Residual limb problems such as infections, wound breakdowns, adherent scars, and skin problems can delay prosthetic fitting and affect final functional level. As with any rehabilitation program, functional goals reflect the patient's own goals, physical and mental status, preamputation level of activity, and level of amputation. The ideal is to have the patient ambulate independently in all types of situations without external support and with as low an expenditure of energy as possible. Elderly patients may like to use a cane when walking outside of the home, but they need to be trained to function without external support if warranted.

ENERGY COSTS

A number of studies have been performed to determine energy expenditures for different types of ambulation. Waters and associates studied the energy costs (as measured by rate of oxygen usage per minute) for prosthetic ambulation in 70 unilateral lower extremity amputees compared with a like group of nonamputees. The older amputees tended to walk at a slower rate than the younger amputees, but all, except for vascular above-knee amputees, maintained a normal rate of oxygen uptake. Above-knee amputees with vascular disease exhibited significantly higher levels of oxygen usage and were unable to adjust their rate of walking to lower energy expenditures. All of the patients who walked with a prosthesis exhibited a lower rate of oxygen consumption than individuals who walked with crutches without a prosthesis. Waters and associates concluded that the higher the level of amputation, the slower the rate of walking and the higher the energy cost.

Traugh and associates studied the energy expenditures of unilateral above-knee amputees who walked with a prosthesis with the prosthetic knee locked and unlocked and those who walked with crutches without a prosthesis. They found that crutch walking and above-knee prosthetic ambulation required the same amount of energy expenditure, which was about 65 percent more than for a nonamputee. Similar results were obtained by Huang and associates, who also determined that the energy cost of ambulating for a bilateral above-knee amputee was 280 percent that of an unimpaired individual of the same sex and age. Dubow and associates reported that bilateral below-knee amputees required 123 percent more $\dot{V}O_2$ (ml/m/kg), had a 26 percent higher heart rate, and walked slower than a similar group of nonamputees.

Generally, research appears to indicate that the higher the level of amputation, the greater the amount of energy required for ambulation and the slower the cadence. Bilateral amputees use considerably more energy than unilateral amputees. Crutch walking without a prosthesis requires at least as much energy as ambulating with an above-knee prosthesis.

PHYSIOLOGIC PROBLEMS

Residual limb problems can delay prosthetic rehabilitation. Skin problems such as dermatitis, furuncles, cysts, and infections usually require avoidance of the prosthesis for a period of time, care in skin hygiene, and, occasionally, medication. Soap residue left on the skin can become an irritant, and the patient must be taught to completely rinse the residual limb, socks, and socket after washing.

Patients with vascular disease must be alert to pressure on the residual limb from the prosthetic socket. Necrosis of distal tissue can occur even after the wound heals. Patients with diabetes who may have decreased sensation need to learn to carefully inspect the residual limb after each wearing to note any areas of redness or pressure. If some of the skin around the incision adheres to the distal end of the bone, the forces created by prosthetic wear may cause pain or abrasions. Care must be taken during the healing period to prevent such adhesions by careful massage and movement of the skin around the bone. Occasionally, bone spurs may develop, causing excessive pressure on the overlying skin. Juvenile traumatic amputees are subject to problems created by the bone continuing to grow through the skin at the end of the residual limb.

Some amputees develop a painful residual limb, which interferes with the ability to wear a prosthesis. Pain may be from physiologic or psychogenic origins or may encompass elements of both. Chronic pain in the amputee can be both difficult to treat and debilitating to the patient. Many of the newer techniques of behavior modification can be used with amputees as with other individuals with chronic pain problems. A painful phantom can be extremely resistant to treatment. Management of the phantom is discussed in greater detail in Chapter 18.

A neuroma is a natural sequela of the transection of a nerve, and all amputees have neuromas. The critical issues are the size and location of the neuroma; if it is small and situated in soft tissue well above the distal end of the residual limb, it will usually not cause problems. Large superficial neuromas may become squeezed between the socket wall and the bone and thus cause pain. Sometimes, relieving the socket wall at the site of the neuroma may resolve the problem. Injecting the neuroma with an analgesic or steroid formula may be necessary; since the relief is only temporary, this may need to be repeated several times. In more stubborn instances, surgery to remove or relocate the neuroma may be indicated. The use of ice or TENS or other electrotherapy measures has been successful on occasion and should be tried before more strenuous measures are employed.

Pain during or following wearing of the prosthesis may be due to some problem with the prosthetic socket. Minor impingement of the socket in areas of superficial tendons or excessive soft tissue may only cause problems after prolonged wearing. Careful inspection of the stump-socket interface is necessary to make sure that the pain is not due to changes in socket pressure or excessive socket pressure in one area.

BASIC GAIT TRAINING

DONNING THE PROSTHESIS

One of the first things that the patient needs to learn is how to correctly put on the prosthesis. There are reference points in each socket, and teaching proper donning is simply a matter of teaching the patient the proper reference points. Patients quickly learn the correct feel of the prosthesis and rarely have difficulty with donning. Most prostheses are worn with a stump sock of appropriate ply which is donned first, taking care that there are no wrinkles.

SYME AND BELOW-KNEE LEVELS

The residual limb in both Syme's and below-knee levels fits snugly into the socket. The distal end of the below-knee residual limb touches the end pad with minimum pressure, while there is some degree of weight-bearing on the end of the Syme's residual limb. In both levels, the patellar bar makes contact with the midline of the patellar tendon.

Some prostheses initially fit rather snugly, and the patient may have to stand to get all the way into the socket. Care must be taken not to create any skin abrasions while donning the prosthesis. On occasion, patients may experience some difficulty donning a PTS prosthesis with the high medial and lateral walls. A slight turning of the residual limb as the prosthesis is being donned will ease the tibial condyles past the wings of the prosthesis. Suspension straps are attached after the residual limb is well into the socket. If a thigh corset is being used, care must be taken to ensure that total contact has been achieved before the corset is attached.

ABOVE-KNEE LEVELS

PELVIC-BAND SUSPENSION

Above-knee prostheses with pelvic-band suspension are usually donned in the sitting position. The adductor longus channel at the anterior medial corner of the socket and the ischial seat on the top of the posterior wall are the major reference points. The patient is taught to palpate the adductor longus tendon to make sure that it is in the channel and to feel the firm pressure of the ischial seat.

SUCTION SOCKET PROSTHESIS

The suction above-knee prosthesis is worn without a sock and is donned in the standing position. A stockinet or elastic bandage is used to pull the residual limb into the socket and push the air out of the socket at the same time. The skin of the residual limb must be dry and free from abrasions. There is some controversy regarding the use of powder on the residual limb prior to donning. If the amputee perspires heavily, the powder and the perspiration will form a paste-like substance after several hours of wear, which may break the suction seal. On the other hand, powder helps dry the skin and makes donning easier. Each person will have to determine the best technique individually.

The wrap is put on the residual limb smoothly and without wrinkles, from the distal end to the inguinal area. The end of the wrap is placed through the valve hole of the socket. The residual limb is placed into the socket; the patient then stands and places the prosthesis slightly in front of the other leg while maintaining all weight on the sound leg. Beginners may control the prosthetic knee by placing one hand on the anterior distal end of the socket. At this time, it is a good idea to check the location of the adductor longus tendon to ensure that the prosthesis is correctly aligned. The patient then pumps the residual limb up and down slightly while pulling downward on the end of the wrap. In this manner, the residual limb is pulled into the socket and the air is pushed out. The process of pumping and pulling is continued until the residual limb is well into the socket and the wrap has been removed. When the residual limb is well seated into the socket, the valve is replaced and any remaining air is expelled by shifting all of the body weight onto the prosthesis while holding the valve stem open. If a Silesian bandage is worn, it is secured at this time. The patient learns to carry a pull wrap at all times in case the prosthesis is removed for any reason.

Donning a suction socket takes balance and coordination; not all patients like the process. In warm, humid climates, perspiration makes donning and maintaining suction difficult. Some individuals prefer to use a combination of suction and auxiliary support such as a Silesian bandage, which allows the wearing of a sock. In this instance, the sock is placed well over the stump and is used to initiate the donning of the prosthesis but is not completely removed. When the residual limb is well seated in the socket, the end of the sock is placed just inside the valve hole.

HIP DISARTICULATION AND HEMIPELVECTOMY

Donning these prostheses can be done in either the sitting or standing position. Most of the body weight is borne on the sound side and the bucket is slipped into place. After standing, straps can be tightened and the bucket adjusted for comfort. The major refer-

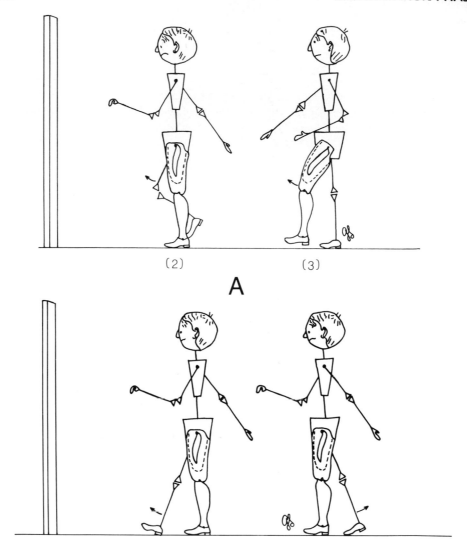

(2)   (3)

A

B

FIGURE 21-1. *A,* Weight-Shifting Exercise. *(1)* Stand facing a mirror. *(2)* Shift weight to the prosthesis by shifting the hips laterally rather than by laterally side bending. Make sure the shoulders and pelvis remain level. Raise the sound foot for a few seconds while balancing on the prosthesis. This teaches the amputee to shift the weight adequately toward the prosthetic side. *(3)* Bend the prosthetic knee, by flexing the hip on the prosthetic side, just enough to raise the heel from the floor. This teaches the amputee how to "break" the prosthetic knee to initiate swing phase. *B,* Weight-Shifting Exercise. *(1)* Stand facing a mirror. *(2)* Shift weight laterally toward the prosthetic side, standing on the prosthesis. *(3)* Keep the prosthetic foot "planted" on one spot as the sound leg is rhythmically moved forward and backward. (Caution: The prosthetic knee may become unstable as the sound leg is moved backward unless the trunk is kept forward, in front of the knee axis.) *(4)* Shift full weight to the sound leg each time the leg is in front of and behind the prosthesis. *(5)* The sound foot should pass close to the prosthetic foot as it moves forward and backward to allow adequate lateral shift to the prosthetic side.

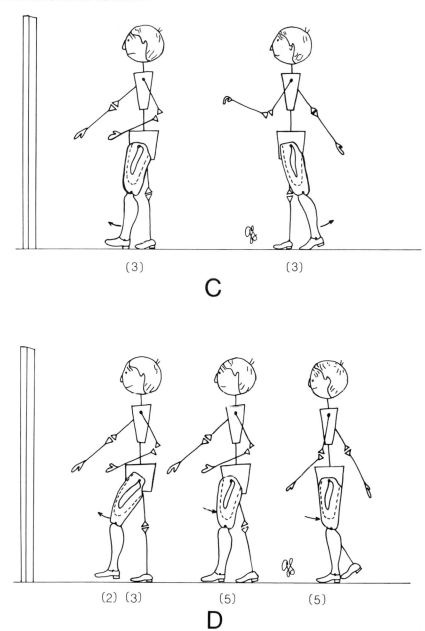

(3)   (3)

C

(2) (3)   (5)   (5)

D

FIGURE 21-1. *Continued.* C, Preliminary Walking Exercise. *(1)* Stand facing a mirror. *(2)* While keeping the prosthetic foot in place, step forward and backward several times with the sound leg. *(3)* Keep the sound foot in place and step forward and backward several times with the prosthesis. *(4)* Complete the step by coming forward with the sound leg. *(5)* Repeat the sequence. *D,* Preliminary Walking Exercise. *(1)* Stand facing a mirror. *(2)* Stand with weight on the sound leg. *(3)* Bend the prosthetic knee by flexing the hip. *(4)* Keep the sound foot in place and step forward and backward with the prosthesis. *(5)* Place full weight on the prosthesis at the end of the forward and backward step. The prosthetic knee is kept in full extension, especially when the prosthesis is forward, by pressing the residual limb against the back of the socket.

ence points are the iliac crest on the amputated side and the ischium on either the amputated or nonamputated side, depending on the level of amputation. Instead of ready-made socks, many patients prefer to sew together the bottom ends of a T-shirt on the amputated side and slide it over the end of the residual limb. This maneuver is reported to limit crinkling and bunching of material, which can cause pressure points.

BALANCING ACTIVITIES

The first thing any amputee has to learn is how to balance and shift weight on the prosthesis and how to interpret the pressures on the residual limb in the different phases of gait. A thorough knowledge of prosthetic biomechanics is necessary to design appropriate training programs, and the time spent in the early parts of the training cycle will enhance the final outcome.

All amputees, regardless of level, need to learn to shift their weight on the prosthesis, balance momentarily in single-leg support phase, and place the prosthesis an appropriate distance in front of the sound leg. The basic training phase for the above-knee amputee (Fig. 21-1) can be adapted for below-knee levels. Below-knee amputees fitted with patellar-tendon-bearing prostheses must learn to let their knee flex from heel-strike to mid-stance in a natural gait pattern.

Above-knee amputees need to learn to control the prosthetic knee as part of the initial balancing activities. During the preliminary exercises, emphasis is placed on knee control until the individual can perform this activity automatically when prosthetic weight-bearing is commenced.

Since amputees cannot feel the floor directly, they tend to look at the floor during initial training. A mirror helps the individual focus on feeling the socket pressures change during the different parts of the gait cycle.

There are numerous activities that enhance balance training and make it more fun. Music helps some people move rhythmically, while others will enjoy playing catch with a large beach-type ball. The importance of the initial balance training cannot be overemphasized. Below-knee amputees more readily learn to shift their weight over the prosthesis, but above-knee amputees often have difficulty learning to trust the prosthesis. Ideally, the above-knee amputee should be able to balance on the prosthesis in single-leg support for 2 to 3 seconds. Once this is accomplished, the rest of the training will be easier. However, if weight shifting and balance are not achieved, the person may never attain a satisfactory gait.

INITIAL WALKING

Initial walking is usually commenced in the parallel bars, with the patient encouraged to use the bars for balance only rather than for weight-bearing. A mirror helps the person assume a better standing position with the weight well distributed over the feet. Figure 21-2 depicts an initial walking sequence for an above-knee amputee. The below-knee amputee will follow a similar sequence but must be reminded to roll over the foot allowing the knee to flex after mid-stance, while the above-knee amputee must be reminded to "lock" the prosthetic knee by extending the residual limb against the posterior wall of the socket at the moment of heel-strike, except with the Henschke-Mauch S-N-S system. Some individuals can be taught outside the parallel bars from the

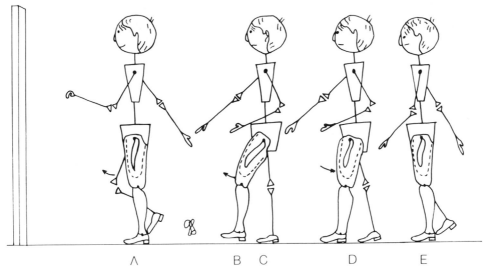

FIGURE 21-2. Walking Forward. *A,* Step with the sound leg. *B,* Shift the weight forward and laterally over the sound leg. *C,* Flex the residual limb to cause the prosthetic knee to flex as the shank follows through into extension. *D,* Step through, making a step of equal length with the prosthetic heel ahead of the toe of the sound foot. As the prosthetic knee reaches full extension, heel-contact is made on the prosthetic side. On heel-contact on the prosthetic side, the residual limb is pressed against the posterior wall of the socket. This motion is necessary to maintain knee stability as long as the weight-bearing line is behind the knee axis, usually until just past mid-stance. *E,* Shift the weight forward and laterally over the prosthetic leg.

outset. Balance exercises may be started with the patient facing a wall, which can be used for support.

Some individuals have difficulty incorporating good weight shifting over the prosthesis into the gait cycle. It may be beneficial to give the patient a cane to use on the involved side as an aid to complete weight shifting. In the parallel bars, the individual can be asked to place the ipsilateral hand on the parallel bars and not use the other hand.

It is strongly recommended that the patient be maintained under supervision in the parallel bars until a smooth, well-coordinated gait has been developed and the person either does not use the parallel bars for support or uses the bars with one hand for light support only. During the initial training period, the person can also be taught the proper way to get up and down from a chair (Fig. 21-3).

ANCILLARY AIDS

Energy expenditure is a major concern to lower extremity amputees. Energy expenditure is directly related to the smoothness of the gait pattern and the use of external devices. It is desirable to train the person to functional ambulation without external devices. A cane may be desired by some elderly people for use outside of the home. On occasion, crutches may be used if the patient has other medical conditions that preclude ambulating with less support. A walker is not indicated in the majority of

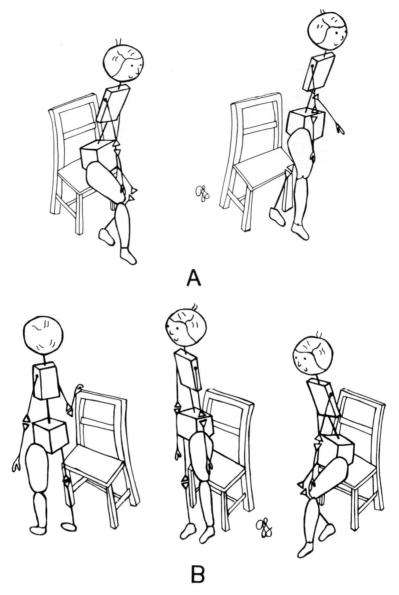

FIGURE 21-3. *A,* Rising From A Chair. *(1)* Slide the hips to the forward edge of the chair. *(2)* Place the sound foot behind the prosthetic foot, close to the front of the chair. *(3)* Lean forward, with the center of gravity over the sound foot. *(4)* Stand by extending the hip and knee of the sound leg while using the prosthesis for balance (not weight-bearing). If a manual lock is being used, it would be engaged before steps are taken. *B,* Sitting Down In A Chair. *(1)* The chair is best approached from the nonprosthetic side. *(2)* Weight is transferred to the sound leg. *(3)* The amputee pivots on the sound foot as the prosthetic leg is brought back into position for sitting. *(4)* The manual lock, if used, is released. The residual limb is extended against the back of the socket to release the hydraulic resistance to flexion if a Henschke-Mauch S-N-S knee is used. The residual limb is then gradually flexed, which flexes the prosthetic knee. The amputee then leans forward and laterally over the sound limb for balance and reaches back to grasp the armrest or chair seat as the weight is lowered to the chair by slowly flexing the sound leg while maintaining trunk flexion.

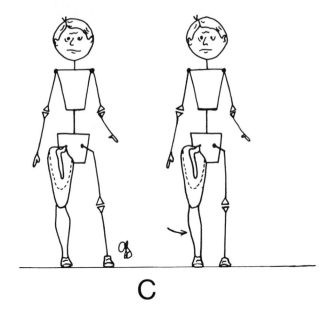

C

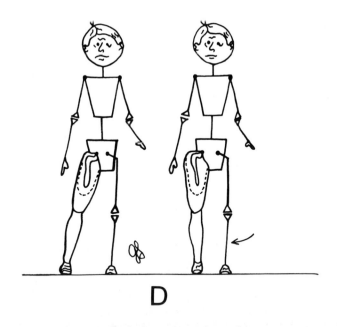

D

FIGURE 21-3. *Continued. C,* Sidestepping Toward The Sound Limb. *(1)* Balance on the prosthesis. *(2)* Step laterally as the sound leg is abducted. *(3)* Shift weight and balance on the sound leg. *(4)* Adduct the residual limb and place the prosthetic foot next to the normal foot. *(5)* Repeat the sequence. *D,* Sidestepping Toward The Prosthetic Side. *(1)* Balance on the sound limb. *(2)* Step laterally as the residual limb is abducted. *(3)* Shift weight to the prosthesis. *(4)* Adduct the sound limb and place the sound foot next to the prosthetic foot. *(5)* Repeat the sequence.

instances and should not be considered as an intermediary training step between the parallel bars and a cane. Prostheses are designed and constructed for maximum function when the individual walks in a smooth step-over-step pattern. A walker does not allow such a pattern and requires a great expenditure of energy. Using the walker as a shortcut to allow the patient to be discharged from treatment early or to use the prosthesis at home before a good gait has been achieved usually leads to gait deviations and a dependency on the walker that may never be overcome. A walker should be used only if it is obvious that the individual will not be able to use the prosthesis with any other form of external support. An elderly amputee who can go to the bathroom independently with a walker is easier to care for at home than one who may be wheelchair dependent. However, the walker should be used sparingly and only after careful evaluation of the individual's potential.

SPECIAL CONSIDERATIONS

HYDRAULIC KNEE MECHANISMS

Training an amputee with a hydraulic knee mechanism is a little different from training one fitted with a mechanical knee joint. In all models, the hydraulic mechanism is designed to adjust the swing of the shank to the amputee's pace to ensure that the foot is ready for heel-strike at the appropriate time. Rather than increasing or decreasing hip flexion force to adjust shank swing, the amputee lets the hydraulic mechanism do the job. Training is simply a matter of letting the amputee get used to the function.

The Henschke-Mauch S-N-S system is a little different and requires different training cycles for knee control. The system has three modes: swing and stance phase control, swing phase control only, and knee flexion lock. A stirrup lever near the top of the piston rod operates as a selector switch. When the lever is in the down position, swing and stance phase control are both operative. This is the most frequently used setting. There is also a button head adjustment control to set stance phase resistance. It is recommended that this be set at maximum resistance during initial training. As the amputee gains competence in walking, the resistance can be reduced; the amputee will eventually find the appropriate balance between swing and stance phase control for daily activities.

For the system to be operational, the amputee must be taught to walk over the ball of the foot. Putting pressure on the ball of the foot and maintaining the hyperextension moment generated about the knee after mid-stance for a tenth of a second reduces stance phase control and allows the knee to flex naturally. Experienced amputees changing to the Henschke-Mauch S-N-S system may experience some difficulty if they were used to transferring weight to the sound leg before rolling over the prosthetic leg. Failure to reduce the stance phase control will result in the knee locking. Active amputees usually encounter little difficulty with this mechanism, but more timid walkers may have some problem generating knee flexion. The stance phase control aspect of the mechanism provides a degree of safety. The hydraulic mechanism does not buckle like mechanical knee units, thereby providing some protection if the individual catches the toe of the prosthesis while walking or transferring weight to the prosthesis before full knee extension has occurred. The mechanism will hold for a moment then slowly let the knee flex, giving the amputee time to catch his or her balance. In the first few degrees of knee flexion, the stance phase control mechanism will provide support for the amputee even if the knee is not fully extended.

The combination of swing and stance phase control and, in particular, the controlled knee flexion, allows the amputee to go down stairs and ramps in a more normal manner. Because of cost, the mechanism is not used prevalently. Individuals who are involved in training a patient fitted with the Henschke-Mauch S-N-S system are encouraged to work with the prosthetist in the training program.

BILATERAL AMPUTEES

The basic gait training activities for a bilateral amputee are similar to those used with a unilateral amputee. If the individual ambulated as a unilateral amputee prior to becoming a bilateral amputee, the process is easier. A bilateral below-knee amputee has a greater potential for becoming a functional walker than someone with an above-knee and a below-knee amputation. It is very difficult for the bilateral above-knee amputee to become a functional walker, although a number of young traumatic amputees have succeeded in this endeavor. Most bilateral amputees need some form of external support, especially for elevation activities.

Considerable time needs to be spent on balance and weight-shifting activities since the individual no longer has any direct contact with the ground. Most bilateral amputees use a somewhat wider base than unilateral amputees, and many bilateral amputees exhibit a tendency to roll a bit from side to side. While these extraneous movements need to be minimized, they usually cannot be completely eliminated. The patient should progress directly from the parallel bars to whatever form of external support will be used at home. A walker is not indicated for bilateral amputees.

Functional outcomes are directly related to the balance, strength, and coordination of the patient and to the levels of amputation. The amount of energy expended must not preclude participation in other activities. The higher the levels of amputation and the more external support needed, the less functional the ambulation.

As all unilateral amputees need crutches for times when they are not wearing a prosthesis, all bilateral amputees need a wheelchair.

PREVIOUS WEARERS

When an experienced amputee receives a new prosthesis, it is a good idea to evaluate both the fit of the prosthesis and the person's ability to use it. While long-standing gait deviations are resistant to change, a careful evaluation may reveal areas where some additional training may be indicated.

ADVANCED ACTIVITIES

IN THE HOME

Once the patient is able to ambulate safely on level ground, there are a number of activities still to be learned. Spending some time teaching these activities is worthwhile, for not everyone benefits from a trial-and-error approach. Because most below-knee amputees can easily perform required activities of daily living, the techniques outlined below are primarily for the above-knee amputee. They may be adapted to individual needs.

SITTING ON THE FLOOR

Place the prosthesis about half a step behind the sound foot, keeping the weight on the sound foot. Bend from the waist and flex at the knees and hips, reaching for the floor with both arms outstretched and pivoting to the sound side. Then, gently lower the body to the floor. This activity is one continuous movement.

GETTING UP FROM THE FLOOR

Get on the hands and knees; place the sound leg forward, well under the trunk, with the foot flat on the floor while balancing on the hands and the prosthetic knee. Then, extend the sound knee while maintaining the weight over the sound leg. Move to an erect position by pushing strongly with the sound leg and the arms, bringing the prosthesis forward when almost erect.

KNEELING

Place the sound foot ahead of the prosthetic foot, keeping the weight on the sound leg. Slowly flex the trunk, hip, and knees until the prosthetic knee can be gently placed on the floor. Above-knee amputees can usually kneel on the prosthetic leg, but below-knee amputees find that the patellar bar creates too much pressure in this position. Below-knee amputees will usually kneel on the sound side. Getting up from a kneeling position is like getting up from the floor.

FALLING

Although it is not appropriate to practice falling with all patients, methods of self-protection should be discussed. In general, the patient needs to be advised to try to fall away from the prosthesis and to put the body weight on the uninvolved side if possible. If the activity is practiced, it is a good idea to practice both forward and backward falling.

FALLING FORWARD

With the toes against the mat, pitch forward, breaking the fall with the arms outstretched and absorbing the shock with slightly flexed elbows. Transfer partial weight to both knees, or roll onto the unaffected hip, then shoulder.

FALLING BACKWARD

Jackknife forward at the waist so that the buttocks strike the mat first, then roll backward onto the rounded back and shoulders.

PICKING UP AN OBJECT FROM THE FLOOR

Place the sound foot ahead of the prosthetic foot, with the body weight remaining on the sound leg. Bend forward at the waist, flexing the hips and knees until the object can be reached. Care must be taken to maintain the weight on the sound leg. Some individuals like to bend sideways rather than forward, while others find it easier to keep the prosthetic knee straight and bend the sound leg until the object can be picked up.

OUTSIDE THE HOME

To be totally functional, each amputee must cope with a world full of obstacles, steps, and hills. Take the amputee outside to walk on uneven surfaces, in crowds, and on different terrains; practice crossing the street on the green light, walking through sand, and getting on a bus or subway. Being able to ambulate in the sheltered environment of the therapy gym is not necessarily equatable with functioning in the more demanding external world. Regardless of the patient's age, balance, or agility, some training time needs to be spent on outside activities. Many elderly amputees who are quite functional without external support in the home will need a cane outside the home for a little extra balance.

Many below-knee amputees can go up and down stairs one leg over the other, depending on the length of the residual limb, the height of the step, and the person's balance and coordination. The process of extending the below-knee residual limb in the socket, which is required by this activity, drives the anterior distal end of the residual limb hard into the anterior socket wall. Individuals with sensitive skin and poor balance should not attempt this maneuver. Not all individuals can tolerate the pressure on the anterior distal end of the residual limb; some will prefer to go up and down steps one leg at a time, leading with the sound leg going up and the prosthesis going down. The amount of advanced training will vary with the level of amputation and the balance and coordination of the patient.

Most below-knee amputees can walk up and down ramps and inclines with little difficulty. The limited dorsiflexion of the SACH foot requires a little more knee flexion going up the incline, and if the hill is steep, a shorter prosthetic step.

Below-knee amputees do not have a great deal of difficulty with most advanced activities such as clearing an obstacle, getting in and out of a car, and even running, although the latter creates considerable rotational forces between the socket and the residual limb. Individuals with limited balance and coordination will need to be taught each of the advanced activities; the more active individuals will quickly develop their own techniques once they have learned the basics and have had some practice.

UP AND DOWN STEPS

Some above-knee amputees can learn to go down steps one leg over the other, buckling the prosthetic knee at each step. However, the majority will probably be safer using one step at a time.

Lead with the sound foot going up, taking one or two steps at a time. To clear the edge of the step with the prosthesis, extend and slightly abduct the hip and place the prosthetic foot next to the sound foot. A handrail may be used for initial practice, but full functional rehabilitation requires the ability to go up and down steps without a handrail. Going down, lead with the prosthetic foot, making sure that the knee is kept locked during weight-bearing. The sound leg is brought down on the same step. To go down one leg over the other, place the heel of the prosthetic foot on the edge of the step; shift the weight over the prosthesis, keeping the knee extended. When the sound leg is in position to recover on the next step, flex the prosthetic hip, allowing the knee to buckle, and let the weight go on the sound leg. Then, extend the prosthetic knee to swing the shin forward over the next lowest step and quickly shift the body weight onto the prosthesis and continue in a rhythmic progression.

UP AND DOWN INCLINES

Lead with the sound leg going up inclines, taking a little longer step than usual. Hike the prosthetic hip enough to prevent the toe from catching, and swing the prosthesis through; avoid abducting it. Take a somewhat shorter step with the prosthetic leg, making sure that the knee is extended during weight-bearing. The shorter prosthetic step compensates for the limited dorsiflexion of the SACH foot. Some trunk flexion may also be needed on very steep hills. Continue up the incline in the line of progression.

On very steep hills or for individuals who have balance problems, the diagonal method may be more effective. Ascend on the diagonal, leading with the sound leg and keeping the prosthetic leg slightly behind the sound leg. On very difficult or slippery inclines, sidestepping leading with the sound leg may be the technique of choice.

Lead with the prosthetic leg going down an incline, taking a somewhat smaller step than usual and taking particular care to keep the knee extended. Shift the weight over the prosthesis, and when the sound foot is in a position to recover, voluntarily flex the prosthetic knee, catching the body weight on the sound leg. Modifications include using shorter steps, using repeated single steps, and descending sideways.

CLEARING OBSTACLES

Face the obstacle with the sound foot slightly in front and the body weight on the prosthesis. Step over the obstacle with the sound leg, then transfer the body weight to the sound leg. Quickly extend the prosthetic hip, then forcefully flex the prosthetic hip, whipping the prosthesis forward over the obstacle. Then step forward with a normal gait pattern. An alternate method is to stand sideways to the obstacle with the sound leg closest to the obstacle. With the weight on the prosthesis, swing the sound leg over the obstacle and transfer the body weight to the sound leg. Then swing the prosthesis forward, up and over the obstacle.

RUNNING

Step forward with the sound leg, then shift the body weight to the sound leg and hop forward on the sound side. Swing the prosthesis forward and shift the body weight onto the prosthesis for momentary support. Immediately transfer the weight to the sound leg and continue the hop-skip running. A soft plantarflexion bumper or heel wedge allows for a faster foot-flat; slight dorsiflexion in foot alignment allows the amputee to take a longer stride on the sound side. Increased knee friction or a hydraulic unit helps control the swing of the shank during running.

SUMMARY

There are many other obstacles in our society which the amputee must learn to overcome. Escalators often pose a problem and probably should be avoided by individuals who have poor balance or who use crutches. In general, one leads with the sound leg both getting on and getting off escalators.

Advanced activities are often left out of amputee training programs, particularly with the elderly. Yet, the ability to perform such routine activities is necessary to a functional lifestyle in our society.

CARE OF THE PROSTHESIS

SOCKS

All lower extremity amputees, except for those fitted with above-knee suction prostheses, will wear one or more socks between the residual limb and the socket. Socks are generally knitted of cotton or wool and come in different thicknesses (called plys), different lengths, and different circumferential sizes. Socks are knitted specifically for the above-knee or the below-knee residual limb. Most patients receive 6 one-ply cotton socks and 6 five-ply wool socks with the prosthesis.

It is generally desirable to fit the socket as snugly as possible, particularly if considerable shrinkage of the residual limb is anticipated. Many individuals will initially be fitted with a one-ply sock; however, those with sensitive skin, mature residual limbs, or bony prominences may be initially fitted with a five-ply wool sock. Regardless of how the person is initially fitted, he or she will need to learn how to adjust the socks as the residual limb changes size. It is important that the patient understand the use of the socks to maintain the proper relationship of the residual limb to the socket. If the amputee wears too few socks or too thin a sock, the residual limb will go too deep in the socket and will create excessive end-bearing. If the amputee wears too many socks or too thick a sock, the residual limb will not go down far enough in the socket and the prosthesis will appear to be too long.

Socks can be made of other materials, and there are regional variations in the types of socks used. For individuals who have a problem with wool next to the skin, a thin nylon sheath may be worn directly over the residual limb. The nylon sheath is particularly smooth and reduces friction between the socket and the residual limb; it is used by many amputees.

Socks need to be changed daily and washed carefully in cool water with a mild soap or detergent. Socks should be rinsed thoroughly because soap residue can cause skin irritations. Socks should also be dried flat and blocked to keep their shape. As socks become worn, they become thinner, and the amputee needs to be aware that an old five-ply sock may actually be only four plys thick. Socks need to be replaced when they are becoming worn.

PROSTHETIC MAINTENANCE

As with any mechanical instrument, the prosthesis will require some maintenance and care. The prosthetic socket should be cleaned daily with a damp cloth and allowed to dry completely. The valve of the above-knee suction socket needs to be cleaned and brushed daily to remove anything that might block the little hole or the threads of the screw. Leather needs to be kept dry and clean. Hydraulic knee units are not serviced by the prosthetist; most are sealed units that have to be returned to the factory for repair. The prosthetist will remove the hydraulic unit and install a loaned unit so that the patient can continue to ambulate while the unit is being repaired.

As the prosthesis is worn, leather may become brittle and frayed, joints may wear and need new parts, and occasionally, cracks may develop in the finish. The prosthetic foot may become worn with use and can be damaged by getting wet. Preventive maintenance and care of the small problems will keep a prosthesis functional for a considerable amount of time. It is recommended that regular recheck visits with the clinic team be scheduled once a patient has completed initial gait training and has taken the prosthesis home. A workable schedule is to have the person initially return within 6 to 9 weeks, then in 6 months, and finally on a yearly basis. It is recommended that all amputees be checked by the clinic team on a yearly basis to make sure that no problems have arisen and that the prosthesis is in good condition.

BIBLIOGRAPHY

AMERICAN ACADEMY OF ORTHOPAEDIC SURGEONS: *Atlas of Limb Prosthetics.* CV Mosby, St Louis, 1981.

BATZDORFF, J AND FRANKEL, B: *Initial gait training of the patient with an above knee amputation.* Phys Ther 58:575–578, 1978.

DUBOW, LL, ET AL: *Oxygen consumption of elderly persons with bilateral below knee amputations: Ambulation vs. wheelchair propulsion.* Arch Phys Med Rehabil 64:255–259, 1983.

HUANG, CT, ET AL: *Amputation: Energy cost of ambulation.* Arch Phys Med Rehabil 60:18–24, 1979.

KEGEL, B, CARPENTER, ML, AND BURGESS, EM: *Functional capabilities of lower extremity amputees.* Arch Phys Med Rehabil 59:109–120, 1978.

KERSTEIN, MD, ET AL: *What influence does age have on rehabilitation of amputees?* Geriatrics 30:67–71, 1975.

LEWIS, E: *Elements of Training with the Mauch S-N-S System for Above Knee Amputees.* Research and Development Division, Prosthetic and Sensory Aids Service, Veterans Administration, New York, 1970.

TRAUGH, GH, CORCORAN, PJ, AND REYES, RL: *Energy expenditure of ambulation in patients with above-knee amputations.* Arch Phys Med Rehabil 56:67–71, 1975.

VAN GRIETHUYSEN, C: *Gait training for the below knee amputee.* Prosthet Orthot Int 3:163–165, 1979.

WATERS, RL, ET AL: *Energy cost of walking of amputees: The influence of level of amputation.* J Bone Joint Surg 58A:42–46, 1976.

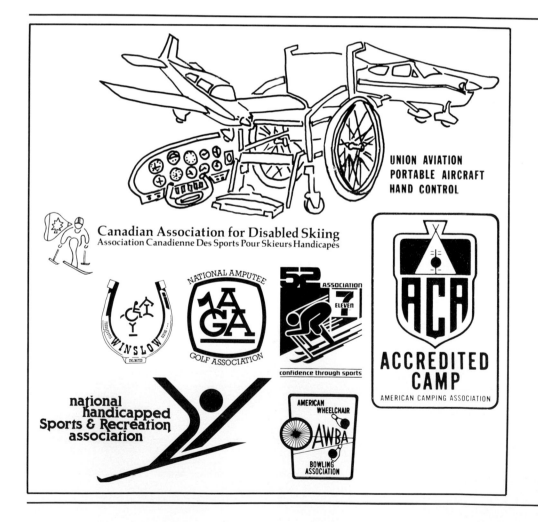

UNION AVIATION
PORTABLE AIRCRAFT
HAND CONTROL

Canadian Association for Disabled Skiing
Association Canadienne Des Sports Pour Skieurs Handicapés

CHAPTER **22**

LIVING WITH A PROSTHESIS

BELLA J. MAY, Ed.D., R.P.T.

PSYCHOSOCIAL ADJUSTMENTS	ACTIVITIES OF DAILY LIVING
VOCATIONAL ADJUSTMENTS	RECREATIONAL ACTIVITIES

Learning how to walk with a prosthesis is only the beginning of the rehabilitative process. Living with a prosthesis requires making some changes in lifestyle and daily habits. The individual must cope with new problems that range from learning how to go to the bathroom in the middle of the night to finding gainful employment. The return to a full, active life is the goal; the dimensions of that life will be differentially defined by each individual. For some, it will include vigorous vocational and recreational activities; for others, it may mean being able to putter in the garden and walk across the street to visit neighbors. Regardless of lifestyle, each amputee must cope with many physical, psychological, social, and financial adjustments.

PSYCHOSOCIAL ADJUSTMENTS

Amputation means the loss of a body part—the loss of a piece of one's self. Adjustment is a complex psychosocial process that takes time, understanding, and support by family and friends. There are many factors that influence the adjustment process, including the person's already established coping mechanisms and degree of emotional maturity. Initial discharge from the rehabilitation facility and re-entry into the world of everyday life can be a most traumatic period, and members of the rehabilitation team can help prepare the individual and the family for the transition.

Individual adjustment is influenced by the reaction of significant others and the amputee's perceptions of that reaction. A sense of inferiority to others, a sense of inadequacy in meeting daily obligations, and a sense of being seen as a freak or as repulsive to others can all contribute to a withdrawal from society and an unwillingness to risk social interactions. The presence of other disabling conditions, such as multiple amputations, blindness, or cardiac disease, influences adjustment and social interactions. If the individual perceives disapproval by group members and experiences self-devaluation, withdrawal may seem justified. It is important for the individual to learn to cope with any feelings of inferiority and rejection as well as with any overprotection by the family. The early reaction of family and friends is a great influence on the person's adjustment. To many nondisabled individuals, physical disability infers inadequacy; family and friends may subtly change in their interactions with the amputee. Some people are uncomfortable around the handicapped—caught in a conflict between talking about or ignoring the disability. It is desirable for people to interact directly with the amputee using a natural tone of voice. Family education needs to be an early and integral part of the total rehabilitation program. As it is valuable for the amputee to have an opportunity to see and talk with other amputees, so it may be valuable for family members to have the opportunity to discuss common problems with family members of other amputees.

There may be financial barriers to social interaction. The amputee who cannot use public transportation and does not have a car is dependent on others for transportation. For many, forced dependency is difficult to accept and increases feelings of inferiority. There are many practical problems that have to be faced and that have the potential of generating anger, guilt, and frustration as family schedules have to be altered to meet the needs of the patient. Family members may be required to assist with therapy in the home, to transport the person to many appointments, and to stretch limited financial resources. Family members can become so involved in the process that the individuality of the amputee is lost as the focus becomes the amputation and not the person. Sometimes, family members make decisions for the amputee, particularly if the amputee is elderly and dependent on family other than a spouse. As roles change, the amputee can become progressively more dependent and isolated.

Health professionals, anticipating such problems, can help all those involved face developing problems openly and empathetically. Written materials can be made available for both the patient and the family. The attitude of rehabilitation team members toward the amputee, as well as toward the family, can set a positive or a negative tone. The patient should be involved in setting goals and making decisions about the rehabilitation program. Team members can create an open environment by listening attentively and by considering the family as much as possible in making appointments. Going home on weekend passes during the rehabilitative phase helps all involved assess different aspects of living with a prosthesis in planned stages.

Some individuals may discover "secondary benefits" from the loss of a limb. They may use the disability to manipulate family and friends or to obtain attention not otherwise available.

The individual's sexual identity also influences adjustment. Adolescents are quite conscious of their bodies and are particularly sensitive to the reactions of others. Young amputees may deny their sexuality rather than face their changed body image. Both men and women may have difficulty adapting to a changed body image and an altered sexual being. Much work has been done in recent years on the sexual problems of the handicapped, resulting in greater recognition of the scope of the problems and greater awareness by rehabilitation workers. Group and individual therapy are useful tools to help with adjustment. An open and understanding attitude by rehabilitation personnel will make it easier for the individual to verbalize fears and concerns.

Problems of psychosexual adjustments are not limited to the young. Elderly amputees face the same problems and have the same need for support and guidance. Additionally, elderly amputees may have to cope with physical changes in coital position, interference with balance, and a painful phantom during orgasm.

The majority of amputees are able to satisfactorily cope with negative feelings and make a positive adjustment to their disability. Emotionally mature individuals recognize that there has been a change in their physical being—a change that needs to be accepted for what it is—but not a change in their essential being. As the people integrate their altered physical state into satisfactory lifestyles, the importance of the physical change will recede. The individuals will come to realize that they can still be worthy and contributing members of society. They will develop mechanisms to cope with intrusive questions and the looks of others as well as with the annoyances that accompany a permanent physical disability.

VOCATIONAL ADJUSTMENTS

A satisfactory psychosocial adjustment to amputation requires a satisfactory vocational adjustment. Many amputees are able to return to their preamputation employment situation. Sometimes a change in assigned work within the same company is required; if not accompanied by a reduction in salary or status, the amputee will adapt easily to the new work. A change that leads to lower job status or a decrease in salary will tend to increase the person's feelings of inadequacy. For some, a return to preamputation employment is not possible, and the individual must seek other vocational placement. Often, it is the individuals from the lower educational and socioeconomic levels who have the most difficulty finding gainful employment after amputation.

The prosthesis must allow the individual to meet the physical demands of the job. The team must be aware of how much lifting, bending, climbing, and carrying of heavy objects is necessary and select components accordingly. Many employers are reluctant to hire handicapped individuals, and visits by counselors from the Division of Vocational Rehabilitation can be educational. Sometimes retraining is necessary before the individual can find suitable employment. Many factors affect the employability of the amputee, including the general economic status of the country and the attitudes of employers in the community.

ACTIVITIES OF DAILY LIVING

There are a number of activities that the individual must learn once basic gait and stairs have been mastered. Depending on where the person lives, he or she will need to learn to walk on various types of surfaces such as sand, city streets, farm land, and the like. Sometimes learning to cross the street within the time frame of the green or walk light can be an adventure. The ability to move from place to place independently is of paramount importance in today's lifestyles. Unanticipated barriers can sometimes lead to panic, and it is the wise therapist who anticipates such barriers and helps the individual learn to surmount them. Escalators can seem like mountains when first encountered. A person with relatively good balance can step on and off the escalator with the sound foot on both ascent and descent. Individuals who use crutches or whose balance is not secure are better advised to use elevators. Theater rows or church pews may represent other unexpected barriers. Sidestepping facing the already seated patrons allows the individual to use arm rests for unexpected losses of balance. The individual needs to be able to step backwards securely as well as sidestep before taking the prosthesis outside.

For many people, independent mobility means driving a car. Depending on the side and level of amputation, the automobile may or may not need to be adjusted. In some instances, switching the gas or brake pedal for use with the other foot may be necessary. Bilateral lower extremity amputees need hand controls, which allow for operation of the accelerator and brake with the hands. Most mechanics can install hand controls or make the necessary adaptations to automobiles. Some individuals, particularly those with above-knee or hip disarticulation amputations, may encounter some difficulty getting in and out of the automobile, particularly if it has bucket seats. Two-door vehicles fitted with bench seats offer a little more room for entry and exit. Individuals who have lost the left leg encounter few problems because they can sit in the car in the usual manner and then bring the prosthesis in after them. Right lower extremity amputees may need to learn to put the prosthesis in the car first.

Public transportation presents other hazards, particularly for elderly and multiple amputees. Some individuals are unable to pull themselves up that high first step. In some communities, adapted busses are available. Independent ambulators will have no particular problems with trains or airplanes other than the limited leg room available between seats. The amputee may want to choose an aisle seat with the prosthesis closest to the aisle. Canes or crutches may be taken by flight attendants during takeoffs and landings. Individuals who cannot ambulate independently will need to make special arrangements with the airlines prior to any flight.

In some instances, the home will need to be adjusted to make it possible for the person to function independently. Multiple amputees or those who use a wheelchair when not wearing the prosthesis may have difficulty getting in and out of the bathroom or moving around a two-story house. Outside steps without a handrail may pose a hazard, particularly in cold or icy weather. Early planning is necessary, and a home visit by the therapist can prevent later problems. Energy expenditures are greater for the amputee than for the nonamputee and are greater for the above-knee amputee than for the below-knee amputee. Elderly individuals may not have the necessary reserves for the energy demands of everyday living with an above-knee prosthesis, and the location of a bedroom or bathroom may need to be altered to allow them to function on one floor of the home.

Living with a prosthesis also means adjusting to numerous minor changes in everyday life. The amputee may not be able to walk as fast as in the past, may need to alter the type of clothing worn and cope with the problem of changing shoes. With the prosthesis aligned to one pair of shoes, both men and women have to cope with the altered prosthetic alignment that results from changing heel height. Often, the team has not prepared the individual for this problem. Many people today wear dress shoes for work, athletic shoes for leisure times, boots in the winter, and sandals in the summer. Each type of footwear has a different height heel and a different configuration, yet the SACH foot is not adaptable to different shoes. Sometimes amputees can change feet to accommodate changes in shoes, but this is expensive and requires a modular prosthesis for easy changes. A felt insert in athletic shoes will moderate the problem of the negative heel, but this does not solve the problem of higher heeled shoes. There are some newer feet that accommodate different heel heights, and it behooves the prosthetist to review the options with each patient prior to the fitting of the first definitive prosthesis. Members of the prosthetic team need to be knowledgeable about changes in components to guide the amputee from the beginning. Satisfactory adjustment will be more likely if the individual is prepared for the many changes that will be required in everyday life.

RECREATIONAL ACTIVITIES

Americans are increasingly involved in leisure and sports activities, and most amputees want to participate as well. A full and satisfying lifestyle includes the ability to participate in avocational activities to improve physical fitness, sociability, self-confidence, and to have fun.

There are a number of activities that require little or no adaptation of the prosthesis or of movement patterns. Even multiple amputees and those who function primarily with a wheelchair can enjoy playing cards, gardening, or even bowling. More athletically inclined unilateral amputees can engage in team or individual sports, including skiing, swimming, and playing basketball.

Kegel and associates surveyed 100 unilateral lower extremity amputees to determine their involvement in sports activities. Sixty percent of the respondents were active in sports that ranged from fishing to jogging. Age rather than level of amputation appeared to be the major factor influencing participation. Most amputees had been able to return to preamputation sports activities, particularly if the activity did not require running or jumping. Most amputees found it difficult to jog or go hunting, as these activities placed considerable stress on the residual limb. The majority of amputees wore their regular prosthesis for recreational activities. Seven individuals had special waterproof prostheses, 8 percent used rotation devices in the shank of the prosthesis, and 7 percent used assistive devices such as crutches or outriggers. Only 28 percent believed that the prosthetist was knowledgeable about available components for sports, and several had designed their own adaptations. Prosthetists who were also surveyed indicated that cost was a major factor in the fabrication of special prostheses for sports, particularly since most third-party payers will not fund recreational limbs.

During the Vietnam War, the United States Army developed a program to teach amputees how to ski. As the program developed, both unilateral and bilateral amputees learned to ski using one ski and two outriggers. The sports program expanded to include many other activities, such as horseback riding, swimming, and even skydiving.

Many unilateral amputees continue with ballroom dancing, bowling, weightlifting, and the like. Many gymnastic activities can be performed by bilateral as well as unilateral amputees with few adaptations. Amputees have also been able to ice- and roller-skate with little difficulty. Care is needed to ensure that the height of the artificial foot can accommodate the height of the skate shoe. Athletically inclined individuals should be encouraged to participate in the vigorous physical activities of their choice.

Outdoor activities such as camping, fishing, swimming, and water-skiing are also fairly easy to perform with little adaptation. Care should be taken around water to protect the prosthesis from dampness. Most amputees swim without the need of special devices, although there are adapted swim fins that may be useful for bilateral lower extremity amputees. Hiking and hunting, which require walking over rough, uneven ground, may prove more stressful on the residual limb. Some individuals use old prostheses that have larger sockets and pad the residual limb to reduce torques and rotational stress.

Adaptations for prostheses that make participation in sports easier are available. There is a rotation component that can be installed in the shank of the prosthesis that enables the individual to turn the body as is required in golf and similar sports. Multiaxial feet enhance walking and movement activities on uneven ground. Some amputees have installed spring components in the shank of the prosthesis to aid in running and jumping activities. Outriggers have been developed for skiers and used successfully for many years. Most amputees ski on the sound leg with one or two forearm crutches to which a short ski fore-section has been attached; this is sometimes referred to as three-track skiing. Bilateral amputees usually use one prosthesis and two outriggers.

Highly motivated amputees have been able to participate in most sports, although sports that require running and jumping are the most difficult. The unilateral lower extremity amputee will run using a combination hop and skip motion. Enoka and associates studied the running gait of 10 physically active unilateral below-knee amputees; 6 were able to run (defined as alternating periods of single support and complete non-support in the stride) at speeds ranging from 2.7 to 8.2 meters (9 to 27 feet) per second. Three additional patients were able to achieve periods of non-support from the intact limb but not from the prosthesis. Only one individual, who had sustained some brain damage, was unable to produce nonsupport from either extremity. Marked differences were found in the components of the gait among patients, some of whom had not run prior to amputation. Over time, each achieved some degree of skill and developed some endurance. Lightweight well-fitted prostheses with some foot mobility were found to be the most advantageous. The authors concluded that although running can be a useful sports activity for unilateral below-knee amputees, more work was needed to develop appropriate prosthetic components.

Amputees can also participate in a number of team sports, although in some instances wearing the prosthesis may not be allowed. The National Federation of State

TABLE 22-1. ORGANIZATIONS INVOLVED IN SPORTS FOR THE HANDICAPPED

Sports Associations Assisting Amputees	Services Provided
Adapted Sports Association, Inc. 6832 Marlette Road Marlette, MI 48453	Activities have been merged with the National Handicapped Sports & Recreational Association (NHSRA).
American Camping Association (ACA) Bradford Woods Martinsville, IN 46151	The ACA works with many groups and professional organizations to assure camping's accessibility to individuals of all ages, including the elderly, the economically disadvantaged, the learning disabled, and those with physical impairments.
American Wheelchair Bowling Association (AWBA) Executive Office N54 W15858 Larkspur Ln. Menomonee Falls, WI 53051	The AWBA was formed in 1962. It is composed of wheelchair bowlers who encourage, develop, and regulate wheelchair bowling under uniform rules and regulations (the American Bowling Congress and their own AWBA Rules and Regulations). AWBA national tournaments are held each year.
Camp Roy-el P.O. Box 973 Traverse City, MI 49684	Camp Roy-el provides a 2-week period of recreational camping for youngsters between the ages of 8 and 17 with all types of physical impairments.
Canadian Association for Disabled Skiing (CADS) Head Office Box 307 Kimberley, BC, V1A 2Y9 Canada	CADS was formed in 1976. It provides a publication called *Skiing is Believing,* assists in the development of Provincial & Territorial Disabled Skiing Associations, and provides clinics to teach ski instructors the latest methods of teaching the disabled how to ski in both alpine and nordic skiing.
Canadian Federation of Sport Organizations for the Disabled (CFSOD) 333 River Road Ottawa, Ontario Canada K1L 8H9	CFSOD serves as a national forum and spokesgroup for the Canadian Blind Sports Association, the Canadian Amputee Sports Association, the Canadian Association for Disabled Skiing, the Federation of Silent Sports of Canada, Inc., and the Canadian Wheelchair Sports Association.
International Sports Organization for the Disabled (ISOD) SHIF Idrottens Hus S-123 87 Farsta, Sweden	ISOD is an international sports federation that was formed by national member associations to promote sports for the disabled.
National Amputee Golf Association (NAGA) 5711 Yearling Court Bonita, CA 92002	NAGA provides (within funding limitations) golf lessons and clubs to amputees who are interested in participating in golf. NAGA conducts regional golf tournaments and sponsors an annual national contest solely for amputees.
National Handicapped Sports and Recreational Association (NHSRA) Farragut Station P.O. Box 33141 Washington, DC 20033	NHSRA started in 1967 with a primary interest in amputee snow skiing. It provides year-round sports and recreational opportunities to persons with mobility and visual handicaps. It also sponsors teaching clinics and competitive sports events.

TABLE 22-1. *Continued.*

Sports Associations Assisting Amputees	Services Provided
The 52 Association, Inc. 441 Lexington Avenue New York, NY 10017	A group of 52 New York business and civic leaders incorporated The 52 Association in the closing days of World War II to assist disabled veterans 52 weeks a year. It owns and operates a 41-acre recreational rehabilitation center in Ossinging, New York. The 52 Association is a nonprofit organization that, with the Southland Corporation (7-Eleven Stores), sponsors ski clinics for amputees and blind persons in the United States and Canada.
Union Aviation, Inc. Sturgis Airport P.O. Box 207 Sturgis, KY 42459	Provides hand controls to fit Cessna and Grumman single-engine aircraft. The control, designed for aircraft with rudder pedals that also incorporate toe brake control, enables the pilot to have full rudder control, independent brake control, and simultaneous brake control.

High School Associations revised its rules in 1977 to allow lower extremity amputees, particularly below-knee amputees, to wear their prostheses while participating in team sports such as football. The rules specify requirements for padding and stipulate that the wearing of the prosthesis must not place the opponent at a disadvantage. Amputees have been able to play football, baseball, volleyball, and even wrestle. Amputees participate on wheelchair basketball teams, and many amputees have participated in the Wheelchair Olympics. The International Sports Organization for the Disabled classifies handicapped individuals for participation in various sports activities. There are also a number of organizations that are involved in sports for the handicapped (Table 22-1).

Living with an amputation requires physical and emotional adjustments. To a great extent, the fullness of the life of an amputee will be determined by the factors that affect most of our lives: family support, financial security, and a healthy body. The presence of an amputation does not mitigate against any of these factors, and each person will have to develop an individual approach to a satisfying life.

BIBLIOGRAPHY

ADAMS, R: *Bowling for the physically handicapped.* Inter-Clinic Info Bull 10:9–13, 1970.

ADAMS, RC, ET AL: *Games, Sports and Exercises for the Physically Handicapped,* ed 3. Lea & Febiger, Philadelphia, 1982.

ALTNER, P, RUSIN, J, AND DEBOER, A: *Rehabilitation of blind patients with lower extremity amputations.* Arch Phys Med Rehabil 61:82–85, 1980.

BOYD, LA: Scuba provides expression. J Rehabil 38:21, 1972.

CAINE, D: *The geriatric amputee.* Bull Prosthet Res 10–17:139–147, 1972.

CHAIKLIN, H AND WARFIELD, M: *Stigma management and amputee rehabilitation.* Rehab Lit 34:162–166, 1973.

CLIFT, S AND JOHNSTON, J: *Instructor's Manual for Disabled Skiers.* Canadian Association for Disabled Skiing, Banff, Canada, 1976.

COMFORT, A: *Sexual Consequences of Disability.* George F Stickley, Philadelphia, 1978.

CUMMINGS, V: *Amputees and sexual dysfunction.* Arch Phys Med Rehabil 56:12–13, 1975.

DIAMOND, M: *Sexuality and Disability.* National Easter Seal Society, Chicago, 1981.

DOERNBERG, N: *Some negative effects on family integration of health and educational services for young handicapped children.* Rehab Lit 39:107–111, 1978.

EDELSTEIN, J: *Optimizing the function of geriatric amputees.* Physical and Occupational Therapy in Geriatrics 1:21–41, 1980.

ENOKA, RM, MILLER, DI, AND BURGESS, EM: *Below-knee amputee running gait.* Am J Phys Med 61:66–84, 1982.

FOORT, J: *How amputees feel about amputation.* Orth Pros 28:21–27, 1974.

FRIEDMANN, L: *The Psychological Rehabilitation of the Amputee.* Charles C Thomas, Springfield, Ill, 1978.

GOLDMAN, F: *Environmental barriers to sociosexual integration.* Rehab Lit 39:185–189, 1978.

GRAVES, J AND BURGESS, E: *The extra-ambulatory limb concept as it applies to the below knee amputee skier.* Bull Prosthet Res 10–20:126–131, 1973.

HAMILTON, EA AND NICHOLS, PJR: *Rehabilitation of the elderly lower limb amputee.* Br Med J 2:95–99, 1972.

HARRIS, PJ, ET AL: *The fate of elderly amputees.* Br J Surg 61:665–668, 1974.

HUGHES, HN AND HELMUTH, G: *A modified prosthetic foot for pilots.* Orth Pros 29:33–34, 1975.

HUTTON, IM AND ROTHNIE, NG: *The early mobilization of the elderly amputee.* Br J Surg 64:267–270, 1977.

KEGEL, B, WEBSTER, JC, AND BURGESS, EM: *Recreational activities of lower extremity amputees: A survey.* Arch Phys Med Rehabil 61:258–264, 1980.

KERSTEIN, M, ET AL: *What influence does age have on rehabilitation of amputees.* Geriatrics 30:67–71, 1975.

KUHLTHAU, L: *Equitation for amputees.* Inter-Clinic Info Bull 10:9–12, 1971.

MACBRIDE, A, ET AL: *Psychosocial factors in the rehabilitation of elderly amputees.* Psychosomatics 21:258–265, 1980.

MALONE, J, ET AL: *Therapeutic and economic inpact of a modern amputation program.* Bull Prosthet Res 10–32:7–17, 1979.

REINSTEIN, L, ASHLEY, J, AND MILLER, K: *Sexual adjustment after lower extremity amputation.* Arch Phys Med Rehabil 59:501–504, 1978.

RUBIN, G AND FLEISS, D: *Devices to enable persons with amputation to participate in sports.* Arch Phys Med Rehabil 64:37–40, 1983.

RULLMAN, L: *A new concept in outriggers for three track skiing.* Inter-Clinic Info Bull 10:13–17, 1971.

SADOUGHI, W, LESHNER, M, AND FINE, HL: *Sexual adjustment in chronically ill and physically disabled populations.* Arch Phys Med Rehabil 52:311–317, 1971.

SHONTZ, F: *Psychological adjustment to physical disability.* Arch Phys Med Rehabil 59:251–254, 1978.

SMITH, JP: *In what sports can patients with amputations and other handicaps successfully and actively participate?* Phys Ther 50:121–126, 1970.

STEINBERG, F, ET AL: *Rehabilitation of the geriatric amputee.* J Am Geriatr Soc 22:62–66, 1974.

VARGO, JW: *Some psychological effects of physical disability.* Am J Occup Ther 32:31–34, 1978.

WEAVER, PC AND MARCHALL, SA: *A functional and social review of lower limb amputees.* Br J Surg 60:732–737, 1973.

UNIT **4**
SPECIAL CONSIDERATIONS

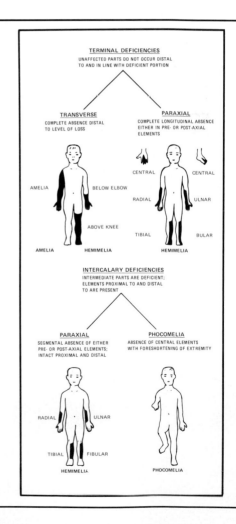

TERMINAL DEFICIENCIES

UNAFFECTED PARTS DO NOT OCCUR DISTAL
TO AND IN LINE WITH DEFICIENT PORTION

TRANSVERSE

COMPLETE ABSENCE DISTAL
TO LEVEL OF LOSS

PARAXIAL

COMPLETE LONGITUDINAL ABSENCE
EITHER IN PRE- OR POST-AXIAL
ELEMENTS

CENTRAL   CENTRAL

AMELIA   BELOW ELBOW

RADIAL   ULNAR

ABOVE KNEE

TIBIAL   BULAR

AMELIA   HEMIMELIA   HEMIMELIA

INTERCALARY DEFICIENCIES

INTERMEDIATE PARTS ARE DEFICIENT;
ELEMENTS PROXIMAL TO AND DISTAL
TO ARE PRESENT

PARAXIAL

SEGMENTAL ABSENCE OF EITHER
PRE- OR POST-AXIAL ELEMENTS;
INTACT PROXIMAL AND DISTAL

PHOCOMELIA

ABSENCE OF CENTRAL ELEMENTS
WITH FORESHORTENING OF EXTREMITY

RADIAL   ULNAR

TIBIAL   FIBULAR

HEMIMELIA   PHOCOMELIA

JUVENILE AMPUTEES

The juvenile amputee is the amputee who still has growth potential or is not yet skeletally mature.

CLASSIFICATION

Juvenile amputations are classified into two broad categories: acquired and congenital. Acquired amputations result from trauma, tumor, infection, or disease. The chief causes of traumatic amputations are vehicular, household, and playground accidents, farm and power tools, gunshots and explosions, burns, and train accidents. Amputations for infections, such as osteomyelitis, tuberculosis, or open fractures, are rare because of the use of antibiotics, but they do occur occasionally. The nomenclature used for acquired amputations is the same as that used for amputations for the adult, described in Chapter 1.

Congenital amputations are the result of a birth defect or anomaly. Many congenital amputations require subsequent surgical amputation for conversion of the anomaly to enable better prosthetic fitting. Limb anomalies may be caused by either genetic or environmental factors. Genetic factors, which presumably arise at the time of conception, have been estimated to cause 90 percent of the malformations: 10 percent by chromosomal aberrations, 20 percent by single-gene (mendelian) disorders, and 60 percent by multiple-gene disorders (polygenic inheritance). Environmental factors such as anoxia, irradiation, hormones, chemicals, and some viral infections are estimated to cause 10 percent of the malformations during the second 25-day (embryonic) period.

One such environmental factor was thalidomide, a synthetic drug that was marketed (initially in 1958) in Germany as Contergan, in England as Distaval, in Portugal as Softenon, in the United States as Kevadon, and in Canada as Kevadon and Talimol. It was used as an antiemetic during pregnancy and was sold widely in West Germany, without prescription, as a sedative and tranquilizer. It was placed on prescription in April 1961 following reports of polyneuritis in adults. By November 1961, several astute observers in Germany showed that thalidomide was a definite cause of limb anomalies when taken 4 to 6 weeks after conception, and it was withdrawn from the market. The number of cases of deformities due to thalidomide has been estimated at 3000 to 4000 in Germany alone.

A different nomenclature is used for congenital amputations than for acquired juvenile amputations. To further complicate the issue, a different system of nomenclature for congenital amputations is used in different parts of the world.

Several commonly used skeletal deficiency classifications are presented in Table 23-1. The Frantz/O'Rahilly terminology was introduced in 1961 and was rapidly adopted in the United States. The two basic types of deficiencies were considered to be terminal and intercalary (Fig. 23-1). Terminal implies absence of distal skeletal elements that are either transverse—extend across the width of the limb—or longitudinal (paraxial)—parallel to the long axis of the limb. Transverse terminal deficiencies are homologues of acquired amputations of the same level. Intercalary denotes the absence of parts ordinarily interposed between the proximal and distal aspects of the remaining limb. Intercalary deficiencies are also further divided into transverse (phocomelia) and longitudinal (paraxial) varieties (Fig. 23-2).

A revision was introduced in 1966 to respond to the foreign objections to the 1961 system of nomenclature. The term hemimelia was eliminated, and meromelia (meros, part) was used to designate all partial absences (see Table 23-1).

TABLE 23-1. CLASSIFICATION OF CONGENITAL SKELETAL LIMB DEFICIENCIES

Frantz & O'Rahilly (1961, USA)	European (originated in Germany)	Revised Frantz & O'Rahilly (1966, USA)	Proposed International Terminology (1974)
	TERMINAL (T) DEFICIENCIES (Absence of all skeletal elements distal to the proximal limit of the deficiency, along the designated axis, longitudinal or transverse)		TRANSVERSE LIMB DEFICIENCIES Lower Limb (LL)
	TRANSVERSE (-) (Absence extending across the width of the limb, including all distal elements)		
Amelia (T-) lower right or left (Complete absence of limb exclusive of girdle)	Amelia, lower right or left (Hip disarticulation)	Amelia (T-) lower right or left	Thigh (Th), Complete Amelia
Hemimelia (T-) (above-knee type) right or left (Absence of some portion of limb, literally, half a limb)	Peromelia, lower right or left, mid-femoral level (Short, above-knee residual limb)	Meromelia (T-): Femur, proximal (P), middle (M), or distal (D), right or left (Partial absence of a limb) P = absence of all or part of proximal third M = absence of all or part of middle third D = absence of all or part of distal third	Thigh (Th) Upper 1/3 Middle 1/3 Lower 1/3
Hemimelia (T-) (knee-disarticulation type), right or left	Peromelia at the level of the right or left knee	Meromelia (T-): Tibiofibular, right or left	Leg (Leg), Complete
Partial hemimelia (T-), right or left (Part of leg is present)	Peromelia at the mid-tibiofibular level, partial aplasia of the right or left tibia and fibula	Meromelia (T-): Tibia, proximal (P), middle (M), or distal (D); fibula P, M, or D; right or left	Leg (Leg) Upper 1/3 Middle 1/3 Lower 1/3

TABLE 23-1. Continued

Frantz & O'Rahilly (1961, USA)	European (originated in Germany)	Revised Frantz & O'Rahilly (1966, USA)	Proposed International Terminology (1974)
Apodia (Absence of foot)		Meromelia (T-) Tarsal	Tarsal (Ta), Complete
Complete adactyly (Absence of all five digits and metatarsals)		Meromelia (T-) Metatarsal	Metatarsal (MT), Complete
Complete aphalangia (Absence of one or more phalanges from all five digits)		Meromelia (T-) Phalangeal	Phalangeal (Ph), Complete
	Longitudinal (Paraxial) (/) (Complete absence extending parallel with the long axis of the limb, either of the pre- or post-axial elements, or central digital rays) Pre-axial = absence of a portion of leg and foot on the great toe side Post-axial = absence of a portion of leg and foot on the lateral side		LONGITUDINAL DEFICIENCIES Lower Limb (LL)
Complete paraxial hemimelia, Tibial (T) or Fibula (F), lower right or left (Complete absence of one of the leg elements and the corresponding portion of the foot)	Ectromelia with axial aplasia, tibial or fibula, metatarsal, and phalangeal, right or left	Meromelia (T/) Tibial or Fibula, right or left	Tibia (Ti), Complete Tarsal (Ta), Partial Metatarsal (MT) 1.2, Complete Phalangeal (Ph) 1.2, Complete — Fibular (Fi), Complete Tarsal (Ta), Partial Metatarsal (MT) 4.5, Complete Phalangeal (Ph) 4.5, Complete
Incomplete paraxial hemimelia, Tibia (T) or Fibula (F), lower right or left	Ectromelia with partial aplasia of the tibia or fibula and complete aplasia of the tarsals, metatarsals,	Meromelia (T/) Tibial or Fibula, proximal (P), middle (M), or distal (D), right or left	Tibia (Ti), Partial Tarsal (Ta), Partial Metatarsal (MT) 1.2, Complete

(Part of the defective leg element is present with absence of the corresponding portion of the foot)	and phalanges, right or left		Phalangeal (Ph) 1.2, Complete
			Fibular (Fi), Partial Tarsal (Ta), Partial Metatarsal (MT) 4.5, Complete Phalangeal (Ph) 4.5, Complete
Partial adactyly (Absence of one to four digits and their metatarsals)		Meromelia (T/) Metatarsal I, II, III	Metatarsal (MT), Partial Phalangeal (Ph), Partial
Partial aphalangia (Absence of one or more phalanges from one to four digits)		Meromelia (T/) Phalangeal, lower right or left I, II, III	Phalangeal (Ph), Partial

INTERCALARY (I) DEFICIENCIES

(Absence of middle parts lying between a proximal-distal series of limb components; elements proximal to and distal to the absent parts are present)

Transverse (-)
(Phocomelia)
(Absence of central segment with foreshortening of the extremity)

Complete phocomelia (I), right or left (Foot attached directly to trunk)	Phocomelia, lower, right or left	Meromelia (I-) Femoral Tibiofibular, right or left	Longitudinal deficiency (combined) Femoral (Fe), Complete Tibia-Fibula (Ti, Fi), Complete
Incomplete (proximal) phocomelia (I), right or left (Leg and foot attached directly to trunk)	Ectromelia, Proximal type	Meromelia (I-) Femoral, right or left	Longitudinal deficiency (proximal) Femoral (Fe), Complete

TABLE 23-1. *Continued*

Frantz & O'Rahilly (1961, USA)	European (originated in Germany)	Revised Frantz & O'Rahilly (1966, USA)	Proposed International Terminology (1974)
Incomplete (distal) phocomelia (I), right or left (Foot attached directly to thigh)	Ectromelia, Distal type	Meromelia (I-) Tibiofibular, right or left	Longitudinal deficiency (distal) Tibia-Fibula (Ti, Fi), Complete
	Longitudinal (Paraxial) (/) (Segmental absence of middle pre- or post-axial elements; intact proximal and distal)		
Complete paraxial hemimelia, Fibular or Tibial, lower right or left (Similar to corresponding terminal defect but foot is more or less complete)	Ectromelia with complete axial aplasia, Fibular or Tibial, right or left	Meromelia (I/) Fibular or Tibial, right or left	Tibia (Ti) or Fibula (Fi), Complete
Incomplete paraxial hemimelia, Fibular or Tibial (I), lower right or left (Similar to corresponding terminal defect but foot is more or less complete)	Ectromelia with partial axial aplasia, proximal third of the fibula or tibia, right or left	Meromelia (I/) Fibula P or Tibia P, right or left	Tibia (Ti) or Fibular (Fi), Partial
Partial adactyly (Absence of all or part of a metatarsal: first or fifth)		Meromelia (I/) Metatarsal I, II, III	Metatarsal (MT), Partial
Partial aphalangia (Absence of proximal and/or middle phalanx from one or more digits: 1, 2, 3, 4, or 5)		Meromelia (I/) Phalangeal, lower left or right, I PP or PM, II PP or PM, etc.	Phalangeal (Ph), Partial

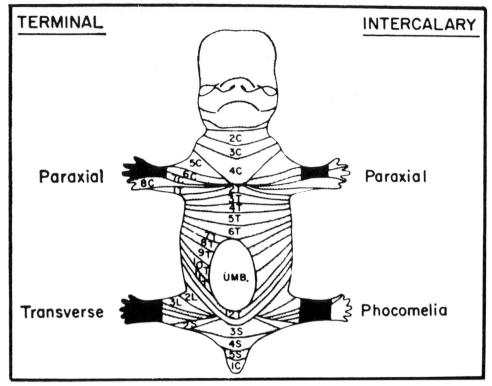

FIGURE 23-1. Dermatome relationships of congenital skeletal limb deficiencies. (From Hall, CB, Brooks, MD, and Dennis, JF: *Congenital skeletal deficiencies of the extremities: Classification and fundamentals of treatment*. JAMA 181:591, 1962, with permission.)

Swanson proposed a system of nomenclature that covers soft tissue as well as skeletal defects (Table 23-2). Such anomalies as duplication (excessive digits), overgrowth (gigantism), and congenital circular constriction band syndrome were included.

In 1974, another terminology was proposed for international classification of deficiencies (see Table 23-1). All limb deficiencies were consolidated into two groups: transverse and longitudinal. The new transverse deficiencies encompassed the old terminal transverse deficiencies. The new longitudinal deficiencies encompassed the terminal longitudinal deficiencies as well as both the longitudinal and transverse intercalary deficiencies.

As with the adult amputations (Chapter 1), the transverse deficiencies are described by the level at which the limb terminates (Fig. 23-3). The longitudinal deficiencies are described by naming the bone(s) affected as well as the degree of absence (completely or partially absent or hypoplastic). Longitudinal deficiencies are subdivided into (1) proximal, (2) distal, and (3) combined, in which both proximal and distal parts of the extremity are affected.

TREATMENT

The treatment of the limb-deficient child is a complex problem, especially if the amputation is congenital, and should be managed by a knowledgeable pediatric amputee

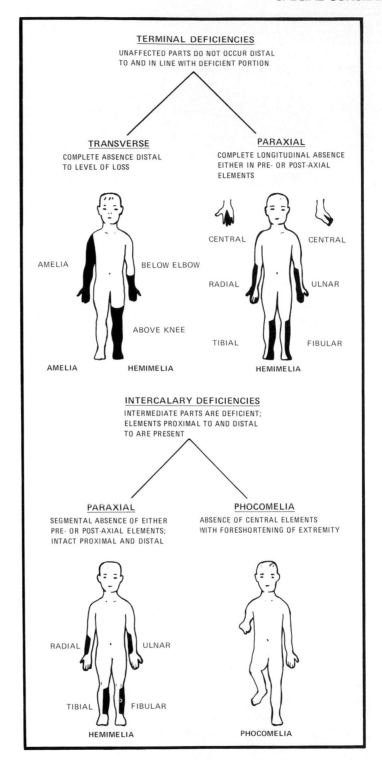

FIGURE 23-2. Subdivisions of terminal and intercalary types of deficiencies. (From Hall, CB, Brooks, MD, and Dennis, JF: *Congenital skeletal deficiencies of the extremities: Classification and fundamentals of treatment.* JAMA 181:591, 1962, with permission.)

TABLE 23-2. SEVEN CATEGORIES SUGGESTED BY DR. ALFRED SWANSON

I. Failure of formation of parts (arrest of development): characterized by either partial or complete failure of limb formation.
   A. Transverse: all congenital amputation-type conditions (e.g., complete aphalangia, apodia, hemimelia, amelia).
   B. Longitudinal: characterized by a deficiency in the longitudinal axis of the skeletal structures and associated tissues. All completely or partially absent bones are named. There may be longitudinal failure of formation of the entire limb (phocomelia) or failure of the preaxial (tibial), postaxial (fibular), or central components.
   Children in this category are often rehabilitated with prosthetic devices.
II. Failure of differentiation (separation) of parts: includes all defects in which the basic anatomic units are present but not completely developed.
III. Duplication: duplication may be of a single bone or an entire limb.
IV. Overgrowth (gigantism): conditions in which either part or all of the limb is disproportionately large.
V. Undergrowth (hypoplasia): may be in the entire limb or its divisions.
VI. Congenital constriction band syndrome: results from focal necrosis along the course of the limb during the fetal stage of development. The necrosis of the superficial tissue heals as a circular scar, creating a band. If the constriction band is severe, intrauterine gangrene may develop, causing a true fetal amputation. (Another theory is that the amputation is caused by amniotic bands that possibly result from insufficient secretion of amniotic fluid, inflammation of the amnion, or anomalous development of the amnion. These bands wrap tightly around the part, causing constriction of circulation with resultant necrosis and eventual amputation.)
VII. Generalized skeletal abnormalities.

---

team. Such a team may be available in only a few specialized centers in each state.

It is generally agreed that the successful habilitation of the child is dependent on the acceptance of the disability by the parents. A prosthesis is fitted when the child is physically ready. It is also important that the parents be psychologically ready for the prosthesis. This may be enhanced by involving the parents in ongoing seminars and small group discussions with members of the staff as moderators. The parents need support and guidance from the medical team.

The aim of amputation surgery, if performed, is to produce a limb that is comfortable and adequate for a prosthesis and that will remain adequate and comfortable through the remaining growth period and for the duration of the person's life. The outcome should allow pain-free weight-bearing, stability, an adequately sensate limb, near-normal gait, maximum bone growth, and satisfactory cosmetic appearance. It is generally agreed that amputation for cosmetic reasons alone should not be done until the child is old enough to share in the decision.

The child who has a traumatic or surgically elected amputation should be placed on a carefully planned postoperative program that includes exercises/activities to prevent contractures and to maintain the function of the residual limb. The parents should be informed of the hazards of contractures and the effect that they may have on the usefulness of the prosthesis. The parents also need instruction in a home program, which may include assisting the child to use a limb to perform functional activities in an atypical manner.

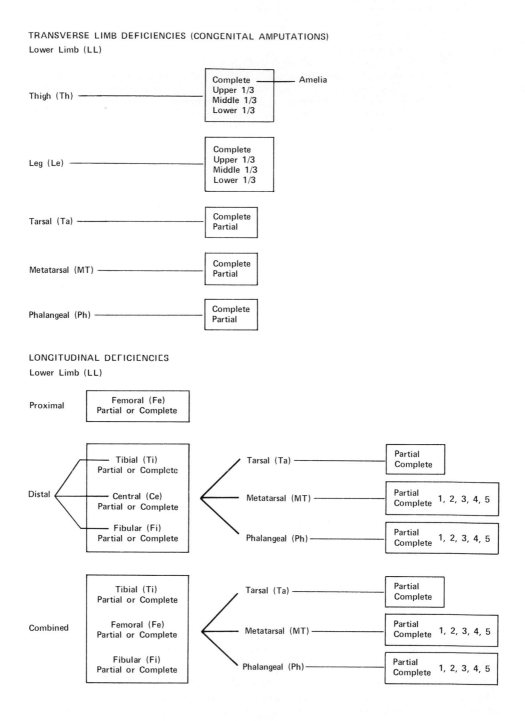

FIGURE 23-3. Failure of formation of parts.

CORRECTIVE SURGERY

FOR BONE OVERGROWTH

In the lower extremity, bone overgrowth occurs most often in the fibula and tibia, especially if the amputation is through the diaphysis. This is one reason that disarticulation amputations are recommended. The overgrowth has been shown to be appositional, not epiphyseal. Radiologically, the overgrowth appears as a sharp spicule of poorly trabeculated bone that extends from the end of the cut bone. Irritation of the soft tissue sometimes produces a bursa. Bone overgrowth occurs more often following acquired amputations or amputations to convert anomalies, and rarely in terminal transverse congenital deficiencies. Bone overgrowth rarely occurs if the primary amputation is after the age of 12 years. Surgical procedures to prevent overgrowth, such as cross-synostosis and capping the end of the bone with various materials, including a Silastic intramedullary plug, are occasionally unsuccessful. With bone overgrowth, the skin becomes attenuated, thin, and shiny. If bone growth exceeds the growth of overlying soft tissue and skin, then pressure necrosis and eventual penetration of the skin are likely, unless the bone is surgically shortened. Multiple surgical revisions may be required before bone maturity if overgrowth does occur and capping is unsuccessful. Full-thickness skin coverage is desirable at the end of growing bones for successful (comfortable) prosthetic use.

FOR SHAPING (CONVERSION)

Corrective surgery may be necessary to shape the limb for a prosthetic socket, but it is usually only done following a trial fitting without conversion. Small appendages may be used to control the prosthesis and thus should not be removed hastily. In general, all epiphyseal growth plates should be preserved to allow the greatest length possible. At times, skin traction, skin grafts, and closure under slight tension may be possible in children when they are not in amputation of the mature adult. Surgical conversion is more often needed for longitudinal rather than transverse deficiencies, to enable comfortable weight-bearing limbs. Even if the distal epiphyseal plate is preserved, the limb will be somewhat shorter at skeletal maturity than the sound leg. Relative shortening of the residual limb is profound with an above-knee amputation but not with a below-knee amputation because the proximal femoral epiphysis contributes only 15 percent to longitudinal growth of the extremity, whereas the proximal tibial epiphysis contributes more than 50 percent. The child may have a minor leg length discrepancy and thus present with a long above-knee residual limb at the time of amputation. At skeletal maturity, the same residual limb may be only of medium length, which is still sufficient for prosthetic control. The discrepancy will be greater the younger the age at amputation.

PROSTHESES

The prosthesis for a congenital amputation is generally fitted as early as possible, consistent with motor development, to enable the child to meet the motor milestones. Thus, a lower extremity prosthesis would be indicated when the child demonstrates the desire to stand, which is usually when the child is between 9 and 12 months old. For an acquired amputation, the prosthesis is fitted as soon after surgery as the residual limb will permit. It is necessary that the limb be comfortable (nontender). The early prosthesis may be a simple brace-like device. The goal should be to provide a prosthesis that is not only functional but also acceptable to touch and sight. Thus, the foot is often eventually amputated to allow more conventional prosthetic fitting. The very young below-knee child amputee may slip out of a patellar-tendon-bearing (PTB) prosthesis and will thus require a more conventional below-knee prosthesis with sidebars and a corset. The PTB prosthesis can usually be fitted by the age of 6 or 7 years.

Roentgenograms are taken prior to prosthetic fitting to determine the bone structure of the incomplete extremity. Subsequent roentgenograms will allow assessment of the developmental patterns to enable the determination of prosthetic modifications for optimum fit as the child grows. The child must be followed closely to avoid skin problems and socket discomfort due to growth. Bone growth in the congenitally deficient limb will likely be uneven or diminished due, at least in part, to abnormal, asymmetric, or reduced muscle pull.

Basically, the most distal joint that has adequate joint stability and function is ascertained. The remaining limb distal to this joint is considered the residual limb. Prosthetic fitting necessitates translating the child's deformity, with subsequent surgical modifications, into the type of conventional amputation the limb most closely resembles.

Alignment techniques for the child's prosthesis are nearly identical to those for the adult's prosthesis. Adjustable legs are available in child's sizes for both above- and below-knee amputees.

TRANSVERSE LIMB DEFICIENCIES

Since terminal transverse limb deficiencies are homologous to acquired amputations, the amputees are fitted with adult-like prostheses that are suitable for the level of amputation. Standard prosthetic components, fabrication techniques, and fit and alignment criteria are used. Variations in the configuration of the residual limb such as vestigial remnants of the digits, invaginations, or redundant skin folds are usual, but they rarely require surgical revision.

APHALANGIA

This defect can involve one or more digits at any level. A shoe filler and spring between the inner and outer soles of the shoe are usually all that is required.

TRANSTARSAL AMPUTATION

Transtarsal defects are similar to Lisfranc amputations. The phalanges, metatarsals, and, usually, the cuneiform and cuboid bones are missing. Talipes equinus is present, along with the underdevelopment of the triceps surae muscle, with resulting genu recurvatum upon ambulation. This rare defect can be treated with a reinforced steel shank and a foam-rubber shoe filler.

APODIA

In cases of complete absence of the foot, the tibia and fibula may initially look normal on roentgenographic examination but will show retarded growth at maturity when compared with the contralateral leg. The toddler may initially be fitted as a Syme amputee, but as an adult, the limb will likely be at the long below-knee level. The prosthesis used is a modified Syme type.

BILATERAL LOWER AMELIA

Amelia of the lower extremities is usually bilateral. Bilateral lower amelia is a homologue of bilateral hip disarticulation (Fig. 23-4A). The pelvis is relatively normal. Osseous remnants of the femoral heads may be present. Prosthetically, these children are fitted with a prosthetic bucket at 4 to 6 months of age, which stabilizes the trunk and pelvis to facilitate the development of independent sitting balance. At about 9 months of age, the bucket may be attached to rocker feet or to a platform on casters to allow limited mobility (Fig. 23-4B). At 18 to 24 months of age, bilateral hip disarticulation prostheses, usually with nonarticulated knees, can be fitted. A swing-to or swing-through gait is taught, as with a paraplegic. The prosthetic knees are articulated when the child's motor skills are adequate (Fig. 23-4C).

QUADRIMEMBRAL (TOTAL) AMELIA

Quadrimembral amelia is a rare condition that has a limited rehabilitation potential. Prosthetically, it is necessary to provide a bucket that is molded snugly over the iliac crests and about the buttocks to enable sitting. Since a large portion of the body surface is missing, the ability to dissipate body heat is so reduced that minimal activity may produce profuse sweating and cause fatigue. The upper limb problem is approached after sitting balance has been established.

LONGITUDINAL (INTERCALARY AND TERMINAL LONGITUDINAL) DEFICIENCIES

Amputations for this group of deficiencies are performed for better prosthetic fitting and function, better cosmetic appearance, or both. Prostheses for this group of amputees

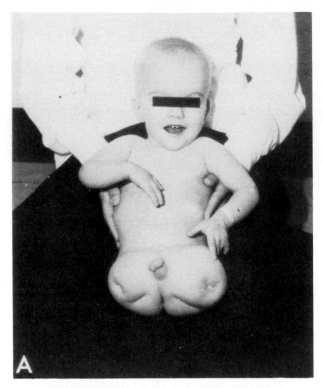

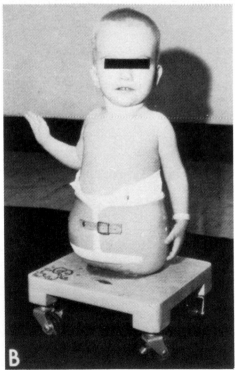

FIGURE 23-4. *(A)* A 13-month-old boy with bilateral lower limb amelia. *(B)* A molded plastic laminate bucket, which provides stability for sitting balance, attached to a platform with casters.

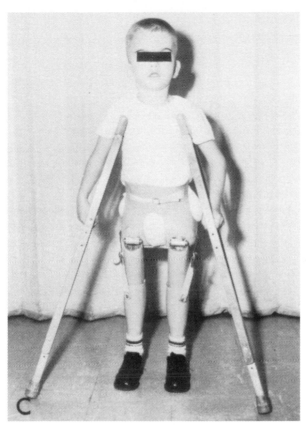

FIGURE 23-4. *Continued.* *(C)* The boy at 5 years old, fitted with bilateral hip-disarticulation prostheses with articulated knees. Crutches allow a swing-to or swing-through gait. (From Aitken, GT: *The child amputee: An overview.* Orthop Clin North Am 3:464, 1972, with permission.)

require individualized design, fabrication, fitting, and alignment because of the wide variety of abnormalities such as malrotation, leg length discrepancy, proximal joint instability, and muscular inadequacies. The most distal stable joint is determined, the presenting deformity is translated into an amputation type, and then the limb is fitted with a nonstandard, comfortable prosthesis. Because most sockets are nonstandard, custom-made nonstandard components are sometimes necessary. Alignment can be altered somewhat to accommodate for malrotation.

The three most common longitudinal deficiencies in the lower limb are first, fibular hemimelia; second, proximal femoral focal deficiency (PFFD); and third, tibial hemimelia.

FIBULAR HEMIMELIA

Paraxial fibular hemimelia is complete or partial absence of the fibula. These children characteristically have a short tibial segment with an anterior bow, usually at the junction of the distal and middle thirds, which has a dimple in the skin at the apex of the bow. The anterior bow resolves with growth in many children. Occasionally, there is medial bowing that does not show spontaneous correction. The foot is usually in an equinovalgus position because of the lack of a lateral malleolus. Commonly associated anomalies are absence of lateral rays with absence of some tarsal bones (usually the talus and cuboid) or fusion of some tarsal bones (usually the calcaneus to the talus) which collectively is called terminal complete paraxial fibular hemimelia. A tight fibrocartilaginous band that extends from the proximal end of the tibia to the calcaneus is probably the underdeveloped fibular analage. Occasionally, there is also congenital shortening of the femur, absence of the femur, or some abnormality of the distal tibial epiphysis, which is slow to ossify. Growth in the affected limb will be proportional to the normal limb; thus, eventual shortening can be estimated. Absence of the fibula occurs more often than partial development. The defect is bilateral in approximately 25 percent of the cases. In unilateral cases, there seems to be a greater incidence of right-sided lesions. Fibular hemimelia occurs more frequently in males than in females.

Therapeutic approaches include: (1) compensation for inequality of leg lengths by a shoe lift with or without a brace; (2) tibial or femoral lengthening as well as contralateral epiphysiodesis, if the anticipated limb length discrepancy will be greater than 7.5 cm (3 in) (usually done for children with some residuum of fibula present, little tibial bowing, a foot with four or five rays, and normal ankle alignment); (3) epiphysiodesis or epiphyseal arrest of the contralateral leg, if the anticipated limb length discrepancy will be 7.5 cm (3 in) or less; (4) excision of the fibrocartilaginous band in the area of the absent fibula, which may decrease the anterior tibial bowing and foot deformity (sometimes performed in conjunction with a tibial osteotomy); and (5) ankle disarticulation with a Syme-type flap closure, a Syme amputation, or a Boyd amputation and fitting with an end-bearing Syme-type prosthesis with a PTB-like proximal socket (usually required for children with no fibula, a bowed tibia, a short femur resulting in an estimated leg length discrepancy of more than 7.5 cm [3 in], and a severe foot deformity).

Some surgeons believe that in a child, the heel pad cannot be preserved in proper position if it is surgically removed from the inferior aspect of the calcaneus, as in the Syme amputation, which will often cause destruction of fascial cells of the pad. Thus, they recommend retaining the plantar pad to a fragment of the calcaneus, which is arthrodesed to the denuded distal surface of the tibia. Kirschner wires are used to hold the pad in place until bony union occurs. This alternate procedure is similar to the Boyd amputation.

Complete excision of the cartilaginous epiphysis of the calcaneus is an important technical detail to avoid growth of a painful ossicle that will require later excision. Amputation may be contraindicated if severe malformations of the upper limbs are present since the toes may be used for grasping and self-care. If the foot is retained, the valgus contracture is corrected and the peroneal tendons are transposed posteriorly. If amputation is selected as the treatment of choice, then it should be performed prior to school age to minimize psychological trauma.

If the femur is short or absent, the knee joint levels will be unequal and there will be severe leg length inequality. Contralateral epiphyseal arrests are not usually adequate. Fitting with a Syme-type prosthesis will equalize total leg length, but the knees will often be unequal.

Genu valgum is an associated problem of fibular hypoplasia. Although it does not significantly limit the child's activity, it is unsightly and does cause a poor gait, with the limb held in external rotation. Therapeutic approaches include insetting the foot of the prosthesis or increasing the height of the lateral wall of the brim of the socket.

PROXIMAL FEMORAL FOCAL DEFICIENCY (PFFD)

This deficiency of the proximal end of the femur is characterized by a very short femoral segment, which is held in flexion, abduction, and external rotation. The quadriceps muscle is frequently hypoplastic with a correspondingly small or vestigial patella. Often, there is associated ipsilateral paraxial fibular hemimelia. The total limb length of the affected side is about the level of the knee joint on the unaffected side. The condition may be bilateral or unilateral. Bilateral PFFD with bilateral paraxial fibular hemimelia is rare. There are four subcategories of PFFD, as described by George Aitken, which can be differentiated radiographically after the child is 9 to 12 months old:

Category A: All proximal components of the femur eventually ossify with severe subtrochanteric varus, often with pseudarthrosis. Short femoral shaft. Well-formed acetabulum.

Category B: The head of the femur is in a competent acetabulum, but there is never bony or cartilaginous continuity between the shaft and head at maturity. Short femoral shaft.

Category C: The femoral head does not ossify; the acetabulum is severely dysplastic. Short femur.

Category D: There is no acetabulum and no head of the femur; the femoral segment is abnormally short and severely flexed, with no proximal femoral apophysis. (Most bilateral cases of PFFD are in this category.)

An alternate classification was proposed by Lange and associates in 1977:

Class I: A subtrochanteric varus deformity and mild to moderate shortening. Commonly confused with developmental coxa vara. Mild form of PFFD. The prognosis is good.

Class II: Acetabulum is present, but there is delayed ossification of the femoral head. The proximal femoral shaft is displaced laterally from the head and appears to extend proximal to the acetabulum. The head and shaft are joined by a cartilage bridge. The prognosis is favorable.

Class III: Intact acetabulum but late ossification of the femoral head. The femoral shaft and head are separated and bridged by amorphous fibrous tissue rather than by bone or cartilage. All are unstable.

Class IV: Aitken Categories C and D. Severe deficiency with absence of the acetabulum and femoral head. Marked femoral shortening. Hips are unstable.

The varus deformity in PFFD differs from developmental coxa vara in that the varus is subtrochanteric.

In most cases, there is no known surgical procedure to equalize femoral lengths. In children with Aitken Category D type PFFD, the difference in leg length may not be marked prior to 2 years of age, and thus a shoe lift may be all that is necessary. At the age of 5 or 6 years, however, the leg length discrepancy is significant. Prosthetically, the child is treated as either a below-knee or an above-knee amputee. If it is decided to treat the child as a below-knee amputee, then a tenomyoplastic Chopart amputation or a

Van Nes, 180-degree rotational osteotomy of the tibia is performed (Fig. 23-5). The rotational osteotomy, previously described by Joseph Borggreve in 1930, allows the ankle joint to be utilized as a knee joint and the foot, which has been turned around, to function as a below-knee residual limb. The calf muscles act as the quadriceps. The procedure may be performed in two stages to avoid ischemia owing to torsion of the vessels. The prosthesis resembles one used for a below-knee amputation (Fig. 23-6). The unstable, unfused knee should be immobilized by the prosthesis.

When the patient is near skeletal maturity, the anatomic knee is fused, which will reduce the fixed flexion deformity, if present. The prosthesis is then changed to a more conventional below-knee prosthesis with a thigh-lacer and external knee joints. The knee joints are aligned posteriorly to ensure adequate knee stability.

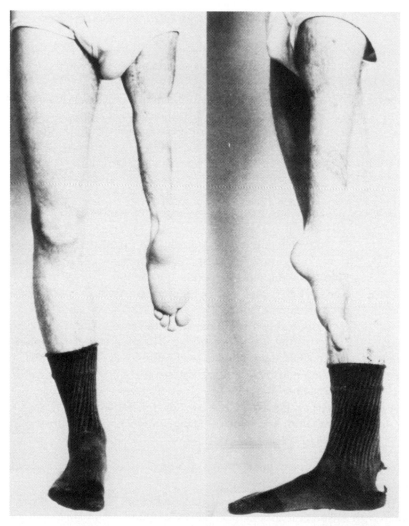

FIGURE 23-5. The Van Nes procedure (first reported in 1930), which consists of a 180-degree tibial rotation-plasty so that the ankle joint can be used as a knee joint, in a young man who had a Category A proximal femoral focal deficiency. Arthrodesis of the knee was performed at the age of 17 years. (From Kritter, AE: *Tibial rotation-plasty for proximal focal deficiency.* **J Bone Joint Surg 59A:929, 1977, with permission.)**

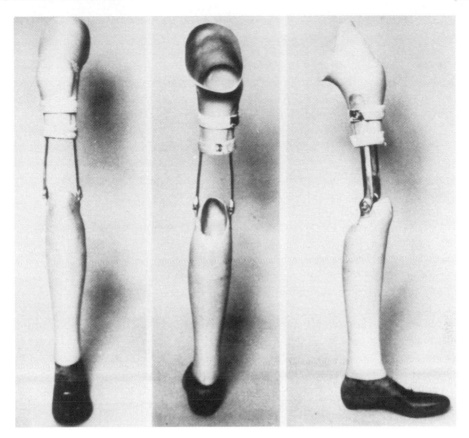

FIGURE 23-6. A prosthesis for a child with proximal femoral focal deficiency following a Van Nes procedure. Note the quadrilateral ischial weight-bearing proximal socket (pelvic band optional), external knee hinges, and distal socket for the foot that has a high anterior trim line over the heel of the rotated foot. (From Kritter, AE: *Tibial rotation-plasty for proximal focal deficiency.* J Bone Joint Surg 59A:928, 1977, with permission.)

Associated paraxial fibular hemimelia with absence of the fourth and fifth rays gives poor results following a tenomyoplastic Chopart disarticulation or a Van Nes reconstruction and is thus a contraindication. The procedures are indicated for children with a normal foot and ankle and, preferably, a stable hip. After tibial rotation-plasty and subsequent knee fusion, the axis of motion of the ankle should be level with the axis of the contralateral knee. If the femoral segment is too long or too short to allow the ankle and contralateral knee axes to be at the same level, then tibial rotation-plasty is contraindicated.

It has been suggested that if the initial rotation is performed before the age of 6 years, rerotation will probably be required twice before skeletal maturity. Muscle forces that tend to derotate the foot postoperatively are the probable cause. The final position of rotation can be adjusted when the knee is arthrodesed. The initial rotation is usually performed when the child is 10 to 12 years of age, which enables a more accurate prediction of limb length at maturity. If the Van Nes rotational osteotomy fails, a Syme amputation can be performed. Improved above-knee prostheses for children have made surgically created knees less desirable.

If the child is managed as an above-knee amputee, then several surgical procedures are considered: (1) ankle disarticulation with a Syme-like end-bearing flap, a Syme amputation, or a Boyd amputation, all of which facilitate end weight-bearing (usually performed when the foot can no longer reach the ground but before the age of 4 to minimize psychological trauma); (2) knee arthrodesis, which will give a single skeletal lever and correct the malrotation somewhat, is primarily advised for Categories A and B (deferred because premature closure will result in a residual limb that is too short); (3) correction of the hip flexion deformity; and (4) reconstructive surgery to increase stability at the hip (usually only considered for Categories A and B, which have an adequate acetabulum with the femoral head in the acetabulum), such as a subtrochanteric valgus osteotomy to reduce the angular and rotational deformity. The decision for an ankle disarticulation is more readily accepted by the parents if there are abnormalities of the foot as well.

If a pseudarthrosis exists, with cartilaginous continuity between the proximal femoral segment and the shaft, the cartilaginous element can be excised. Fixation is obtained by a small rod or nail-and-plate to hold the bony elements in contact or by a bone graft across the cartilage. Surgical management of the pseudarthrosis is particularly indicated if proximal migration of the distal femoral segment occurs. Exploration in early life will enable treatment before weight-bearing causes upward displacement of the femoral shaft. Surgical reconstruction for instability of the hip offers little prospect if the acetabulum is absent.

The above-knee or knee-disarticulation type of prosthesis has a proximal socket designed for ischial weight-bearing. For children with Category A or B involvement, the proximal thigh is normal enough to use a modified quadrilateral socket. For children with Category C or D involvement, the socket has more of a cylindrical shape. The socket may have a flexible inner wall, which allows entry of the bulbous end of the limb and provides suspension. A Silesian bandage may be used for secondary suspension. The correct prosthetic length is assumed if the child's spine is straight. The iliac crests are not always symmetric and are thus not always a reliable reference point.

In cases of bilateral PFFD, if the limbs are approximately the same length, then the child may walk without prostheses, but the height will be significantly short. For a more natural height, the child can be fitted with modified above-knee prostheses in which the feet are positioned in plantarflexion or are amputated at the ankle. Factors that favor ablation of the feet are: (1) feet that are badly deformed and do not function well for ambulation, (2) a significant leg length discrepancy, and (3) the potential to provide a more cosmetic prosthesis. The main factor against foot ablation is that without the procedure, the child is often able to ambulate when not wearing a prosthesis. Also, if the upper limbs are either absent or severely deformed, both feet must be saved because they are necessary for self-care activities. The Van Nes rotational osteotomy is not recommended for bilateral PFFD.

TIBIAL HEMIMELIA

Tibial hemimelia (Fig. 23-7) is characterized by complete or partial absence of the tibia and, frequently, central aphalangia of the hands ("lobster-claw" hands). This condition is unusual in that it is seen in siblings, and thus the parents of children with tibial hemimelia should receive genetic counseling. The proximal end of the fibula, which is flat and bowed, usually overrides the transverse axis of the knee joint owing to a lateral

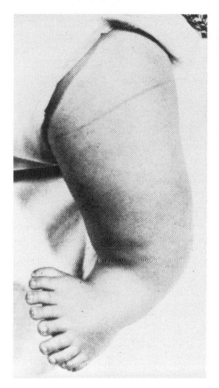 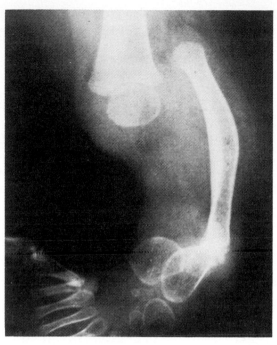

FIGURE 23-7. Photograph *(Left)* and radiograph *(Right)* of the leg of a child, showing complete absence of the tibia, posterolateral dislocation of the fibula at the knee, varus of the foot, and supernumerary digits. (From Jones, D, Barnes, J, and Lloyd-Roberts, GC: *Congenital aplasia and dysplasia of the tibia and intact fibula: Classification and management.* J Bone Joint Surg 60B:33, 1978, with permission.)

and posterior dislocation, resulting in a very short leg with malrotation on the affected side. The foot is in severe varus. Knee flexion with popliteal webbing and diplopodia (reduplication of a number of rays) or polydactyly is characteristic. Other associated deformities include: fusion of tarsal bones (usually talocalcaneal or talocalcaneonavicular); shortness or partial absence of the fibula; malformation of the distal femoral condyle and intercondyloid fossa (in cases of partial defect of the tibia where the upper end is present, the femur is usually normal); absence of the femur or congenital dysgenesis of the proximal femur and subluxation or dislocation of the hip and absence of one or more rays of the foot. The talus, navicular, medial and intermediate cuneiforms, and medial two or three metatarsals and digits are the most common absences. The thigh muscles that normally attach to the tibia are frequently abnormal or absent, resulting in a smaller thigh, in both length and circumference, than on the opposite side. The patella, which is usually present, may be small and have delayed ossification. Associated upper limb deformities, in addition to partial aphalangia (split-ray or lobster-claw hands), include supernumerary digits and partial adactyly (floating thumb). Muscles may be absent; these are usually, but not always, muscles that would have no bony attachment. Occasionally, muscles develop an extraordinary transposition of the insertion, and they function in the reverse of normal. Unilateral absence of the tibia occurs more often than bilateral absence. Of the unilateral cases, the right limb is involved more frequently than the left and total absence of the tibia occurs more often than partial absence. There seems to be a slight preponderance of occurrence in males over females. In cases of a partial tibial defect, the distal end is the part that is almost invariably absent (Table 23-3). Except in uncommon cases of slight partial absence, the leg is useless for normal ambulation, although crawling or walking on the knees is sometimes possible.

For complete tibial hemimelia, the conversion surgery used is usually either disarticulation or reconstruction. A knee disarticulation amputation and fitting with a knee disarticulation type of prosthesis, which will equalize leg length and eliminate the malrotation and knee joint instability, is more commonly done. In select cases, the child may be treated as a below-knee amputee by transplantation of the proximal end of the fibula under the distal end of the femur to articulate with the femoral condylar notch, construction of a knee joint, foot ablation by ankle disarticulation with a Syme-type flap, and fitting with a below-knee prosthesis; this is usually recommended during the first year of life. Construction of a knee joint between the femoral condyles and the head of the fibula and, in a second operation, fusion of the distal end of the fibula to the

TABLE 23-3. TYPES OF CONGENITAL APLASIA AND DYSPLASIA OF THE TIBIA*

Type	Radiologic Description	Occurrence
1 — a	• Tibia not seen (tibia is, in fact, totally absent) • Hypoplastic lower femoral epiphysis (femoral epiphysis translucent) • Proximal dislocation of fibula	Most frequent early finding
1 — b	• Tibia not seen (proximal part of tibia is present but, as yet, is an unossified, translucent, cartilaginous anlage which is misleading) • Normal lower femoral epiphysis • Proximal dislocation of fibula	Most frequent early finding
2	• Distal tibia not seen, but proximal tibia is visible • Proximal dislocation of fibula	More common than Type 3
3	• Proximal tibia not seen, but distal tibia is visible • Lower femoral epiphysis is well developed • Proximal dislocation of fibula • No true knee joint	
4	• Distal tibiofibular diastasis with a complete but shortened tibia • Proximal dislocation of fibula • Foot normal in structure	

*Adapted from Jones, D, Barnes, J, and Lloyd-Roberts, GC: *Congenital aplasia and dysplasia of the tibia with intact fibula: Classification and management.* J Bone Joint Surg 60B:31, 1978.

talus or calcaneus is another option. Adaptive changes that may occur with weight-bearing include flaring of the proximal end of the fibula and formation of a true knee joint. The prosthesis needs to be designed to provide mediolateral stability at the knee. Because these surgical procedures are very complex and instability with poor voluntary control at the fibulofemoral joint often continues after surgical correction, knee disarticulation is usually preferred. Also, knee flexion is often less in the reconstructed joint than in the prosthesis.

In partial tibial hemimelia, synostosis of the fibula to the remnant of the tibia can be performed, followed, after healing, by an ankle disarticulation with a Syme-type flap closure. A below-knee type of prosthesis that provides stability at the knee joint is used.

PHOCOMELIA

The term phocomelia is derived from the Greek terms phoke (seal) and melos (limb). It may be complete (the foot is attached to the trunk), proximal (the foot attaches to the lower leg which attaches to the trunk), or distal (the foot attaches to the thigh). Complete lower limb phocomelia (Fig. 23-8A and B) where the foot is at the hip, usually with no bony elements of the femur, tibia, or fibula, is functionally a homologue of a hip disarticulation. Removal of the foot is contraindicated. The foot provides sensory feedback and an excellent weight-bearing surface and enhances suspension. A modified Canadian-type hip-disarticulation prosthesis is used (Fig. 23-8C).

For children with complete phocomelia of all four extremities, the initial treatment is aimed at developing adequate head and trunk control. The child is next placed in a pelvic bucket that is mounted on a suitable base to comfortably support the child in the vertical position. A rocker base later replaces the stable platform so that the child can develop a sense of balance (Fig. 23-9A). At about 2 years of age, the child progresses to a swivel walker with a socket similar to bilateral Canadian hip-disarticulation prostheses (Fig. 23-9B). The feet of the swivel walker are tilted 6 degrees so only the medial edges touch the floor. If the body is shifted laterally, then the ipsilateral foot will be flat on the floor and the contralateral foot will clear the floor so it can swing forward. After the child masters the device, the height can be increased gradually, usually in 4-cm (1 1/2-in) increments. To walk backward, the child must lean backward to get the center of gravity behind the axis of the swivel unit and then move in a side-to-side rocking motion.

The child eventually progresses to wearing articulated prostheses (Fig. 23-9C). A power cart can be used for mobility on slopes and rough terrain and for greater distance indoors or outdoors (Fig. 23-9D).

In proximal lower limb phocomelia, the femur and acetabulum are absent. The tibia slides up and down against the pelvis because the ligaments are loose.

In distal lower limb phocomelia, the foot, which articulates with the distal femur, often has just one digit. The femoropelvic joint is usually quite unstable.

SACRAL AGENESIS

Sacral agenesis is characterized by absence of the sacrum. Lumbosacral agenesis is absence of the sacrum and lumbar vertebrae. Associated symptoms include: vertebral-pelvic instability resulting in a collapsing kyphoscoliotic spine; urologic and gastroin-

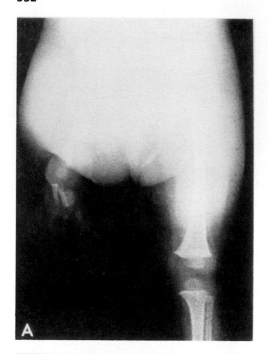

FIGURE 23-8. *(A)* Roentgenogram of lower limb phocomelia. *(B)* Clinical appearance in a 6-year-old boy. *(C)* Fitting with a modified Canadian-type hip-disarticulation prosthesis. (From Aitken, GT: *The child amputee: An overview.* Orthop Clin North Am 3:454, 1972, with permission.)

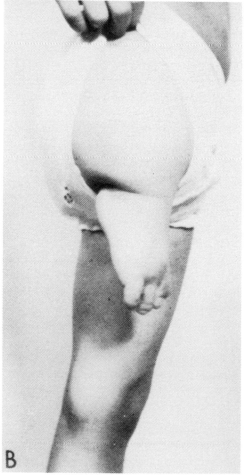

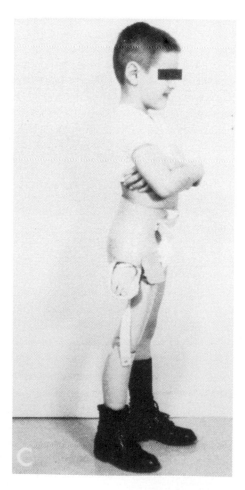

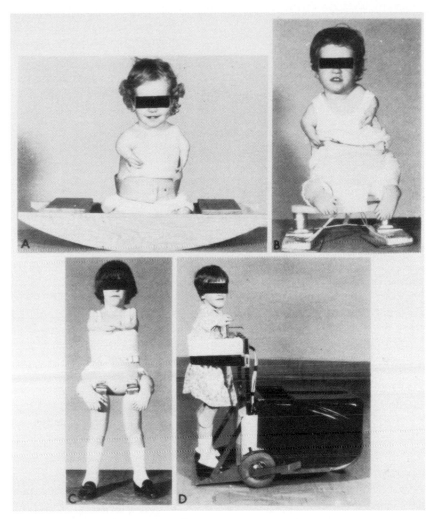

FIGURE 23-9. *(A)* A rocker base allows the child with phocomelia to touch the rudimentary lower limbs to the floor and rock from side to side. *(B)* A swivel walker allows forward progression by side-to-side motion. *(C)* Articulated, bilateral Canadian-type hip-disarticulation prostheses. *(D)* A custom-made power cart. (From Sauter, WF: *Prosthesis for the child amputee.* Orthop Clin North Am 3:487, 1972, with permission.)

testinal anomalies, which may be life-threatening; paralysis of the lower extremities, which are subject to pressure sores; feet in equinovarus or calcaneovalgus; congenital fusion of ribs; bilateral hip dislocation; spina bifida with myelomeningocele; hemivertebrae; and hip and knee flexion contractures, usually with a wide popliteal web. The buttocks are flat with a short intergluteal cleft and a depressed dimpling lateral to the gluteal cleft. Genital involvement is infrequent. The ilia approximate posteriorly, resulting in a small diameter of the pelvic ring.

Therapeutic approaches include: (1) surgical procedures, such as colostomy or ileal diversion, to manage the urologic and gastrointestinal problems; (2) establishment of a stable vertebral-pelvic complex by halo-femoral traction, followed by vertebral iliac fusion before thoracopelvic or lumbopelvic flexion becomes fixed and irreversible renal changes occur; (3) stretching or surgical release of contractures; (4) osteotomies to align the lower extremities for better sitting balance or use of prostheses; and (5) subtrochanteric amputation of the lower extremities to allow the use of prostheses for ambulation.

If bilateral subtrochanteric amputations are performed, prosthetic training begins in a thoracopelvic socket with stubbies to obtain sitting balance and trunk control. Leg length can be gradually increased with progression to Canadian-type hip-disarticulation prostheses.

TRAINING

Most children require minimal training in the use of lower extremity prosthetic devices. The parents should be given systematic instruction in the therapy program and should be supervised at regular intervals since they will continue with it at home. Since young children are primarily involved with play, play will usually serve as the primary motivation for desired movements and activity.

Therapists must be careful not to expect more from child amputees than from their counterparts with normal extremity function. The normal child does not establish heel-to-toe gait until about 2 years of age. At about 20 months, the normal child can stand on one foot with help, at 3 years on one foot momentarily, at 4 years for several seconds, and at 5 years of age stance on one leg is indefinite. Allowances are made for the congenital amputee.

In above-knee amputees, the knee is nonarticulated (locked) until the child is secure in stiff-legged walking. Prosthetic heel-strike to toe-off gait is not usually attained until the child is about 5 years old or can demonstrate sustained one-legged standing. Efforts to develop a smooth alternating progression should follow. The major causes of gait deviations are growth or wear of prosthetic parts from use.

In cases of bilateral involvement, when one or both limbs terminate at or above the knee, stubbies may be used in the transitional stage. Stubbies consist of quadrilateral sockets with foot pieces that usually have a rocker bottom that is slightly elongated posteriorly. A Silesian bandage is usually sufficient for suspension unless the residual limbs are short, in which case a pelvic band with hip joints is used. Shoulder straps may be used prior to 5 years of age since bilateral pelvic bands limit hip motion. The socket is preflexed a few degrees to prevent an excessive lumbar lordosis. Stubbies are indicated as an initial prescription when the child is too young for a secure balance on conventional articulated prostheses as a primary fitting.

The juvenile amputee should be expected to grow both longitudinally and circumferentially. A new prosthesis is indicated when the old prosthesis is more than 1 cm (2/5 in) short. A delay in the replacement of a short prosthesis may result in the development of scoliosis. A new prosthesis is required about every 1 to 2 years for circumferential growth. Follow-up is usually necessary every 3 to 6 months but may need to be more frequent during adolescent growth spurts. Parents must be instructed in and responsible for the care of the residual limb and prosthesis for the young child.

The child amputee's prosthetic needs are primarily for comfort and mechanical function. When the child becomes a teenager and social activities become a very important aspect of life, then the cosmetic appearance of the prosthesis becomes important. Often, female amputees are given two prosthetic feet, one in the neutral position and one in equinis to accommodate high-heeled shoes.

BIBLIOGRAPHY

ACKER, RB: *Congenital absence of femur and fibula: Report of two cases.* Clin Orthop 15:203–207, 1959.

ADDISON, J: *Sacro-coccygeal agenesis.* Proc R Soc Med 48:163–164, 1955.

AITKEN, GT: *Amputation as a treatment for certain lower-extremity congenital abnormalities.* J Bone Joint Surg 41A:1267–1285, 1959.

AITKEN, GT: *Hazards to health: Etiology of traumatic amputations in children.* N Engl J Med 265:133–134, 1961.

AITKEN, GT: *Current concepts in the management of the juvenile amputee.* Orthop Pros Appl J 16:257–262, 1962.

AITKEN, GT: *Overgrowth of the amputation stump.* Inter-Clinic Info Bull 1:1–8, 1962.

AITKEN, G: *Surgical amputation in children.* J Bone Joint Surg 45A:1735–1741, 1963.

AITKEN, GT: *Prosthetic fitting following amputation for bone tumor: A preliminary report.* Inter-Clinic Info Bull 3:1–2, 10, 1964.

AITKEN, GT: *The child with an acquired amputation.* Inter-Clinic Info Bull 7:1–15, 1968.

AITKEN, GT: *Proximal femoral focal deficiency.* In SWINYARD, CW (ED): *Limb Development and Deformity: Problems of Evaluation and Rehabilitation.* Charles C Thomas, Springfield, Ill., 1969, pp 456–476.

AITKEN, GT: *The child amputee: An overview.* Orthop Clin North Am 3:447–472, 1972.

AITKEN, GT: *Congenital short femur with fibular hemimelia.* J Bone Joint Surg 56A:1306, 1974.

AITKEN, G (ED): *Selected Lower Limb Anomalies: Surgical and Prosthetic Management.* National Academy of Sciences, Washington, DC, 1971.

AITKEN, GT AND FRANTZ, CH: *The juvenile amputee.* J Bone Joint Surg 35A:659–664, 1953.

AITKEN, GT AND FRANTZ, CH: *Prostheses for the juvenile amputee.* Am J Dis Child 89:137–143, 1955.

AITKEN, GT AND FRANTZ, CH: *The juvenile amputee: A fourteen-year follow-up.* J Bone Joint Surg 46A:1376, 1964.

AJINKYA, YN: *Intra-uterine amputations and annular constrictions in a living infant, now a child of 4, due to amniotic adhesions resulting from oligohydramnios.* J Obstet Gynecol 45:692–694, 1928.

ALEXANDER, J: *The child amputee: Summary of a forum.* Arch Phys Med Rehabil 56:169–172, 1975.

AMSTUTZ, HC: *Natural history of treatment of congenital absence of the fibula.* J Bone Joint Surg 54A:1349, 1972.

ANDERSON, RJ: *Notes of a case of intra-uterine amputation.* Br Med J 2:78, 1881.

ASHHURST, APC: *Congenital absence of the fibula.* Ann Surg 63:378–380, 1916.

BADGER, VM: *Evaluation of foot conversions for congenital anomalies: Syme, Boyd, and Chopart.* Inter-Clinic Info Bull 8:1–17, 1969.

BARBER, CG: *Amputation of the lower leg with induced synostosis of the distal ends of tibia and fibula.* J Bone Joint Surg 26:356–362, 1944.

BARENBERG, LH AND GREENBERG, B: *Intrauterine amputations and constriction bands: Report of a case with anesthesia below the constriction.* Am J Dis Child 64:87–92, 1942.

BEAL, LL: *The impact of an anomalous child on those concerned with his welfare.* Orthop Pros Appl J 16:144–147, 1962.

BEEKMAN, F: *Amputations during childhood.* Surg Clin North Am 18:425–431, 1938.

BERMAN, W: *Congenital absence of the sacrum and coccyx complicating pregnancy.* Am J Obstet Gynecol 50:447–450, 1945.

BEVAN-THOMAS, WH AND MILLAR, EA: *A review of proximal focal femoral deficiencies.* J Bone Joint Surg 49A:1376–1388, 1967.

BLUMEL, J, EVANS, EB, AND EGGERS, GWN: *Partial and complete agenesis or malformation of the sacrum with associated anomalies: Etiologic and clinical study with special reference to heredity: A preliminary report.* J Bone Joint Surg 41A:497–518, 1959.

BOCHMANN, D AND THOMSON, HG: *The slip-socket prosthesis for juveniles: A new clinical application.* Inter-Clinic Info Bull 8:1–6, 1969.

BROOKS, MB AND MAZET, R, JR: *Prosthetics in child amputees.* Clin Orthop 9:190–204, 1957.

BROOKS, MB AND SHAPERMAN, J: *Infant prosthetic fitting: A study of the results.* Am J Occup Ther 19:329–334, 1965.

BROOKS, MB, ET AL: *The child with deformed or missing limbs: His problems and prostheses.* Am J Nurs 62:88–92, Nov 1962.

BROWN, FW: *Construction of a knee joint in congenital total absence of the tibia (paraxial hemimelia tibia): A preliminary report.* J Bone Joint Surg 47A:695–704, 1965.

BURLEY, DM: *Thalidomide and congenital abnormalities.* Lancet 1:271, 1962.

BURTCH, RL: *A study of congenital skeletal limb deficiencies.* Inter-Clinic Info Bull 2:1–6, 1963.

BURTCH, RL: *The classification of congenital skeletal limb deficiencies: A preliminary report.* Inter-Clinic Info Bull 3:4–9, 1963.

BURTCH, RL: *Nomenclature for congenital skeletal limb deficiencies: A revision of the Frantz and O'Rahilly classification.* Artificial Limbs 10:24–35, 1966.

BUTTRUP, E: *Parents of child amputees.* Prosthet Int 2:10–12, 1964.

BUTTRUP, E: *The child amputee and his parents.* Rehabil Lit 33:139–141, 1972.

CAESAR, RT: *Case of amelus or limbless monster.* Br Med J 1:525, 1889.

CAINE, D AND REEDER, AJ: *The problem of the congenital amputee.* Med J Aust 50:301–305, 1963.

CARY, JM: *Traumatic amputation in childhood: Primary management.* Inter-Clinic Info Bull 14:1–10, 1975.

CHITTENDEN, RF: *The use of prosthesis for limb defects in children.* Am J Surg 86:128–138, 1953.

CHITTENDEN, RF: *Problems related to prosthesis in childhood.* Clin Orthop 8:197–208, 1956.

COMER, JF: *The juvenile amputee.* J Med Assoc State Ala 21:81–86, 1951.

CORNER, EM: *The clinical picture of congenital absence of the fibula.* J Bone Joint Surg 1B:203–206, 1913.

COVENTRY, MB AND JOHNSON, EW, JR: *Congenital absence of the fibula.* J Bone Joint Surg 34A:941–955, 1952.

CRAFT, AWJ: *Prostheses for children.* Lancet 1:639–642, 1944.

CRISTINI, JA: *Surgical management of the proximal femoral deficient extremity.* J Bone Joint Surg 55A:424–425, 1973.

DAMSBO, AM: *Habilitation of a two-year-old bilateral above-knee amputee.* J Am Phys Ther Assoc 43:584–587, 1963.

DANKMEIJER, J: *Congenital absence of the tibia.* Anat Rec 62:179–194, 1935.

DAVIDSON, WH AND BOHNE, WHO: *The Syme amputation in children.* J Bone Joint Surg 57A:905–909, 1975.

DAVIES, EJ, FRIZ, BR, AND CLIPPINGER, FW, JR: *Children with amputations.* Inter-Clinic Info Bull 9:6–19, 1969.

DEL DUCA, V, DAVIS, EV, AND BARROWAY, JN: *Congenital absence of the sacrum and coccyx: Report of two cases.* J Bone Joint Surg 33A:248–253, 1951.

DEMOPOULOS, JT AND LANE, ME: *Prosthetic restoration in phocomelia: Case presentation.* Bull Hosp Joint Dis 32:215–234, 1971.

DEMOPOULOS, JT, ET AL: *Prosthetic restoration in congenital lower limb deficiency: A case study.* Bull Hosp Joint Dis 36:150–158, 1975.

DOCK, G: *Intra-uterine amputations.* Trans Assoc Am Physicians 29:528–534, 1914.

DOIG, WG: *Proximal femoral phocomelia.* J Bone Joint Surg 52B:394, 1970.

DRESHER, CS AND MACDONELL, JA: *Total amelia.* J Bone Joint Surg 47A:511–516, 1965.

DUER, C: *Case of spontaneous amputation of both lower extremities in a newborn infant.* Br Med J 2:1179, 1897.

DURAISWAMI, PK: *Experimental causation of congenital skeletal defects and its significance in orthopaedic surgery.* J Bone Joint Surg 34B:646–698, 1952.

EASSON, WM: *Psychopathological environmental reaction to congenital defect.* J Nerv Ment Dis 142:453–459, 1966.

EDVARDSEN, P: *Resection osteosynthesis and Boyd amputation for congenital pseudarthrosis of the tibia.* J Bone Joint Surg 55B:179–182, 1973.

EILERT, RE AND JAYAKUMAR, SS: *Boyd and Syme ankle amputations in children.* J Bone Joint Surg 58A:1138–1141, 1976.

ELMSLIE, RC: *Case of congenital absence of sacrum, with associated dislocation of one hip and talipes calcaneo-valgus.* Proc R Soc Med 15:8, 1921.

ELTING, JJ AND ALLEN, JC: *Management of the young child with bilateral anomalous and functionless lower extremities.* J Bone Joint Surg 54A:1523–1530, 1972.

EPPS, CH, JR AND BRENNECKE, FE: *Juvenile amputee program.* Med Ann D C 31:295–298, 307, 1962.

EVANS, EL AND SMITH, NR: *Congenital absence of tibia.* Arch Dis Child 1:194–229, 1926.

FARMER, AW AND LAURIN, CA: *Congenital absence of the fibula.* J Bone Joint Surg 42A:1–12, 1960.

FITCH, FP: *Case of malformation and spontaneous amputation of one of the lower extremities of a foetus in utero.* Am J Med Sci 18:90–91, 1836.

FITCH, RR: *Congenital absence of vertebrae below the first sacral, and malformation of the lower cervical and upper dorsal vertebrae.* Am J Orthop Surg 7:540–543, 1910.

FRANTZ, C: *An evolution in the care of the child amputee.* Artificial Limbs 10:1–4, 1966.

FRANTZ, CH: *Prosthetic problems in the juvenile amputee.* Orth Pros Appl J 6:13–18, 1952.

FRANTZ, CH: *Child amputees can be rehabilitated.* Children 3:61–65, 1956.

FRANTZ, CH: *The child amputee.* Med Times 87:615–631, 1959.

FRANTZ, CH: *The upsurge in phocomelic congenital anomalies.* Inter-Clinic Info Bull 1:1–2, 1962.

FRANTZ, CH: *Increased incidence of malformed infants in West Germany during 1959–1962.* IMJ 123:27–39, 1963.

FRANTZ, CH AND AITKEN, GT: *The juvenile amputee.* J Michigan State Med Soc 57:233–241, 1958.

FRANTZ, CH AND AITKEN, GT: *Management of the juvenile amputee.* Clin Orthop 9:30–47, 1959.

FRANTZ, CH AND AITKEN, GT: *Complete absence of lumbar spine and sacrum.* J Bone Joint Surg 49A:1531–1540, 1967.

FRANTZ, CH AND O'RAHILLY, R: *Congenital skeletal limb deficiencies.* J Bone Joint Surg 43A:1202–1224, 1961.

FREEDMAN, B: *Congenital absence of sacrum and coccyx: Report of a case and review of literature.* Br J Surg 37:229–303, 1950.

FREEHAFER, AA AND SCHWAB, W: *Management of partial tibial absence resulting from infection.* Inter-Clinic Info Bull 16:1–6, 16, 1977.

FUSSEL, MH: *Intra-uterine amputation.* JAMA 29:25–26, 1897.

GILCHRIST, MI AND DUNCAN, MF: *Deb's delight: Fitting an infant's prosthesis.* Nurs Times 66:654–655, May 1970.

GILLIS, L: *Thalidomide babies: Management of limb defects.* Br Med J 2:647–651, 1962.

GILLIS, L: *Amputations including congenital abnormalities.* Practitioner 193:626–633, 1964.

GILPIN, RE: *Habilitation of patients with congenital malformations associated with thalidomide: Prosthetic aspects.* Can Med Assoc J 88:973–979, 1963.

GINGRAS, G, ET AL: *Habilitation of patients with congenital limb malformation: Present and future.* Can J Public Health 55:472–479, 1964.

GINGRAS, G, ET AL: *Congenital anomalies of the limbs. I. Medical aspects.* Can Med Assoc J 91:67–73, 1964.

GIRARD, PM: *Congenital absence of the sacrum.* J Bone Joint Surg 17:1062–1064, 1935.

GLESSNER, JR, JR: *Spontaneous intra-uterine amputation.* J Bone Joint Surg 45A:351–355, 1963.

GOUIN-DÉCARIE, T: *The mental and emotional development of the thalidomide children and the psychological reactions of the mothers: A follow-up study.* Inter-Clinic Info Bull 7:1–6, 1968.

GRAVELY, H: *Case of amelus or limbless monster.* Br Med J 1:1289, 1889.

GRAY, JE: *Congenital absence of the tibia.* Anat Rec 101:265–273, 1948.

GURNEY, W: *Parents of children with congenital amputation.* Children 5:95–100, 1958.

HALL, CB: *Recent concepts in the treatment of the limb-deficient child.* Artificial Limbs 10:36–51, 1966.

HALL, CB, BROOKS, MB, AND DENNIS, JF: *Congenital skeletal deficiencies of the extremities: Classification and fundamentals of treatment.* JAMA 181:590–599, 1962.

HALL, JE: *Habilitation of patients with congenital malformations associated with thalidomide: Surgery of limb defects.* Can Med Assoc J 88:964–972, 1963.

HALL, JE: *Rotation of congenitally hypoplastic lower limbs to use the ankle joint as a knee: A preliminary report.* Inter-Clinic Info Bull 6:3–9, 1966.

HAMILTON, RC: *A vocational evaluation of juvenile amputees who have attained the age of twenty-one years: A preliminary report.* Inter-Clinic Info Bull 3:8–9, 1964.

HAMSA, WR: *Congenital absence of the sacrum.* Arch Surg 30:657–666, 1935.

HARE, DR: *Case of a boy, aged five years and a-half, born without legs, and with each arm only about two inches in length.* Trans Pathol Soc London 10:308–310, 1859.

HARMON, PH AND FAHEY, JJ: *The syndrome of congenital absence of the fibula: Report of 3 cases with special reference to pathogenesis and treatment.* Surg Gynecol Obstet 64:876–887, 1937.

HARTMAN, LA: *Functional habilitation of a phocomelus.* Phys Ther 52:514–517, 1972.

HAUGE, AL, ECKHARDT, AL, AND CAMPBELL, P: *Evaluation of the patellar-tendon-supracondylar prosthesis for children.* Inter-Clinic Info Bull 11:1–6, 1971.

HAWKES, TA AND MESSNER, DG: *Management of bilateral congenital absence of the fibula with associated abnormalities.* Inter-Clinic Info Bull 17:1–15, 1979.

HAYHURST, DJ AND ECKHARDT, A: *Treatment of the patient with bilateral proximal femoral focal deficiency.* Inter-Clinic Info Bull 15:5–9, 17, 1976.

HENKEL, L AND WILLERT, HG: *Dysmelia: A classification and a pattern of malformation in a group of congenital defects of the limbs.* J Bone Joint Surg 51B:399–414, 1969.

HEPP, O: *Frequency of the congenital defect-anomalies of the extremities in the Federal Republic of Germany.* Inter-Clinic Info Bull 1:3–12, 1962.

HIGGS, SI: *Specimen of congenital absence of the sacrum.* Proc R Soc Med 17:39, 1921.

HOOTNICK, D, ET AL: *The natural history and management of congenital short tibia with dysplasia or absence of the fibula: A preliminary report.* J Bone Joint Surg 59B:267–271, 1977.

HORNSBY, W: *Intrauterine amputation of left leg.* Br Med J 1:865–866, 1926.

HOWARD, RG AND HURT, OJ: *Aglossia-adactylia.* Inter-Clinic Info Bull 15:17–20, 1976.

JANELLE, C: *The role of the social service worker in the rehabilitation of the juvenile amputee.* Inter-Clinic Info Bull 7:20–21, 1968.

JARAMILLO, S AND LEHNEIS, HR: *A therapeutic program for children with limb deformities: Preservation of rudimentary appendices and prosthetic design.* Inter-Clinic Info Bull 9:1–7, 1970.

JENDRZEJCZYK, DJ: *Prosthetic management for children with knee disarticulations.* Inter-Clinic Info Bull 17:9–16, 1980.

JONES, D, BARNES, J, AND LLOYD-ROBERTS, GC: *Congenital aplasia and dysplasia of the tibia with intact fibula: Classification and management.* J Bone Joint Surg 60B:31–39, 1978.

JORRING, K: *Amputation in children: A follow-up of 74 children whose lower extremities were amputated.* Acta Orthop Scand 42:178–186, 1971.

KATZ, JF: *Congenital absence of sacrum and coccyx.* J Bone Joint Surg 35A:398–402, 1953.

KAY, H: *A proposed international terminology for the classification of congenital limb deficiencies.* Orth Pros 28:33–48, 1974.

KAY, HW: *The children's prosthetics and orthotics program.* Artificial Limbs 15:6–10, 1971.

KAY, HW: *Clinical application of the new international terminology for the classification of congenital limb deficiencies.* Inter-Clinic Info Bull 14:1–24, 1975.

KAY, HW, KRUGER, LM, AND SWANSON, AB: *An international terminology for the classification of congenital limb deficiencies: Recommendations of a working group of the international society for prosthetics and orthotics.* Arch Orthop Trauma Surg 93:1–19, 1978.

KILLINGSWORTH, WP AND ENGLEDOW, R: *Congenital absence of the four extremities.* Am J Dis Child 63:914–918, 1942.

KING, RE: *Surgical correction of proximal femoral focal deficiency.* Inter-Clinic Info Bull 4:1–10, 1965.

KING, RE: *Providing a single skeletal lever in proximal femoral focal deficiency: A preliminary case report.* Inter-Clinic Info Bull 2:23–28, 1966.

KING, RE: *Some concepts of proximal femoral focal deficiency.* J Bone Joint Surg 49A:1470, 1967.

KING, RE AND MCCRANEY, T: *Proximal femoral focal deficiency: Quo vadis?* Inter-Clinic Info Bull 12:1–8, 1973.

KITABAYASHI, B: *The physical therapist's responsibility to the lower extremity child amputee.* Phys Ther Rev 41:722–727, 1961.

KLEIN, R: *An experimental prosthesis for lower extremity amelia.* Med J Aust 1:476–478, 1964.

KLEIN, RW: *An experiment in ambulation of lower extremity amelia.* Prosthet Int 2:6–7, 1964.

KNAPP, K, LENZ, W, AND NOWACK, E: *Multiple congenital abnormalities.* Lancet 2:725, 1962.

KOSTUIK, JP, ET AL: *Van Nes rotational osteotomy for treatment of proximal femoral focal deficiency and congenital short femur.* J Bone Joint Surg 57A:1039–1046, 1975.

KRITTER, AE: *Tibial rotation-plasty for proximal femoral focal deficiency.* J Bone Joint Surg 59A:927–934, 1977.

KRITTER, A AND BECKER, D: *Proximal femoral focal deficiency and amelia: A case report.* Inter-Clinic Info Bull 14:1–6, 1975.

KRITTER, AE AND GILLESPIE, T: *Bilateral proximal femoral focal deficiency and bilateral paraxial fibular hemimelia.* Inter-Clinic Info Bull 11:1–8, 1972.

KRUGER, LM: *Classification and prosthetic management of limb-deficient children.* Inter-Clinic Info Bull 7:1–25, 1968.

KRUGER, LM: *The use of stubbies for the child with bilateral lower-limb deficiencies.* Inter-Clinic Info Bull 12:7–15, 1973.

KRUGER, LM: *Decision making for the child with multiple limb deficiency.* Inter-Clinic Info Bull 15:13–19, 1976.

KRUGER, LM AND TALBOTT, RD: *Amputation and prosthesis as definitive treatment in congenital absence of the fibula.* J Bone Joint Surg 43A:625–642, 1961.

KURTZ, AD AND HAND, RC: *Bone growth following amputation in childhood.* Am J Surg 43:773–775, 1939.

LAMB, DW, SIMPSON, DC, AND PIRIE, RB: *The management of lower limb phocomelia.* J Bone Joint Surg 52B:688–691, 1970.

LAMB, DW, SIMPSON, DC, AND PIRIE, RB: *The management of lower limb phocomelia.* Inter-Clinic Info Bull 12:11–15, 1972.

LAMBERT, CN: *The juvenile amputee.* Ill Med J 123:514–517, 1963.

LAMBERT, CN: *Applicability of the patellar tendon bearing prosthesis to skeletally immature amputees.* Inter-Clinic Info Bull 3:7, 1964.

LAMBERT, CN: *The juvenile amputee.* Archiv fur Orthopadische und Unfallchirurgie 56:378–384, 1964.

LAMBERT, CN: *Early evaluation and prosthetic fitting of juvenile amputees.* Proc Inst Med Chic 27:54, 1968.

LAMBERT, CN: *Amputation surgery in the child.* Orthop Clin North Am 3:473–482, 1972.

LAMBERT, CN, HAMILTON, RC, AND PELLICORE, RJ: *The juvenile amputee program: Its social and economic value: A follow-up study after the age of twenty-one.* J Bone Joint Surg 51A:1135–1138, 1969.

LAMBERT, CN, ET AL: *Twenty-three years of clinic experience.* Inter-Clinic Info Bull 15:15–20, 1976.

LAMBERT, CN AND SCIORA, J: *A questionnaire survey of juvenile to young-adult amputees who have had prostheses supplied them through the University of Illinois Division of Services for Crippled Children.* J Bone Joint Surg 41A:1437–1454, 1959.

LAMBERT, CN AND SCIORA, J: *The incidence of scoliosis in the juvenile amputee population.* Inter-Clinic Info Bull 11:1–6, 1971.

LANGE, DR, SCHOENECKER, PL, AND BAKER, CL: *Proximal femoral focal deficiency: Treatment and classification in forty-two cases.* Clin Orthop 135:15–25, 1978.

LANGSTON, HH: *Congenital defect of the shaft of the femur.* Br J Surg 27:162–165, 1939.

LATTA, JS: *Spontaneous intrauterine amputations.* Am J Obstet Gynecol 10:640–648, 1925.

LAURIN, CA, FAVREAU, JC, AND LABELLE, P: *Bilateral absence of the radius and tibia with bilateral reduplication of the ulna and fibula.* J Bone Joint Surg 46A:137–142, 1964.

LENZ, W: *Thalidomide and congenital abnormalities.* Lancet 1:45, 1962.

LEVY, JL: *Girl born without legs and without arms: Report of a case.* South Med J 34:1085, 1941.

LICHTOR, A: *Sacral agenesis: Report of a case.* Arch Surg 54:430–433, 1947.

LINEBERGER, MI: *Habilitation of child amputees.* J Am Phys Ther Assoc 42:397–401, 1962.

LLOYD-ROBERTS, GC AND STONE, KH: *Congenital hypoplasia of the upper femur.* J Bone Joint Surg 45B:557–560, 1963.

LYTTLE, D, SPENCER, D, AND PERRY, R: *Satisfaction and self-esteem in patients attending a juvenile amputee clinic.* Inter-Clinic Info Bull 15:1–8, 14, 1976.

MARCOVE, RC, ET AL: *Osteogenic sarcoma under the age of twenty-one: A review of one hundred and forty-five operative cases.* J Bone Joint Surg 52A:411–423, 1970.

MARQUARDT, E: *The operative treatment of congenital limb malformation. I.* Prosthet Orthot Int 4:135–144, 1980.

MARQUARDT, E: *The operative treatment of congenital limb malformation. II. Case study.* Prosthet Orthot Int 5:2–6, 1981.

MARQUARDT, E: *The operative treatment of congenital limb malformation. III.* Prosthet Orthot Int 5:61–67, 1981.

MARTIN, JK: *Congenital malformations associated with thalidomide and their management.* Am Heart J 67:284–285, 1964.

MARTIN, JK AND RATHBUN, JC: *Habilitation of patients with congenital malformations associated with thalidomide: Pediatric aspects.* Can Med Assoc J 88:959–962, 1963.

MAZET, R, JR: *Syme's amputation: A follow-up study of fifty-one adults and thirty-two children.* J Bone Joint Surg 50A:1549–1563, 1968.

MAZET, R, JR AND CAMPBELL, H: *Selected case reports from the child amputee prosthetics project, University of California, Los Angeles.* Orth Pros Appl J 13:49–53, 1959.

MCBRIDE, WG: *Thalidomide and congenital abnormalities.* Lancet 2:1358, 1961.

MCCOLLOUGH, NC, ET AL: *Early opinions concerning the importance of bony fixations of the heel pad to the tibia in the juvenile amputee.* Inter-Clinic Info Bull 3:1–16, 1964.

MCKENZIE, DS: *The prosthetic management of congenital deformities of the extremities.* J Bone Joint Surg 39B:223–247, 1957.

MCKENZIE, DS: *Children: Medical and psycho-social considerations.* Prosthet Int 2:7–9, 1964.

M'LAREN, JS: *A case of congenital absence of the tibia.* J Anat Physiol Lond 23:598–605, 1888–89.

MEYER, H AND CUMMINS, H: *Severe maternal trauma in early pregnancy: Congenital amputations in infant at term.* Am J Obstet Gynecol 42:150–153, 1941.

MEYER, LC: *Congenital hypoplasia of the tibia with deficiency of the distal tibial epiphysis.* Inter-Clinic Info Bull 12:1–8, 1973.

MEYER, LC, FRIDDLE, D, JR, AND PRATT, RW: *Problems of treating and fitting the patient with proximal femoral focal deficiency.* Inter-Clinic Info Bull 10:1–4, 15, 1971.

MEYER, LC, SEHAYIK, RI, AND DAVIS, H: *The telescoping bifurcation synostosis in the treatment of incomplete longitudinal tibial deficiency.* Inter-Clinic Info Bull 17:1–8, 17, 1980.

MITAL, MA: *Limb deficiencies: Classifications and treatment.* Orthop Clin North Am 7:457–464, 1976.

MONGEAU, M: *An approach to the rehabilitation of the child amputee.* Inter-Clinic Info Bull 6:1–2, 34, 1967.

MONGEAU, M, ET AL: *Medical and psychological aspects of the habilitation of thalidomide children.* Can Med Assoc J 95:390–395, 1966.

MUNRO, HL: *A case of congenital absence of one tibia.* Lancet 2:526–527, 1904.

MURAT, JE, GUILLEMINET, M, AND DESCAMPS, R: *Long-term results of rotation-plasty in two patients with subtotal aplasia of the femur.* Am J Surg 113:676–679, 1967.

NICHOLS, PJR, ET AL: *Swivel walkers: Experiences in fitting swivel walkers to children with severe lower-limb deformities.* Ann Phys Med 10:106–111, 1969.

NICHOLS, PJR, ET AL: *The acceptance and rejection of prostheses by children with multiple congenital limb deformities.* Artificial Limbs 12:1–13, 1968.

NUTT, JJ: *Congenital fibular defects: With the report of a case of bilateral congenital total absence of fibulae.* Surg Gynecol Obstet 37:475–479, 1923.

NUTT, JJ AND SMITH, EE: *Total congenital absence of the tibia.* Am J Roentgen 46:841–849, 1941.

O'BRIEN, HR AND MUSTARD, HS: *An adult living case of total phocomelia.* JAMA 77:1964–1967, 1921.

OGG, HL: *Physical therapy for the pre-school child amputee.* Orth Pros Appl J 16:148–150, 1962.

OGG, HL: *Gait analysis for lower-extremity child amputees.* J Am Phys Ther Assoc 45:940–945, 1965.

O'RAHILLY, R: *Morphological patterns in limb deficiencies and duplications.* Am J Anat 89:135–193, 1951.

O'RAHILLY, R: *The nomenclature and classification of limb anomalies.* Inter-Clinic Info Bull 10:11–15, 17, 1971.

PANITCH, V: *The bilateral lower-extremity amputee.* Inter-Clinic Info Bull 8:5–12, 1969.

PANTING, AL AND WILLIAMS, PF: *Proximal femoral focal deficiency.* J Bone Joint Surg 60B:46–52, 1978.

PEARSON, FA AND SPIERS, BW: *Teamwork in the management of dysmelic children.* Physiotherapy 52:197–200, 1966.

PELLICORE, RJ, ET AL: *Incidence of bone overgrowth in the juvenile amputee population.* Inter-Clinic Info Bull 13:1–8, 1974.

PERRY, J, BONNETT, CA, AND HOFFER, MM: *Vertebral pelvic fusions in the rehabilitation of patients with sacral agenesis.* J Bone Joint Surg 52A:288–294, 1970.

PFEIFFER, RA AND KOSENOW, W: *Thalidomide and congenital abnormalities.* Lancet 1:45–46, 1962.

PHIPPEN, W, HUNTER, JM, AND BARAKAT, AR: *The habilitation of a child with multiple congenital skeletal limb deficiencies.* Inter-Clinic Info Bull 10:11–16, 1971.

PIRKEY, EL AND PURCELL, JH: *Agenesis of lumbosacral vertebrae: A report of two cases in living infants.* Radiology 69:726–729, 1957.

POMERANCE, HH AND SOIFER, H: *Amelia: Review of literature and report of a case.* J Pediatr 34:465–469, 1949.

PRICE, MD: *Baby without arms or legs: Brief history with photograph.* J Indiana State Med Assoc 21:250, 1928.

RADFORD, J AND STEENSMA, J: *The lower extremity toddler amputee: Training procedures.* Phys Ther Rev 37:32–37, 1957.

REED, JM: *A case of intra-uterine amputation.* JAMA 87:1213, 1926.

RICHARDS, JF, JR AND MELTZER, LN: *Prosthetic suspension in a case of "tibial kyphosis."* Inter-Clinic Info Bull 15:21–25, 1976.

RING, PA: *Congenital short femur: Simple femoral hypoplasia.* J Bone Joint Surg 41B:73–79, 1959.

ROMANO, RL AND BURGESS, EM: *Extremity growth and overgrowth following amputation in children.* Inter-Clinic Info Bull 5:11–12, 1966.

ROSENFELDER, R: *Infant amputees: Early growth and care.* Clin Orthop 148:41–46, 1980.

RUSSELL, HE AND AITKEN, GT: *Congenital absence of the sacrum and lumbar vertebrae with prosthetic management: A survey of the literature and presentation of five cases.* J Bone Joint Surg 45A:501–507, 1963.

RUSSELL, JE: *Tibial hemimelia: Limb deficiency in siblings.* Inter-Clinic Info Bull 14:15–23, 1975.

RUSSELL, JE: *Congenital absence of sacrum and lumbar vertebrae: A case report.* Inter-Clinic Info Bull 16:7–12, 1977.

SAUTER, WF: *Prostheses for the child amputee.* Orthop Clin North Am 3:483–494, 1972.

SCHEER, GB: *Treatment of proximal focal femoral deficiencies.* Clin Orthop 85:292, 1972.

SCHUTT, WH: *Dysmelia and its management: Habilitation of children with severe limb deformities presents a great challenge.* Clin Pediatr 4:717–720, 1965.

SHAW, IB: *Treatment of children with proximal femoral focal deficiency.* Inter-Clinic Info Bull 14:9–12, 17–20, 24–25, 1975.

SIMMEL, ML: *The absence of phantoms for congenitally missing limbs.* Am J Psychol 74:467–470, 1961.

SMITH, ED: *Congenital sacral anomalies in children.* Aust NZ J Surg 29:165–176, 1959.

SOLNIT, AJ AND STARK, MH: *Mourning and the birth of a defective child.* Psychoanal Study Child 16:523–537, 1961.

SPRING, JM AND EPPS, CH, JR: *The juvenile amputee: Some observations and considerations.* Clin Pediatr 7:76–79, 1968.

STAMP, WG, MAHON, S, AND MORGAN, HC: *Problems of management of the child with multiple amputations.* Arch Phys Med Rehabil 46:354–368, 1965.

STEELE, S: *Children with amputations.* Nurs Forum 7:411–423, 1968.

STEENSMA, J: *Training the juvenile amputee.* Orth Pros Appl J 6:18–26, 1952.

STEENSMA, J: *Problems of the adolescent amputee.* J Rehabil 25:19–20, 27, 1959.

STEWART, SF: *Absence of sacrum: With report of a case, and a review of the literature.* Arch Surg 9:647–652, 1924.

STOWELL, WL: *Intrauterine amputations and amniotic bands.* Arch Pediatr 22:342–345, 1905.

STREET, DM AND CUNNINGHAM, F: *Congenital anomalies caused by intra-uterine bands.* Clin Orthop 37:82 97, 1964.

SULLIVAN, RA AND CELIKYOL, F: *An ongoing seminar for parents of amputee children.* Inter-Clinic Info Bull 15:9–14, 1976.

SVETZ, CP, WAGNER, C, AND CLARK, MW: *A young hemipelvectomy patient.* Inter-Clinic Info Bull 15:9–13, 1976.

SWANSON, AB: *Phocomelia and congenital limb malformations: Reconstruction and prosthetic replacement.* Am J Surg 109:294–299, 1965.

SWANSON, AB: *Classification of limb malformations on the basis of embryological failures: A preliminary report.* Inter-Clinic Info Bull 6:1–15, 1966.

SWANSON, AB: *Bone overgrowth in the juvenile amputee and its control by the use of Silicone rubber implants.* Inter-Clinic Info Bull 8:9–18, 1969.

SWANSON, AB: *Silicone-rubber implants to control the overgrowth phenomenon in the juvenile amputee.* Inter-Clinic Info Bull 11:5–8, 1972.

SWANSON, AB: *A classification for congenital limb malformations.* J Hand Surg 1:8–22, 1976.

SWANSON, AB: *Congenital limb defects: Classification and treatment.* Clin Symp 33:3–32, 1981.

SWANSON, AB, BARKSKY, AJ, AND ENTIN, MA: *Classification of limb malformations on the basis of embryological failures.* Surg Clin North Am 48:1169–1179, 1968.

SYPNIEWSKI, BL: *The child with terminal transverse partial hemimelia: A review of the literature on prosthetic management.* Artificial Limbs 16:20–50, 1972.

TABLADA, C: *A technique for fitting converted proximal femoral focal deficiencies.* Artificial Limbs 15:27–45, 1971.

TAFT, CB: *Survival and prosthetic fitting of children amputated for malignancy.* Inter-Clinic Info Bull 5:9–28, 1966.

TALBOT, D AND SOLOMON, C: *The function of a parent group in the adaptation to the birth of a limb-deficient child.* Inter-Clinic Info Bull 17:9–10, 17, 1978.

TAUSSIG, HB: *A study of the German outbreak of phocomelia: The thalidomide syndrome.* JAMA 180:1106–1114, 1962.

THOMPSON, TC, STRAUB, LR, AND ARNOLD, WD: *Congenital absence of the fibula.* J Bone Joint Surg 39A:1229–1237, 1957.

TIPPY, LV, KELLER, KM, AND SCHOENECKER, PL: *Management of a child with multiple congenital anomalies.* Inter-Clinic Info Bull 17:11–16, 17, 1979.

VAN NES, CP: *Rotation-plasty for congenital defects of the femur: Making use of the ankle of the shortened limb to control the knee joint of a prosthesis.* J Bone Joint Surg 32B:12–16, 1950.

VAN NES, CP: *Congenital pseudarthrosis of the leg.* J Bone Joint Surg 48A:1467–1483, 1966.

VITALI, M: *Management of congenital deformities, including thalidomide children, in Great Britain.* Inter-Clinic Info Bull 2:7–12, 1963.

VOLLRADT, G: *Physiotherapeutic treatment of dysmelic children.* Inter-Clinic Info Bull 10:1–14, 16, 1970.

VOM SAAL, F: *Epiphysiodesis combined with amputation.* J Bone Joint Surg 21:442–443, 1939.

VOM SAAL, F: *Amputations in children.* Surg Gynecol Obstet 76:709–710, 1943.

VORCHHEIMER, H: *1018 children with skeletal limb deficiencies.* Inter-Clinic Info Bull 6:12–15, 1967.

VOÛTE, PA, ET AL: *Amputations in children: Clinical indications and psychological implications.* Arch Chir Neerl 25:427–433, 1973.

WALLACE, MT: *Group therapy for parents of congenital amputees.* Inter-Clinic Info Bull 5:10–15, 1965.

WEINSTEIN, S AND SERSEN, EA: *Phantoms in cases of congenital absence of limbs.* Neurology 11:905–911, 1961.

WESTIN, GW, SAKAI, DN, AND WOOD, WL: *Congenital longitudinal deficiency of the fibula: Follow-up of treatment by Syme amputation.* J Bone Joint Surg 58A:492–496, 1976.

WHITE, C: *A foetus with congenital absence of the sacrum.* Proc R Soc Med 4:279–280, 1911.

WILLIAMS, DI AND NIXON, HH: *Agenesis of the sacrum.* Surg Gynecol Obstet 105:84–88, 1957.

WILSON, AB, JR: *Limb prostheses for children.* Prosthet Int 2:2–5, 1964.

WOOD, WL, ZLOTSKY, N, AND WESTIN, GW: *Congenital absence of the fibula: Treatment by Syme amputation, indications and technique.* J Bone Joint Surg 47A: 1159–1169, 1965.

YELTON, CL: *Femoral deficiencies.* Inter-Clinic Info Bull 2:1–5, 1963.

ZELIGS, IM: *Congenital absence of the sacrum.* Arch Surg 41:1220–1228, 1940.

ZETTLE, JH, BRUNNER, H, AND ROMANO, RL: *Knee disarticulation socket design for juvenile amputees.* Inter-Clinic Info Bull 16:11–15, 1977.

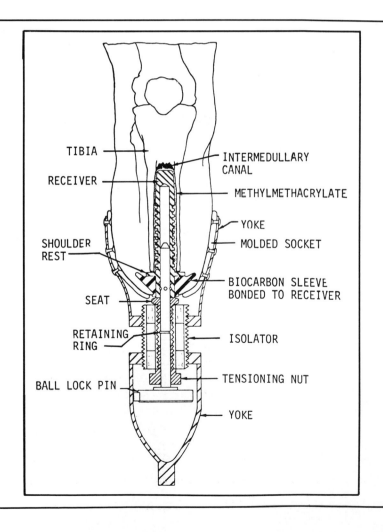

TIBIA

RECEIVER

SHOULDER
REST

SEAT

RETAINING
RING

BALL LOCK PIN

INTERMEDULLARY
CANAL

METHYLMETHACRYLATE

YOKE

MOLDED SOCKET

BIOCARBON SLEEVE
BONDED TO RECEIVER

ISOLATOR

TENSIONING NUT

YOKE

CHAPTER 24

RESEARCH AND DEVELOPMENT

SKELETAL ATTACHMENT OF A PROSTHESIS

The conventional method of coupling a prosthesis to the residual limb via a socket, corset, or straps has cosmetic and functional (control) limitations. Loads carried through the soft tissue may result in abrasions where excessive external pressure or friction exists. Direct skeletal attachment (DSA) offers the possibility of load-bearing directly from the skeleton to the prosthesis so that soft tissue is not compromised by prolonged excessive pressures (Fig. 24-1). Skeletal fixation and transcutaneous interface must be successful, however.

Ideally, the mechanical joints of a prosthesis should be powered by the amputee's existing muscles. For this to be successful, the muscles have to move the lever arm in an efficient manner. An artificial tendon needs to be developed that could be attached strongly to the existing skeletal muscles and could pass through the skin without allowing bacterial invasion. Other problems that have to be solved are the biocompatibility of the living bone and skin with the prosthetic material, the biomechanical problem of the distribution of forces (in vivo dynamic loading) at the bone-prosthesis interface, and the development of a matrix suitable for bone ingrowth at the interface (stabilization of DSA with controlled bone ingrowth). There are many problems associated with the development of viable, long-term bonding of bone to prosthesis and a drainage-free perforation of the skin by prosthetic material. The prosthesis secured by DSA should not impede circulation to the bone or soft tissue, and should permit motion and weight-bearing without pain.

The first DSA was a below-knee prosthesis to the tibia, performed by Dr. G. Dümmer in Germany and independently by Elliott Cutler and James Blodgett at Harvard during and just after World War II. Dr. John B. Esslinger began animal experimentation in the mid-1950s in Detroit, Michigan, utilizing skeletally attached prostheses on dogs.

SKIN INTERFACING

The successful, long-term transcutaneous passage of a prosthetic device is a very difficult problem to solve. A perforated carbon collar below the skin was used by Esslinger to create an interface between the skin and the prosthesis. The medullary canal was plugged with a device that had a distal attaching mechanism.

Various materials that pass through the skin have been studied. Rigid materials cause infection more readily than flexible materials. Some of the materials that have been used to provide the gradual transition of stiffness from the inert material to the bone are flexible plastic, coiled steel springs, perforated collars (Fig. 24-2) of tapered flexibility, and Dacron or nylon velour fabric bonded to a solid surface to form an impervious laminate. The implant is successful only if no drainage occurs at the interface and there is epithelial downgrowth along the neck of the percutaneous conduit.

BONE INTERFACING (SKELETAL FIXATION)

Prosthetic-bone fixation (Fig. 24-3) must be secure for unlimited periods of time in DSA. Non-cemented skeletal fixation devices tend to gradually loosen with constant

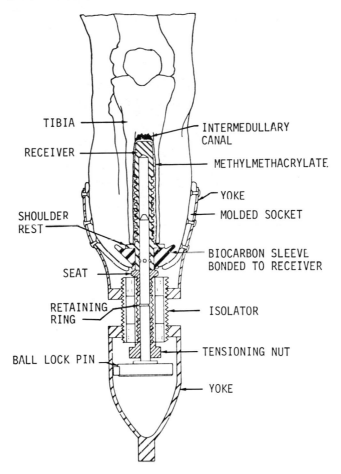

FIGURE 24-1. A system for direct attachment of a prosthesis to the bone of the amputation limb. (From *A dream about to come true?* Newsletter . . . Amputation Clinics 7:6, 1975, with permission.)

mechanical stress. Methyl methacrylate, functioning as a bone cement, has been used successfully as a stress transfer mechanism from prosthesis to bone.

Orthopedic implant materials such as stainless steel, Vitallium, and titanium achieve acceptable levels of tissue reaction for relatively short periods of time and are thus satisfactory for temporary needs. Metallic fixation has been questioned for long-term use. Plastic material that totally conforms to the interface surfaces has been tried with success as a stress transfer mechanism. Porous ceramics are tolerated well by living tissue and allow bone ingrowth, thus providing a successful interface. Although the bone-prosthetic bond may be adequate, the skin interface may be inadequate, resulting in chronic drainage secondary to progressive inflammation and infection about the prosthesis. Grooved surfaces rather than porous ceramic surfaces have been tried to enable better vascular support to bone ingrowth. Vitreous carbon is well accepted by skeletal tissue, with no evidence of tissue toxicity. It is also successfully accepted at the skin interface.

The attachment of a prosthesis to bone can present a problem unless a broad area of support is used. Stress concentrations that can be destructive to living tissue are thus avoided. The major portion of the cortex of the shaft of long bones receives its blood

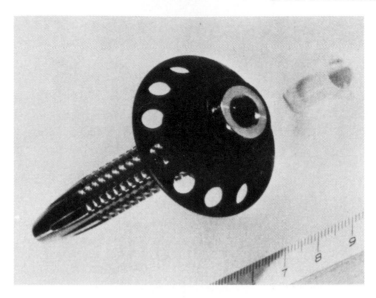

FIGURE 24-2. Femoral implant for skeletal prosthetic attachment. The hollow metal intramedullary pin (developed by NASA) is cemented into the bone. The collar is coated with low-temperature isotropic carbon (developed by Gulf General Atomic Corporation). (From *A dream about to come true?* Newsletter . . . Amputation Clinics 7:6, 1975, with permission.)

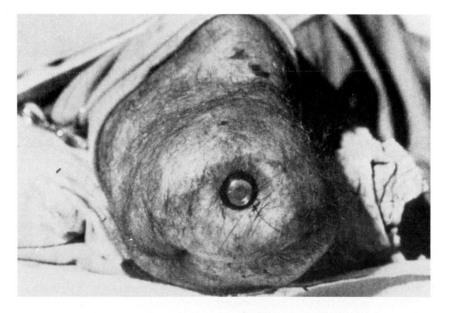

FIGURE 24-3. Skin closure around the carbon collar for a bacteriologic seal. The bore of the carbon collar implant, which receives the quick-disconnect rod of the prosthesis, is visible. (From *A dream about to come true?* Newsletter . . . Amputation Clinics 7:6, 1975, with permission.)

supply from the medullary vessels rather than from the periosteal blood supply. Intra-medullary rods used as a skeletal extension disrupt the blood supply via the nutrient artery within the medullary canal, resulting in bone necrosis and/or osteomyelitis. As an alternative, supracortical extensions, which do not disturb the intramedullary canal, have been developed.

MUSCULOTENDINOUS INTERFACING

Skin-penetrating artificial tendons are also under experimentation. This system would allow existing musculature to control an external articulating joint.

The attachment of an artificial tendon in a way that will withstand repeated stress is a problem. Nylon or Dacron velour has been used to obtain a strong attachment to the musculotendinous portion of an existing skeletal muscle. Tissue ingrowth can be obtained over a wide surface of the velour.

To prevent tissue from growing to both sides of the velour, Silastic is bonded to the back of the velour. In that way, tissue ingrowth is possible only at the tendon-velour interface, and the tendon will have mobility.

A skin-to-velour interface, to seal the wound, tears under repeated stress. This problem has yet to be solved.

SUMMARY

The utilization of DSA continues to be investigated because it offers several advantages over existing prosthetic devices. Skeletal extension would provide more prosthetic sta-bility than an interface through a socket to soft tissue. The amputee would experience a more natural kinesthetic perception due to the increased stability. Soft tissue problems would be minimized by eliminating weight-bearing through the soft tissue. If artificial tendons could be attached to the musculotendinous portion of large skeletal muscles and brought through the skin to attach to an external articulating prosthetic device, then the amputee would have better control of the prosthetic device. The amputee would not have to rely so heavily on gravity and momentum for movement of prosthetic parts. Although there have been some positive results with this approach to prosthetic man-agement, DSA is still, for all practicality, in the experimental stage.

BELOW-KNEE SUCTION SOCKET

A patellar-tendon-bearing (PTB) suction prosthesis was developed in Sweden, with clin-ical trials beginning in 1969. This prosthesis was designed for patients who sustain contact sores and skin irritation on the amputation limb while wearing the ordinary PTB prosthesis or who experience a sensation of instability. By attempting to immobi-lize the skin, it was hoped to avoid these skin problems in those who are prone to them (the physically very active and those with sensory disturbance, excessive soft tissue distally, frail scar tissue, and eczema) and to actually promote healing in already dam-aged skin. This method of suspension is still under investigation.

RIGID SOCKET

In the early design, the socket and the rest of the prosthesis were one unit, with the socket being rigid. Skin lesions in the popliteal area and loss of suction during extreme flexion (when walking on stairs) led to the development of the semirigid detachable suction socket.

DETACHABLE SEMIRIGID SOCKET (SEMIRIGID INSERT SUCTION SOCKET–PTB PROSTHESIS [SISS–PTB PROSTHESIS])

A later design made the socket detachable and semirigid. The donning procedure for this prosthesis is as follows. A tubular stockinet is put on over the limb. The semirigid insert suction socket (the actual socket) is put on over the stockinet, with the stockinet being pulled through the valve (Fig. 24-4a). The soft tissue is pulled to the bottom of the socket. The valve is closed while the limb is pressed into the socket (Fig. 24-4b). The semirigid inner socket, which contains the limb, is next placed into the hard socket of the prosthesis (Fig. 24-4c, d, e). The inner surface of the hard socket is rough and thus holds the semirigid socket in place by friction.

The PTB suction socket is less suited to extremely slender residual limbs with prominent skeletal parts and to limbs that are shorter than 12.7 cm (5 in). Soft tissue distal to the bony end of the limb makes adapting to the PTB-suction prosthesis easier; excessive soft tissue (> 3 cm [1.2 in]) below the distal bony end causes difficulty with the ordinary PTB prosthesis.

Patients report that the PTB suction prosthesis feels more like a real leg. This may be due to less piston action than with the strap-suspended PTB prosthesis. Roentgenographic studies show that there is better limb-socket contact and less soft tissue movement in the socket with the suction rather than the strap suspension of the PTB prosthesis, which should reduce the tendency toward skin lesions. The suction socket is more attractive than strap or corset suspension devices. It is considerably more complicated and difficult to fit the below-knee limb, however, than the above-knee limb with a suction socket because the surface is smaller, there is less soft-tissue in relation to skeletal tissue, and the limb changes shape with flexion and extension at the knee. If a suction socket does become loose, it is more trouble to don than a nonsuction socket because the residual limb has to be pulled down in the socket with a stockinet.

ADVANTAGES

1. Knee joint is free from constrictions.
2. Relatively better cosmetic appearance because proximal trim lines of the prosthesis are lower.
3. Should reduce skin abrasions because of less soft tissue movement than with strap suspension.
4. Intimate fit causes better awareness of the prosthesis (better position sense and control).
5. Less interference with clothing because no cuff or corset is required.
6. Improved circulation because of cyclic variation of pressure.

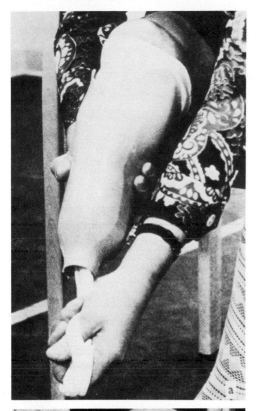

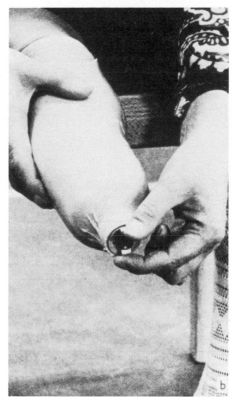

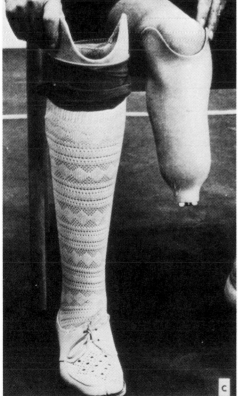

FIGURE 24-4. Donning procedure for the PTB prosthesis. *(a)* The residual limb is assisted into the semirigid insert suction socket by pulling the stockinet through the valve hole. *(b)* The valve is screwed into place while pressure is still being applied to the socket. *(c)* The semirigid insert suction socket is now ready to go into the hard socket component of the PTB prosthesis.

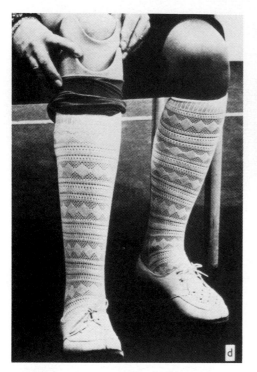
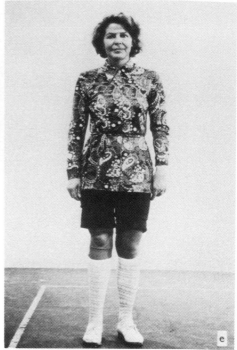

FIGURE 24-4. *Continued.* *(d)* **After donning the prosthetic limb, the rubber sleeve will be pulled up around the socket opening to reduce air leakage into the socket. *(e)* The prosthesis is ready for ambulation. (From Grevsten, S:** *Patellar-tendon-bearing suction prosthesis: Clinical experiences.* **Ups J Med Sci 82:2–3, 1977, with permission.)**

DISADVANTAGES

1. Does not add stability at the knee.
2. Difficult to fit.
3. More trouble to don if it becomes loose.
4. More difficult to maintain a pressure seal than with the above-knee residual limb (extreme maneuvers can cause a loss of suction, resulting in noise or instability).

INDICATION

1. Excessive soft tissue below the distal bony end.

CONTRAINDICATIONS

1. Amputees with mental or personality derangements owing to alcoholism, drug addiction, or senility, because the prosthesis must be put on with care to function properly.

2. Extremely slender residual limb with prominent skeletal parts.
3. Extremely short residual limb.

COMPUTER-PROGRAMMED PROSTHESIS

Research is being conducted at the Massachusetts Institute of Technology (MIT) by Robert W. Mann and Woodie C. Flowers toward the development of an artificial knee and leg that is computer-programmed to more closely imitate the sound leg. Central to this research is an instrument developed in Sweden called the Selspot, an acronym for "selective light spot recognition." The Selspot cameras monitor movement of the sound leg so precisely that the computer is able to precisely direct the movement of the prosthesis. Thus, data recorded by the Selspot cameras are used by the computer to pattern the movements of the prosthesis after those of the sound limb.

BIBLIOGRAPHY

SKELETAL ATTACHMENT

A dream about to come true?, Newsletter . . . Amp Clinics 7:5–7, 1975.

BECHTOL, CO: *The biomechanics of the epiphyseal lines as a guide to design considerations for the attachment of prosthesis to the musculoskeletal system.* J Biomed Mater Res 4:343–362, 1973.

FERNIE, GR, KOSTUIK, JP, AND LOBB, RJ: *A percutaneous implant using a porous metal surface coating for adhesion to bone and a velour covering for soft tissue attachment: Results of trials in pigs.* J Biomed Mater Res 11:883–891, 1977.

HALL, CW: *Developing a permanently attached artificial limb.* Bull Prosthet Res 10–22:144–157, 1974.

HALL, CW, COX, PA, AND MALLOW, WA: *Skeletal extension development: Criteria for future designs.* Bull Prosthet Res 10–25:69–96, 1976.

HALL, CW, ET AL: *A permanently attached artificial limb.* Trans Am Soc Artif Intern Organs 13:329–331, 1967.

HULBERT, SF, MORRISON, SJ, AND KLAWITTER, JJ: *Tissue reaction to three ceramics of porous and non-porous structures.* J Biomed Mater Res 6:347–374, 1972.

KROUSKOP, TA, TRONO, R, AND ADAMSKI, AJ: *The effects of pylon shape on bone-pylon interface performance in direct skeletal attachment.* J Biomed Mater Res 10:345–369, 1976.

LUSSKIN, R, ET AL: *Bone contouring under silicone polymer implants.* Clin Orthop 83:300–316, 1972.

MOONEY, V, ET AL: *Skeletal extension of limb prosthetic attachments: Problems in tissue reaction.* J Biomed Mater Res 2:143–159, 1971.

MURPHY, EF: *History and philosophy of attachment of prostheses to the musculoskeletal system and passage through skin with inert materials.* J Biomed Mater Res 4:275–295, 1973.

NEWELL, PH, ET AL: *Establishment of a theoretical base design of a lower extremity prosthesis.* J Biomed Mater Res 8:331–341, 1974.

BELOW-KNEE SUCTION SOCKET

GALDIK, J: *The below knee suction socket.* Orth Pros Appl J 9:43–46, 1955.

GREVSTEN, S: *Studies of the suspension of below-knee (BK) prostheses.* Acta Orthop Scand 45:971–972, 1974.

GREVSTEN, S: *Patellar tendon bearing suction prosthesis: Clinical experiences.* Ups J Med Sci 82:209–220, 1977.

GREVSTEN, S AND ERIKSSON, U: *Stump-socket contact and skeletal displacement in a suction patellar-tendon-bearing prosthesis.* J Bone Joint Surg 56A:1692–1696, 1974.

GREVSTEN, S AND ERIKSON, U: *A roentgenological study of the stump-socket contact and skeletal displacement in the PTB-suction prosthesis.* Ups J Med Sci 80:49–57, 1975.

GREVSTEN, S AND MARSH, L: *Suction-type prosthesis for below-knee amputees: A preliminary report.* Artificial Limbs 15:78–80, 1971.

GREVSTEN, S AND STALBERG, E: *Electromyographic study of muscular activity in the amputation stump while walking with PTB- and PTB-suction prosthesis.* Ups J Med Sci 80:103–112, 1975.

PEARSON, JR, ET AL: *Pressure variation in the below-knee, patellar tendon bearing suction socket prosthesis.* J Biomech 7:487–496, 1974.

COMPUTERS

BAJD, T AND KRALJ, A: *Simple kinematic gait measurements.* J Biomed Eng 2:129–132, 1980.

MANN, RW: *Cybernetic limb prosthesis: The ALZA distinguished lecture.* Ann Biomed Eng 9:1–43, 1981.

MANN, RW, ET AL: *Precise, Rapid, Automatic 3-D Position and Orientation Tracking of Multiple Moving Bodies.* Department of Mechanical Engineering, Massachusetts Institute of Technology, Cambridge, 1983.

PATRIARCO, AG, ET AL: *An evaluation of the approaches of optimization models in the prediction of muscle forces during human gait.* J Biomech 14:513–525, 1981.

WOLTRING, HJ AND MARSOLAIS, EB: *Optoelectric (Selspot) gait measurement in two- and three-dimensional space: A preliminary report.* Bull Prosthet Res 10–34:46–52, 1980.

INDEX

A "t" following a page number indicates a table. A page number in *italics* indicates a figure.